Interpreting Laboratory Tests in Intensive Care

This book incorporates a wide variety of clinical conditions requiring admission to the intensive care unit that necessitate timely performance of diagnostic tests and their correct interpretation to guide the best treatment. It tries to translate complex physiological principles and diagnostic algorithms into a clinically relevant format that can be easily understood by clinicians. It also explains at length the key clinical inputs to be acquired by laboratory physicians before reporting the results and tries to solve the common dilemmas leading to misinterpretation. The importance of every detail, from sample collection and dispatch to correlation of clinical state report, has been adequately explained with suitable examples and proper explanations.

Interpreting Laboratory Tests in Intensive Care

Edited by
Anirban Hom Choudhuri and Barnali Das

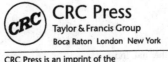

CRC Press
Taylor & Francis Group
Boca Raton London New York

CRC Press is an imprint of the
Taylor & Francis Group, an **informa** business

Designed cover image: shutterstock.com/image-photo/genetic-research-biotech-science-concept-human

First edition published 2025
by CRC Press
2385 NW Executive Center Drive, Suite 320, Boca Raton FL 33431

and by CRC Press
4 Park Square, Milton Park, Abingdon, Oxon, OX14 4RN

CRC Press is an imprint of Taylor & Francis Group, LLC

ISBN: 9781032583549 (hbk)
ISBN: 9781032583532 (pbk)
ISBN: 9781003449713 (ebk)

DOI: 10.1201/9781003449713

Typeset in Palatino
by Deanta Global Publishing Services, Chennai, India

The book is dedicated to Swami Vivekananda for guiding us in the path of service and to our parents and family whose love, care and blessings have been a constant source of inspiration to realize our dream.

Contents

Foreword by Padma Shri (Honorary) Brigadier Dr. Arvind Lal

It gives me immense pleasure to write a foreword for this unique book titled *Interpreting Laboratory Investigations in Intensive Care* edited by Dr. Anirban Hom Chaudhuri and Dr. Barnali Das and published by CRC Press/Taylor and Francis.

Laboratory medicine plays an immense role in intensive care and the advent of newer technologies in laboratory medicine has significantly enhanced the diagnostic tools available in the hand of the intensivists for improving patient monitoring, early diagnosis and patient outcomes. It is thus a great idea to put together the two disciplines and their synergistic uses for achieving the best of patient care in the intensive care unit.

I congratulate the internationally and nationally acclaimed experts, who have integrated the subjects in depth and comprehensively covered the integral areas of emergency medicine and intensive care in this book. With my vast experience in laboratory medicine, I can affirm that this book will be an indispensable source for clinicians to consult in their everyday practice, particularly in emergency care. I commend the authors and the editors who have contributed to this book.

My best wishes for the continued success of this endeavour to enhance patient care through a deeper understanding of the laboratory diagnosis available at the hands of the treating clinician.

With best wishes,
Padma Shri (Honorary) Brig Dr Arvind Lal

Foreword by Dr. Atul Mohan Kochhar

Best wishes:

I applaud the publication of the book *Interpreting Laboratory Tests in Intensive Care edited* by Dr. Anirban Hom Choudhuri and Dr. Barnali Das and published by CRC Press/Taylor and Francis.

This book serves as a comprehensive guide through the intricate landscape of diagnostic testing within the intensive care unit (ICU). It meticulously details the applications and interpretations of a wide range of tests, equipping clinicians and diagnosticians with the knowledge required to navigate the most challenging of clinical scenarios.

I commend the editors for their dedication and expertise in compiling this invaluable resource. I congratulate the internationally and nationally acclaimed authors who have contributed to enriching this work. My compliments also to CRC Press/Taylor & Francis for understanding this much-needed initiative.

This book will undoubtedly serve as an essential companion for intensivists, diagnosticians and all healthcare professionals.

Lastly, it is with great enthusiasm that I introduce this book to the readers, confident that it will enhance the quality of patient care and address patient safety concerns which are key to the NABH vision and mission.

Dr. Atul Mohan Kochhar
MD, DNB, MNAMS, FAAD
CEO, NABH

Preface

The journey of critical care medicine started during the Crimean War in the 1850s when Florence Nightingale chose to segregate the sicker patients from the less sick ones and place them closer to the nursing station so that they were monitored with extra attention and care. With time came ventilators and real-time hemodynamic monitoring devices. This further improved the quality of patient care and aroused interest among medical professionals to acquire expertise in their use. However, in the 21st century, things no longer remained confined to the ventilatory and hemodynamic management alone. The most important determinant for good outcomes after critical care was recognized to be the speed of diagnosis and early appropriate intervention. The catch-line "Time is tissue" was coined to highlight the importance of this approach. However, for early intervention, early and correct diagnosis is necessary. Therefore a lot of research has been accomplished, and many studies are underway to attain seamless integration of diagnostic tests and therapeutic strategies in the intensive care unit. This approach has not only improved outcomes by reducing deaths but also by reducing length of stay and overall costs.

In this regard, point-of-care (POC) diagnostic techniques are fast emerging as popular and indispensable tools in the hands of intensive care physicians. The POC approach is performed at the bedside, i.e. at the site of patient care, and can guide the immediate modification of an ongoing treatment. No doubt, the application of POC has still a lot to unveil and will open new vistas in raising care and improving the outcome of the critically ill. But to adopt POC, diagnostic stewardship is an essential requisite. In the true sense, the best outcome can be achieved not by the timely performance of the appropriate test alone but by its judicious interpretation and action following interpretation. Moreover, it is all the more important to avoid performing tests repeatedly, unnecessarily, and in an untimely manner.

There is a lacuna in understanding the importance of the tests with regard to time, necessity, and order amongst clinicians in their routine practice. Some confusion also prevails amongst the laboratory physicians while interpreting the clinical picture of the patient during reporting. In this book, the authors have made a sincere attempt to harmonize the diagnostic and therapeutic domains of critical care and address the concerns of both laboratory physicians and intensivists to guide them in the best practice for the benefit of patients. This book will be a handy guide at the bedside to refer to appropriate tests and interpret them correctly and cautiously based upon the clinical findings of the patient and is suitable for both the trainees and practicing physicians alike.

The editors will feel content and grateful if the book is appreciated and found useful by readers in their day-to-day practice. The editors thankfully acknowledge all suggestions and comments from readers and will try to resolve their queries, if any.

Acknowledgment

We sincerely acknowledge the contribution of all authors and express our thanks and gratitude for reposing faith in our abilities. We also acknowledge the support and help from family, friends, colleagues, fellows, students, and well-wishers in different matters from time to time. Our sincere thanks to Padma Shri Dr. Arvind Lal and Dr. Atul Mohan Kochhar for their encouraging words and support. The editors would like to thank the publisher for unfailing consideration and unwavering support. We are grateful to Shivangi, Lavanya, Daniel Andrew and the publication team of Taylor & Francis for their continuous support and guidance in making our dream a reality.

Editor Biographies

Dr. Anirban Hom Choudhuri is Director Professor in the Department of Anaesthesiology & Intensive Care and an expert in Critical Care Medicine at Vardhman Mahavir Medical College & Safdarjung Hospital in New Delhi, India. He has nearly 20 years of experience in the practice of critical care medicine and is an avid researcher, teacher, guide, and examiner. He has published many original research, systematic reviews, meta-analyses, and chapters in textbooks and holds a patent with the Government of Australia (patent number: 2021106431). He was the recipient of the Sarvapalli Radhakrishnan Distinguished Professor Award in 2021. His book *Imaging in Critical Care* (1st edition) was published by Taylor & Francis in 2023.

Dr. Barnali Das is a Lead Consultant in the Biochemistry, Immunology, and Toxicology Divisions of the Laboratory Medicine Department at Kokilaben Dhirubhai Ambani Hospital & Medical Research Institute in Mumbai, India. She is Chair of the Association for Diagnostics and Laboratory Medicine (formerly American Association of Clinical Chemistry), India section. She is a Fellow of the Academy of Diagnostics & Laboratory Medicine. She has been invited as adjunct faculty at Kasturba Medical College, Manipal, MAHE. She is a core committee member of the ICMR Taskforce on Establishment of Reference Intervals in Indian Population (TERIIP). She is associated with the IFCC Committee for Reference Interval and Decision Limits (C-RIDL) and was an Executive Member of the Scientific Division of the International Federation of Clinical Chemistry and Laboratory Medicine (IFCC). Dr. Barnali is the recipient of three oration awards and seven international and ten national awards. She has many original research publications in international and national journals.

List of Contributors

Rahul Kumar Anand
Additional Professor, Department of Anesthesiology and Intensive Care
All India Institute of Medical Science (AIIMS)
New Delhi, India

Urmila Anandh
Senior Consultant and Head, Department of Nephrology
Amrita Institute of Medical Sciences and Research Centre
Faridabad, India

Divya Bajpai
Additional Professor, Department of Nephrology
Seth GS Medical College and KEM Hospitals
Mumbai, India

Anirban Bhattacharjee
Assistant Professor, Department of Anesthesia, Pain and Intensive Care
All India Institute of Medical Science (AIIMS)
Guwahati, India

U.D. Bindal
Head, Department of Biochemistry, Post Graduate Institute of Child Health
Noida, India

Rahul Chaurasia
Additional Professor, Transfusion Medicine
All India Institute of Medical Science (AIIMS)
New Delhi, India

Anil K. Chokkalla
Clinical Chemistry Fellow, Department of Pathology and Immunology
Baylor College of Medicine and Texas Children's Hospital
Texas, USA

Michael Christian
Associate Professor of Emergency Medicine
University of Missouri-Kansas City School of Medicine; and Clinical Assistant Professor of Pediatrics
Children's Mercy Hospital, Kansas City
University of Missouri-Kansas City School of Medicine
Kansas City, USA

Paul O. Collinson
Professor of Cardiac Biomarkers
St George's University of London
London, UK

Sridevi Devaraj
Medical Director, Clinical Chemistry and POCT, Department of Pathology and Immunology
Baylor College of Medicine and Texas Children's Hospital
Houston, USA

Uttam Garg
Division Director, Clinical Pathology; Director, Clinical Chemistry, Toxicology
Department of Pathology and Laboratory Medicine, Children's Mercy Hospital; and Professor of Pathology
University of Missouri-Kansas City School of Medicine; Professor of Pathology, University of Kansas School of Medicine
Kansas City, USA

Parshotam Lal Gautam
Professor and Head, Critical Care Medicine
Dayanand Medical College and Hospital
Ludhiana, India

David C. Gaze
Senior Lecturer in Chemical Pathology
School of Life Sciences, University of Westminster
London, UK

Manoj Goel
Principal Director, Pulmonology and Critical Care
Fortis Memorial Research Institute
Gurugram, India

Binita Goswami
Professor, Department of Biochemistry
Maulana Azad Medical College
New Delhi, India

Nikhil Gupta
Professor, Department of Surgery
Atal Bihari Vajpayee Institute of Medical Sciences and Dr Ram Manohar Lohia Hospital (ABVIMS and Associated RML Hospital)
New Delhi, India

A. Zara Herskovits
Assistant Director, Koch Laboratory; Director, Evelyn H. Lauder Breast Center, Department of Pathology and Laboratory Medicine
Memorial Sloan Kettering Cancer Center
New York, USA

Santvana Kohli Arora
Associate Professor, Department of Anesthesiology and Intensive Care
VMMC and Safdarjung Hospital
New Delhi, India

Arun Koul
Professor Neurology
GB Pant Institute of Post graduate medical
education and training
New Delhi, India

Souvik Maitra
Additional Professor
Department of Anaesthesiology, Pain Medicine
and Critical Care
All India Institute of Medical Sciences (AIIMS)
New Delhi, India

Manju Mathew
Associate Professor Critical Care
Pushpagiri Medical College Hospital
Tiruvalla, Kerala, India

Sayan Nath
Consultant, Critical Care Medicine
Manipal Hospitals
Mukundapur, Kolkata, India

Jayram Navade
Consultant Critical Care
S.L. Raheja Hospital – A Fortis Associate
Mumbai, India

Shaik Arif Pasha
Professor and Head, Critical Care Medicine
NRI Medical College
Guntur, India

Magesh Parthiban
Consultant Intensivist
Department of Critical Care Medicine, Kovai Medical
Center and Hospital (KMCH) Main centre
Coimbatore, India

Ankit Patowary
Consultant Rheumatologist
Apollo Hospital (International)
Guwahati, India

Lakshmi V. Ramanathan
Chief, Department of Pathology and
Laboratory Medicine
Memorial Sloan Kettering Cancer Center
New York, USA

Pradeep Rangappa
Consultant, Critical Care
Manipal Hospital
Bangalore, India

Nina Raoof
Intensitivist (Former), Department of
Anesthesiology and Critical Care Medicine
Memorial Sloan Kettering Cancer Center
New York, USA

Bikash Ranjan Ray
Additional Professor, Department of
Anaesthesiology, Pain Medicine and Critical Care
All India Institute of Medical Sciences (AIIMS)
New Delhi, India

Sanjith Saseedharan
Head of the Department of Critical Care
S.L. Raheja Hospital – A Fortis Associate
Mumbai, India

R. Saxena
Associate Professor, Department of Paediatrics
Maulana Azad Medical College and associated
LN Hospital
New Delhi, India

Amrita Shah
Associate Consultant, Critical Care
Manipal Hospital Yeshwanthpur
Bangalore, India

Sweta Shah
Lead Consultant, Microbiology and Infection
Prevention
Kokilaben Dhirubhai Ambani Hospital and Medical
Research Institute
Mumbai, India

Rakupathy Shanmugam
Senior Resident, Department of Anesthesiology
and Intensive Care
All India Institute of Medical Sciences (AIIMS)
New Delhi, India

Shashikant Sharma
Associate Consultant, Critical Care Medicine
Jayprabha Medanta Hospitals
Patna, India

Abha Sharma
Professor, Microbiology
GB Pant Institute of Post graduate medical
education and training
New Delhi, India

Surendra Shingnapurkar
Chief of Laboratory
S.L. Raheja Hospital
Mumbai, India

Aditi Singh
Assistant Professor, Biochemistry
Hindu Rao Hospital
New Delhi, India

Tanu Singhal
Consultant, Pediatrics and Infectious Disease
Specialist, Kokilaben Dhirubhai Ambani Hospital
and Medical Research Institute
Mumbai, India

Kapildev Soni
Professor, Critical Care Medicine, JPNA Trauma
    Centre
All India Institute of Medical Sciences (AIIMS)
New Delhi, India

Anuupama Suchiita
Assistant Professor, Department of Biochemistry
Maulana Azad Medical College
New Delhi, India

Kannan Vaidyanathan
Professor and Head
Dept of Biochemistry, Believers Church
    Medical College Hospital
Tiruvalla, Kerala, India

Siva Prabodh Vuddandi
Professor and Head, Department of Biochemistry
NRI Medical College
Guntur, India

1 Shock

Bikash Ranjan Ray and Rakupathy Shanmugam

Shock is one of the most common indications for intensive care unit (ICU) admission. It indicates an imbalance between oxygen delivery and utilization, leading to multi-organ dysfunction. It is associated with higher morbidity and mortality if not treated early. The diagnosis of the underlying etiology of shock determines the modality of management. The laboratory tests are important not only in their diagnosis and prognostication but also in their classification.

DEFINITION

Shock is defined as a clinical condition in which cellular and tissue hypoxia secondary to tissue hypoperfusion is caused by either decreased oxygen delivery or impaired oxygen extraction.

CLASSIFICATION OF SHOCK [1]

In clinical scenarios, most patients with acute circulatory failure present with a combination of the above-mentioned mechanisms. The most common type of shock is distributive shock, among which septic shock is the predominant type (Table 1.1). Sometimes patients have hypotension, but the etiology is difficult to ascertain, which is termed undifferentiated shock.

Clinically, shock is identified by one of three indications: altered mental status, decreased urine output, and prolonged capillary refill time. The markers of tissue hypoperfusion are serum lactate, Scvo2, and CO2 gap. Once the shock is diagnosed, the etiology of the shock is further evaluated by other laboratory parameters. The basic laboratory tests are complete blood count, renal function test, liver function test, coagulation studies, blood sugar, urine microscopy; point-of-care tests like procalcitonin, D-dimer, troponin, and NT-proBNP; advanced lab tests like CRP, IL-6, blood, urine, sputum cultures, fungal biomarkers, and serological tests; and point-of-care tests like dengue, malaria, scrub card tests, ROTEM, TEG, and viral PCR tests.

BASIC LABORATORY TESTS

Serum Lactate

Lactate is the end product of anaerobic metabolism due to impaired oxygen delivery or oxygen utilization and is a marker of tissue hypoperfusion (type A lactic acidosis). The guidelines for surviving sepsis recommend measuring lactate levels (normal lactate levels are < 2 mmol/L) in the diagnosis of sepsis. Lactate clearance within 48 hours correlates with improved survival in septic shock. In cardiogenic shock, reduced cardiac output leads to insufficient oxygen reaching vital organs and tissues, resulting in anaerobic metabolism and lactate production. Persistent elevation or failure to normalize lactate levels despite interventions may indicate ongoing inadequate perfusion and a poor prognosis. Serial measurements of serum lactate help monitor the response to interventions aimed at improving tissue perfusion. Integration with hemodynamic data, clinical assessment, and other laboratory tests provides a comprehensive understanding of the patient's condition. [2]

COMPLETE BLOOD COUNT [3]

White Blood Cell Count/Differential Count

Leucocytosis/neutropenia: Septic shock causes leukocytosis (elevated total white cell [TWC] count) or leucopenia (absolute neutrophil count < 500/mm3; maturation arrest), which are signs of severe infections. Leukemoid reactions are also signs of sepsis (TWC > $50*10^9$/L).

Bands/left shift: The release of cytokines triggers the circulation of immature granulocytes (left shift) from bone marrow, called bands. Bandemia > 10% is highly specific (85%) for sepsis but usually manifests in a delayed fashion. The main limitations in recognizing bandemia are a requirement for a manual count and high inter/intra-observer variability. [4]

Peripheral smear: Morphological changes such as Döhle bodies, vacuolations, and toxic granules are indicators of bacterial infections, and parasites such as malaria are also seen in peripheral blood smear microscopy. The presence of schistocytes is caused by microangiopathic hemolysis due to sepsis.

Neutrophil-to-lymphocyte ratio (NLR): Acute stressful conditions will increase the neutrophil–lymphocyte ratio (increased neutrophils; decreased lymphocytes). Sepsis has a profound effect

Table 1.1   Classification of Shock

S. no.	Type	Incidence	Pathophysiology	Mechanism
1.	Hypovolemic	16%	Internal or external volume/blood loss	Low cardiac output and inadequate oxygen transport
2.	Cardiogenic	16%	Decreased cardiac contractility/increased filling pressures	
3.	Obstructive	2%	Internal/external blockage of circulation	
4.	Distributive	62%	Inflammation and peripheral vasodilation	Low systemic vascular resistance and impaired oxygen extraction

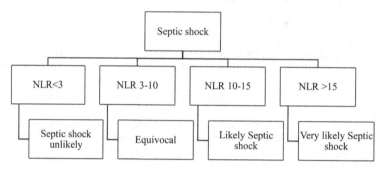

Figure 1.1   Septic shock classification based on NLR (neutrophil-lymphocyte ratio).

on the increment. NLR helps to differentiate acute severe illness from milder stress response (Figure 1.1) with a sensitivity of 96%, but it may not differentiate the etiology of stress response with poor specificity of about 10% (cut-off value for NLR > 3). The main advantage is that it will rise within 6 hours compared to the total white cell count/bands. NLR is superior to CRP and equivalent to procalcitonin in resource-limited settings for diagnosing septic shock. The fall in NLR predicts the adequacy of therapeutic response. The limitations in using NLR are that it is not validated in immunocompromised states like HIV and hematological disorders. In addition, exogenous steroids increase NLR, whereas adrenal insufficiency decreases it.

MDW (monocyte distribution width): MDW is an estimated measure of change in monocyte volume in whole blood, calculated by an automated analyzer through VCS technology (dispersion around the population mean). It is considered a marker of innate immunity activation and helps in early detection and prognosis of sepsis (AUC [0.79; CI 95% 0.73 to 0.84]. Crouser et al; cut-off value for sepsis > 20). MDW is comparable to procalcitonin and better than CRP and WBC in the ICU. [5]

Eosinophilia: Suggestive of anaphylactic shock.

Ongoing inflammation due to stress response from trauma or heart failure also results in elevation of white cell counts. The differential count, other supportive parameters, and clinical correlation help in guiding the diagnosis of the etiology of shock.

Red Cell Count

Hemoglobin level reflects the oxygen-carrying capacity of the blood. Anemia may be due to either acute or chronic conditions. The platelet count also helps in the etiology of anemia. Septic shock causes both hemoconcentration, due to capillary leak of plasma fluids, and anemia, due to hemolysis secondary to DIC in severe septic shock. Hypovolemic shock secondary to trauma or volume causes anemia (fall in all hemoglobin indices like MCV, MCH, and MCHC) and trauma-induced coagulopathy. Anemia in chronic diseases like heart failure, renal failure, and autoimmune conditions can be diagnosed by additional iron studies. Dengue shock syndrome treatment is guided by the trend of hematocrit values.

RDW (red blood cell distribution width): RDW is an automated calculated measure of variation in red cell size. The reference interval of RDW is around 11.5% to 15% and varies with age, gender, and race. Inflammation leads to delayed maturation of RBCs and is a marker of chronic inflammation. Elevated RDW indicates organ dysfunction in sepsis. It is shown to have good prognostic value, but the diagnosis of sepsis by RDW is not validated. [6]

PLATELET COUNT

Platelet count is increased in chronic inflammation and decreased in severe sepsis. Although thrombocytopenia is present in 40% of septic shock, it is not specific, but the severity determines the outcome of sepsis. Sepsis-induced thrombocytopenia is caused by increased platelet adhesion by the release of endotoxins and cytokines, in addition to phagocytosis by the reticuloendothelial system.

MPV (mean platelet volume) and MPV/P ratio: The ratio of MPV and the absolute platelet count (MPV/P ratio) is a measure of the severity of organ dysfunction in sepsis. The decreasing trend within 72 hours of antibiotic therapy is a predictor of outcome in sepsis, especially in low-resource settings.

RENAL FUNCTION TESTS

At least 50% of patients with undifferentiated shock usually have some degree of acute kidney injury with both pre-renal azotemia and acute tubular necrosis as the possible underlying mechanisms of AKI. The magnitude of elevation of urea and creatinine depends on the duration of tissue hypoperfusion. Sepsis-associated AKI, cardiorenal syndrome, and hepato-renal syndrome are different entities with different underlying mechanisms causing renal failure.

Urea: a creatinine ratio of > 20:1 is possibly secondary to pre-renal azotemia in hypovolemic shock, whereas a UCR < 10:1 may be due to a combination of both pre-renal and acute tubular necrosis in septic shock. The older classification of mechanisms is often arbitrary because multifactorial mechanisms usually coexist. Arterial blood gas analysis in AKI reveals metabolic acidosis and hyperkalemia.

Urine microscopy: This is used to differentiate between pre-renal azotemia and ATN. The presence of granular casts and renal tubular epithelial cells are suggestive of ATN. Pus cells, WBC, and nitrite indicate the presence of urosepsis. Hematuria and RBC are increased in glomerulonephritis. [7]

Urine biochemistry: Urine sodium, FeNa, and FeU are some of the advanced parameters used for the discrimination of the mechanism of AKI. False positivity is high in patients with septic shock and on diuretics.

LIVER FUNCTION TESTS

- The magnitude of hepatic dysfunction [8] depends on the duration of the shock (Figure 1.2)

- Hyperbilirubinemia (Table 1.2)

- Parenteral nutrition-associated acute liver dysfunction (PNALD) – manifests after 1–3 weeks of parenteral nutrition initiation

- Complications of hypoxic hepatitis: hepatopulmonary syndrome and spontaneous hypoglycemia [9]

COAGULATION STUDIES

Fibrinogen: This is the final substrate for clot formation and stabilization. Fibrinogen levels < 100 mg/dl result in poor clot formation and increased bleeding. Severe trauma with a high injury severity score causes acquired fibrinogen deficiency (low levels in acute DIC) and increased bleeding and risk of mortality (Figure 1.3). Fibrinogen is an acute phase reactant and is significantly increased in inflammatory conditions, malignancy, and sepsis (Tables 1.3 and 1.4).

Table 1.2 Causes of Hyperbilirubinemia

Direct hyperbilirubinemia	Indirect hyperbilirubinemia
Cholestasis/hypoxic hepatitis	Blood transfusion/hematoma

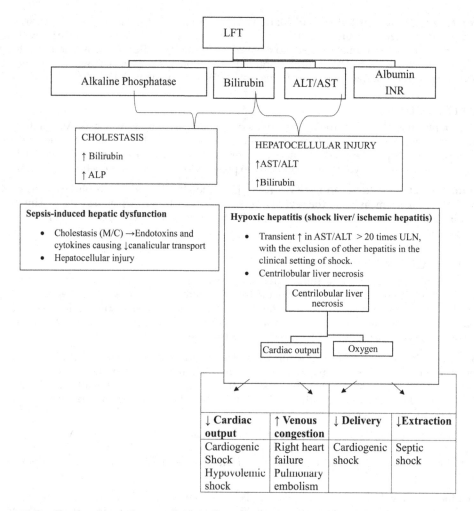

Figure 1.2 Shock-related abnormalities in liver function tests.

Table 1.3 Interpretation of Coagulation Pathway by Laboratory Parameters

Extrinsic Pathway	Intrinsic Pathway	Clot Formation	Fibrinolysis
PT/INR	aPTT	Fibrinogen	D-dimer

POINT-OF-CARE TESTS

Procalcitonin: Procalcitonin is a precursor of calcitonin hormone, used in the recognition of bacterial infections and guiding the antibiotic treatment duration. The normal procalcitonin levels are in the range of 0.5–1 μg/L and fall in > 80% of the absolute value. Alternatively, a cut-off value < 0.5 mcg/L is considered for de-escalation of antibiotic treatment in sepsis. A procalcitonin value > 5 mcg/L is usually suggestive of severe bacterial infections. Trauma, surgery, and fungal infections also cause high procalcitonin levels. Elevation is comparable to CRP in sensitivity and has better specificity compared to CRP. [12]

Bleeding time (BT) and clotting time (CT): Hemorrhagic shock and DIC. Normal bleeding time is in the range of 2–7 minutes. The International Society on Thrombosis and Haemostasis (ISTH) recommends the use of a bleeding assessment tool (BAT) with a score of > 6 in females and > 4 in males with significant bleeding history. Clotting time is in the range of 8–15 minutes (capillary tube method).

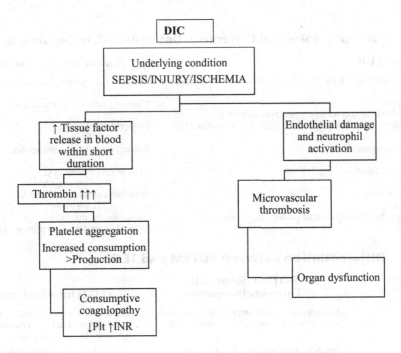

Figure 1.3 Pathophysiology of DIC in shock and organ dysfunction.

D-dimer: This is a degradation product of fibrin polymer and is clinically used as a marker of fibrinolysis. It is elevated in any acute critical illness like thromboembolic conditions, sepsis, trauma, surgery, pregnancy, and liver and renal disorders, with a sensitivity of 96% and poor specificity of 40–60%.

Obstructive shock (DVT and pulmonary embolism): It is recommended to use highly sensitive D-dimer (ELISA) with a cut-off value of ≤ 500 ng/ml (fibrinogen equivalent units; FEU) or ≤ 250 ng/ml (D-dimer unit; DDU). It has a negative predictive value of 98%, and a value ≤ 500 ng/ml (FEU) can be used to rule out DVT and pulmonary embolism in the setting of low clinical probability. However, a value of ≥ 500 ng/ml (FEU) in the setting of intermediate or high clinical probability requires further diagnostic testing.

Troponin: AHA/ACC 2021 recommendation (class 2a): For patients with NST-ACS with < 3 hours of presentation, a normal hs-cTn can rule out myocardial injury. It is specific for myocardial injury but also increased in cardiac conditions other than MI, especially in older patients, AKI, and critical illness. An increase in hs-cTn more than the 99th percentile and an increasing trend in delta change (0/1 hr or 0/2 hr) of cTn values will reliably identify high-risk patients with myocardial injury. [13]

NT-proBNP: If the diagnosis of heart failure in patients with dyspnea is uncertain and there is an intermediate probability of heart failure, the measurement NT-proBNP helps establish the diagnosis. A cut-off value of < 400 pg/ml in patients < 50 years of age can reliably exclude heart failure. It should be correlated with other clinical parameters before concluding the diagnosis.

ROTEM and TEG: These rapid, point-of-care tests will assess the viscoelastic measures of coagulation in real-time by including all the parameters of coagulation like PT, APTT, platelets, fibrinogen, and D-dimer. The main advantage is that it assesses the kinetics of clot initiation, formation, and lysis, and provides a graphical representation of hemostasis, which helps in diagnosing DIC and guiding massive transfusion protocols in hemorrhagic shock (Table 1.5).

Platelet functional assay (PFA-100): This is a screening test used to identify the in-vivo platelet function by an automated analyzer. It monitors the decrease in the flow rate of blood when platelets are combined with an agonist to form a plug. The advantages are that it is rapid, easy to use, and inexpensive.

Table 1.4 Pathophysiological Difference Between DIC in Sepsis and Trauma

Sepsis-induced DIC	Trauma-induced Coagulopathy
Definition: International Society on Thrombosis and Haemostasis (ISTH)	Profound endothelial damage
1. Severe sepsis	↓
2. Mucosal bleeding and multi-organ dysfunction	↑Tissue plasminogen activator
3. Consumption of thrombocytopenia and coagulopathy [10]	↓
	Hyperfibrinolysis
	↓Shock
Endotoxin/hypoperfusion	Thrombin + thrombomodulin
↓	↓
TNF and IL-1 activation	Activation of protein C
↓	↓Anticoagulation
Tissue factor release	Inhibition of factors V and VIII
↓	↓Late stage
Microangiopathic hemolysis and platelet aggregation	Hypercoagulable state (activated protein C depletion) [11]

Table 1.5 Differentiation Between ROTEM and TEG

Feature	ROTEM (Rotational Thromboelastometry)	TEG (Thromboelastography)
Test principle	Measures the viscoelastic properties of clot formation by rotating the sample cup	Measures the viscoelastic properties of clot formation by oscillating a pin within the sample cup
Activation	Uses activators specific for different pathways (e.g., INTEM, EXTEM, FIBTEM)	Typically uses kaolin for initiation of the intrinsic pathway and tissue factor for the extrinsic pathway
Parameters measured	* Clotting time (CT)	* R-time (reaction time)
	* Clot formation time (CFT)	* K-time (kinetics time)
	* Alpha angle	* Alpha angle
	* Maximum clot firmness (MCF)	* Maximum amplitude (MA)
	* Lysis onset and extent (LY30, LY60)	* Lysis at 30 minutes (LY30)

ADVANCED LABORATORY TESTS

Gram staining and culture: Patients with septic shock require additional testing for further management. The isolation of microbial organisms in sterile specimens like blood, urine, CSF, and sputum by culture in an appropriate medium will establish the definitive diagnosis and guide treatment.

PCR assays: Multiplex assays detect rapid and specific amplification of regions of DNA and RNA molecules of bacteria, viruses, and fungal elements with very high sensitivity. False positivity is common because it detects dead pathogens and contamination.

MALDI-TOF (matrix-assisted laser desorption ionization-time of flight): This helps in the rapid and accurate diagnosis of different species of bacteria and fungi by comparing them with the database.

Serological tests: An indirect fluorescent antibody (IFA) assay determines the antibody titers of specific infections, and the seroconversion helps in the prognosis and adequacy of treatment response.

Rapid diagnostic tests: This is based on the identification of antigen/infectious particles in the plasma of patients, and is rapid and low-cost. For malaria and dengue, histidine-rich protein 2 (HRP2) and NS1 antigens, respectively, are commonly used in screening tests. Further confirmation is done by serology or PCR.

Toxicology screen: Useful in suspected shock from drug intoxication.

Amylase and lipase: Obtained in suspected pancreatitis.

Table 1.6 Interpretation of CRP

CRP Levels	Clinical Implications
< 3 mg/L	Normal
3–10 mg/L	Low-grade inflammation
>10 mg/L	Clinically significant inflammation

Tryptase and histamine levels: Useful in suspected anaphylaxis.

Cortisol level: Helpful in suspected adrenal crisis.

Thyroid function tests: Identifies those with suspected myxedema coma.

Interleukin-6 (IL-6): This is a multifunctional cytokine that acts both as a pro-inflammatory and anti-inflammatory mediator, and regulates both innate and adaptive immunity. IL-6 is produced by fibroblasts and endothelial cells, and stimulates acute phase reactant production in the liver. It is involved in neuroprotection and energy metabolism during acute stress. It is elevated in inflammatory conditions like SLE, rheumatoid arthritis, pancreatitis, and in infections like COVID-19.

CRP: CRP is generally a family of pattern recognition molecules involved in innate immune response and complement activation. It is a sensitive marker of acute and chronic inflammation and is elevated in metabolic stresses like ketoacidosis, trauma, and surgery (Table 1.6).

REFERENCES

1. Sign in – UpToDate [Internet]. [cited 2024 Feb 26]. Available from: https://www.uptodate.com/login.

2. Casserly B, Phillips GS, Schorr C, Dellinger RP, Townsend SR, Osborn TM, et al. Lactate measurements in sepsis-induced tissue hypoperfusion: Results from the Surviving Sepsis Campaign database. *Crit Care Med*. 2015 Mar;43(3):567–73.

3. Farkas JD. The complete blood count to diagnose septic shock. *J Thorac Dis*. 2020 Feb;12(Suppl 1): S16–21.

4. Fan S-L, Miller NS, Lee J, Remick DG. Diagnosing sepsis – The role of laboratory medicine. *Clin Chim Acta*. 2016 Sep;460:203–10.

5. Wu J, Li L, Luo J. Diagnostic and prognostic value of monocyte distribution width in sepsis. *J Inflamm Res*. 2022 Jul;15:4107–17.

6. Hu Z-D, Lippi G, Montagnana M. Diagnostic and prognostic value of red blood cell distribution width in sepsis: A narrative review. *Clin Biochem*. 2020 Mar;77:1–6.

7. Bagshaw SM, Bellomo R. Urine abnormalities in acute kidney injury and sepsis. *Contrib Nephrol*. 2010 Apr;165:274–83.

8. Patel JJ, Taneja A, Niccum D, Kumar G, Jacobs E, Nanchal R. The association of serum bilirubin levels on the outcomes of severe sepsis. *J Intensive Care Med*. 2015 Jan;30(1):23–9.

9. Fuhrmann V, Jäger B, Zubkova A, Drolz A. Hypoxic hepatitis – epidemiology, pathophysiology and clinical management. *Wien Klin Wochenschr*. 2010 Mar;122(5–6):129–39.

10. Iba T, Levi M, Levy JH. Sepsis-induced coagulopathy and disseminated intravascular coagulation. *Semin Thromb Hemost*. 2020 Feb;46(1):89–95.

11. Brohi K, Cohen MJ, Davenport RA. Acute coagulopathy of trauma: Mechanism, identification and effect. *Curr Opin Crit Care*. 2007 Dec;13(6):680–5.

12. Schuetz P, Wirz Y, Sager R, Christ-Crain M, Stolz D, Tamm M, et al. Procalcitonin to initiate or discontinue antibiotics in acute respiratory tract infections. *Cochrane Database Syst Rev.* 2017 Oct 12;10(10):CD007498.

13. Sandoval Y, Apple FS, Mahler SA, Body R, Collinson PO, Jaffe AS, et al. High-sensitivity cardiac troponin and the 2021 AHA/ACC/ASE/CHEST/SAEM/SCCT/SCMR guidelines for the evaluation and diagnosis of acute chest pain. *Circulation.* 2022 Aug;146(7):569–81.

2 Sepsis and Septic Shock

Pradeep Rangappa and Amrita Shah

INTRODUCTION

Sepsis is defined as life-threatening organ dysfunction characterized by a Sequential Organ Failure Assessment (SOFA) score of 2 points or more and is caused by a dysregulated host response to infection (sepsis-3) [1]. A SOFA score ≥ 2 points is associated with in-hospital mortality of more than 10%. The clinical presentation, etiology, and differential diagnosis of sepsis exhibit wide variations. Clinical signs/symptoms and laboratory data including blood lactate, complete blood count with differential (CBC), chemistry panel, and liver function tests (LFT) are used in the diagnosis, early recognition of severity (Figure 2.1), risk stratification, and prognosis of sepsis [2, 3].

SEVERITY OF DISEASE: Why Do We Need Early Investigation?

Sepsi-related deaths encompassed 19.7% of all global deaths in 2017 according to a study by The Global Burden of Disease, with the highest burden being noted in low- and middle-income countries [4, 5]. Case fatality ranges from 22.5 to 26.7% [6]. The mortality of ICU-treated sepsis can be estimated to be up to 41.9% at hospital discharge [2]. Prompt diagnosis is crucial, as every hour of delay in antibiotics reduces survival chances by 7.6% [7]. Identification of the pathogen – bacterial, viral, fungal, or protozoal – narrows down the appropriate therapy and antibiotic stewardship for treatment [8]. An evaluation of the source of infection can include samples like blood cultures, urine and stool specimens, respiratory swabs, and endotracheal cultures, and is crucial to confirm the source of infection [2]. Inappropriate empirical antibiotic therapy can lead to an eight-fold higher hospital-related mortality in 24 hours and a 74% higher progression in the inflammatory response [9].

The various laboratory methods are elucidated in Table 2.1 [10].

BASIC LABORATORY AND POINT-OF-CARE TESTS
Conventional Methods

1. **Microbiological method**

Blood culture

■ This is the most popular method to date to identify the etiology of suspected bloodstream infection.

■ Has high sensitivity and is easy to execute.

■ Sets of blood cultures up to 20 mL are used to inoculate two bottles (one aerobic bottle and one anaerobic bottle). In a "paired blood culture," two individual blood culture sets (a total of four bottles) are drawn from two different sites.

■ Studies have shown that sensitivity increases for a single bottle (20 ml), two-bottle sets (40 ml), and three-bottle sets (60 ml) by 65–75.7%, 80–89.2%, and 95–97.7%, respectively [11, 12].

■ Blood culture positivity is followed by gram staining. It is rapid (<15 min), economical, and helps us to categorize pathogens into gram-positive, gram-negative, or gram variable. Studies have demonstrated that for therapeutic interventions, the reporting of gram stain was more impactful than reporting final antimicrobial susceptibility testing (AST) results [13].

2. **Identification through BACTEC FX/VITEK 2 [14, 15]**

Type of system	Example	Working principle and components	Special remarks
Automated/ continuous monitoring blood culture system	BacT/ALERT BACTEC VersaTREK	Have inbuilt sensors to • Detect any change in pressure within the blood culture bottle or track the CO_2 emitted by actively metabolizing species • A fluorescent dye sensor is present, and the level of fluorescence is measured by a photodetector (Figure 2.2).	No need for manual checking of blood culture

DOI: 10.1201/9781003449713-2

| Automated antimicrobial susceptibility testing (AST) system | Phoenix MicroScan WalkAway system VITEK2 | • Works on broth microdilution coupled with/without growth curve algorithm
• It continuously monitors microbial growth every 15 minutes and detects the growth by turbidity measurement in terms of raw transmittance units (RTU)
• It comes up with MIC values and compares growth patterns of test isolate with that of large numbers of reference isolate already in the VITEK database. | It has both a microbial identification (ID) and AST component; gives rise to MIC |

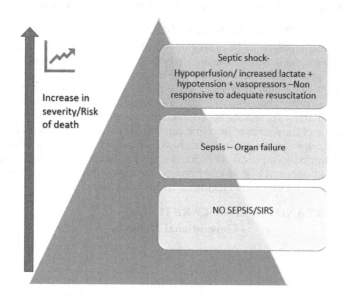

Figure 2.1 Continuum of severity of sepsis.

Table 2.1 Schematic Overview of Diagnostic Methods

Conventional Methods	Microbiological Methods Biochemical Test	Blood Culture/Gram Staining Bactec Fx/VITEK 2
Modern methods	Molecular tests	Polymerase chain reaction (PCR)
		Real-time PCR
		Surface-enhanced Raman spectroscopy (SERS)
		MALDI TOF-MS
	Broad-spectrum genomic detection of AMR (antimicrobial resistance)	High-resolution melting analysis technology (HRM)
		Whole-genome sequencing (WGS)/ next-generation sequencing
		DNA microarray
Advanced methods	Biosensors	Biomarkers
	Point-of-care testing	Biomarkers
	"Omics"	Genomics, proteomics, transcriptomics, metabolomics

(DNA: Deoxyribonucleic acid; MALDI-TOF MS: Matrix-assisted laser desorption ionization-time of flight mass spectroscopy)

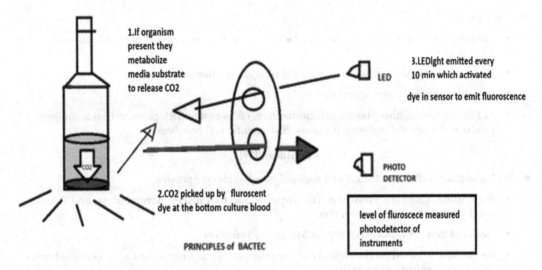

Figure 2.2 Working principle of BACTEC.

Table 2.2 Serological Methods

Functional Assays	Binding Assays
Plaque reduction neutralization assay	Rapid diagnostic tests
Pseudovirus neutralization assay	Fluorescent microarray-based assay
Pathogen receptor inhibitor assay	Indirect enzyme-linked immunosorbent assay (ELISA)
Serum bactericidal assay	Capture ELISA

Drawbacks of Conventional Diagnostic Methods [16, 17]

Blood culture

Long turnaround time (36–72 hours)
Fastidious organism – difficult to grow
Can be a biohazard during the handling of the sample/inoculation for subculturing
False-negative results
High contamination rate

Microscopy (gram staining/ZN staining)

Low sensitivity
Inter-observer high variation
High false-positive results

SEROLOGICAL IDENTIFICATION AND ANTIGEN DETECTION (TABLE 2.2) [18]

In the case of viruses, antibody neutralization is assayed, while in bacteria, detection is done by measuring the antibody-dependent killing of bacteria. Histoplasmosis and coccidioidomycosis can also be detected using serological tests. Immunoassays can be done to identify antibodies to fungal polysaccharides, or proteins like glucuronoxylomannan (GXM) for cryptococcosis. Lateral flow immunoassay (dipstick) for cryptococcal antigen is also possible.

Galactomannan [19]

- The test for serum galactomannan – a polysaccharide in the cell wall of most *Aspergillus* spp. – is an enzyme immunoassay.

- *H. capsulatum* galactomannan can be detected in body fluids, especially urine. Polyclonal rabbit antibodies are used in the antigen capture ELISA.

- Recognizes β (1→5)-linked galactofuranose using rat monoclonal antibodies.

- Limitations:
  - False-positive reactions (patients on β lactam antibiotics or infusion of gluconate-containing Plasma-Lyte)
  - Cross-reactivity with other disseminated fungal infections
  - Variable sensitivity and specificity
  - ELISA, capturing histoplasma galactomannan, cross-reacts with polysaccharide antigens produced by several endemic mycoses (*B. dermatitidis, P. brasiliensis*)

β-Glucan [19]

- (1→3)-β-d-glucan (BG) is a fungal cell wall polysaccharide component.
  - Aspergillus, Candida, Fusarium, Trichosporin, Saccharomyces, Acremonium, and P. jiroveci release this during infection.
  - Does not detect *Cryptococcus* spp. or Mucorales infection.
  - Its measure is based on the capacity of the polysaccharide to activate Factor G of the horseshoe crab coagulation cascade.
  - Used as a screening tool for presumptive diagnosis of invasive fungal infection.
  - Has a strong negative predictive value and high false positives.

Modern Methods

Molecular detection for the identification of pathogens is done using PCR (polymerase chain reaction), real-time PCR, surface-enhanced Raman spectroscopy (SERS), and matrix-assisted laser desorption ionization-time of flight mass spectroscopy (MALDI-TOF MS) [10]. Figure 2.3 shows the showing working principles of MALDI TOF- MS, and its advantages and disadvantages. Culturing of the sample is not required, but a highly precise thermal cycler is needed [20].

Antimicrobial resistance (AMR) detection includes high-resolution melting analysis technology, DNA microarray, and sequencing [10].

Molecular methods are discussed in the following sections (Table 2.3) [21].

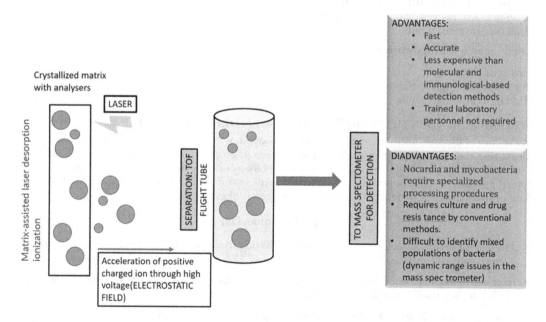

Figure 2.3 The working principles of MALDI TOF-MS, and its advantages and disadvantages.

Table 2.3   Molecular Techniques in Sepsis Diagnosis

Hybridization technique	FISH
	Arrays
	Probe hybridization
Amplification technique	PCR
	Multiplex PCR
	Broad-range PCR
Post-amplification detection technique	PCR + hybridization
	PCR + sequencing
	PCR + MALDI TOF-MS
Non-nucleic acid-based tests	Proteomics
	Spectrometry
	Phage assays

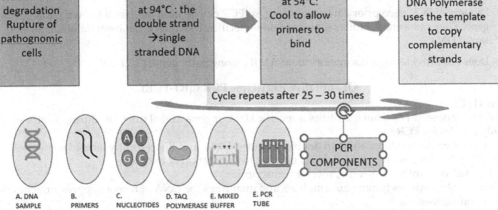

Figure 2.4   Flow of PCR: Uses key components of DNA template molecule, two synthetic primers, synthetic deoxynucleotides, and DNA polymerase enzymes. The three-step process of denaturation, annealing, and extension is carried out in repeated cycles.

Polymerase Chain Reaction (PCR)

Working Principle

This uses gene-specific primers or probes for amplification of the pathogen's target nucleic acid region. Using this purification method, a particular bacterial DNA from whole blood can be identified with samples inoculated with a minimum of 4 CFU/mL [12].

It requires the presence of DNA, primers, nucleotides, and DNA polymerase and helps to detect bacteremia using the 16S rRNA gene, followed by sequencing of amplicons. It comprises a three-step process – denaturation, annealing, and extension – which are carried out in repeated cycles to form a final PCR product (Figure 2.4).

Uses [10]:

■ Detects gram-positive and gram-negative bacteria, and fungi in samples from febrile, neutropenic patients.

■ It can diagnose and serotype pneumococcal bacteremic community-acquired pneumonia in children.

■ Among people with S. aureus bacteremia, PCR can identify patients with methicillin-susceptible S. aureus, allowing reductions in vancomycin use, hospital stays, and costs.

■ Can be used to analyze tumors, and isolate and amplify the DNA of tumor suppressor genes or proto-oncogenes.

Sensitivity and specificity:

It has advantages over blood culture in the case of probable invasive candidiasis, with a positivity rate of 85% compared with 38% for blood culture, and specificity of > 90% [22].

Advantages:

- Simple, easy to understand, and produces rapid results.

- Highly sensitive technique with the potential to produce millions to billions of copies of a specific product for sequencing, cloning, and analysis.

- Can be useful even in culture-negative cases (previous antibiotic therapy) or where the source cannot be identified [10, 21–23].

Disadvantages:

- Analyzation is done only after the completion of the PCR cycle.

- Contamination can lead to misleading results.

- Sensitivity and specificity are affected by the method of template preparation and quality.

- Primers of PCR need prior data sequencing, so PCR can be used only for a known pathogen or gene. They can anneal similar sequences non-specifically, which is not essentially identical to target DNA.

- Does not provide any information about AMR among pathogens [12, 21–23].

Quantitative Real-Time PCR (qRT-PCR)

Uses [24]:

It not only detects DNA but quantifies a specific DNA or gene in real time, i.e., during synthesis, unlike endpoint PCR.

Fluorescent dyes intercalate with double-stranded DNA, and fluorescently labeled sequence-specific DNA probes are used for detection after hybridization of the probe.

It can also quantify cDNA (i.e., reverse transcription).

It not only analyzes tumors but amplifies and quantifies the DNA of tumor suppressor genes or proto-oncogenes.

HYBRIDIZATION: Fluorescent In Situ Hybridization (FISH) [21, 25]

Working Principle

After a positive blood culture, slides are hybridized with fluorochrome-labeled oligonucleotide probes to target 16s rRNA, and visualized microscopically.

Time to detection: 2.5–3 hours.

Sensitivity: 94–99%; specificity: 99–100%.

Advantages:

Used to study the location of targeted organisms with complex environments like biofilms, co-localization, and specific interactions with other organisms.

Organisms studied include Candidatus Nitrotoga fabula (Betaproteobacteria), E. coli (Gammaproteobacteria), B. subtilis (Firmicutes), Niabella soli (Bacteroidetes), Nitrospira inopinata (Nitrospirae), Nitrososphaera gargensis (Thaumarchaeota), and Saccharomyces cerevisiae (Ascomycota).

Disadvantages:

Test limited by the availability of specific antigens for detection.

MATRIX-ASSISTED LASER DESORPTION IONIZATION-TIME OF FLIGHT MASS SPECTROSCOPY (MALDI-TOF MS) [22]

Working Principle

The samples embedded in a matrix are struck by a laser. Some energy is absorbed while others get transferred to the sample, which ionizes as a result. These sample ions are identified using a time-of-flight analyzer (TOF), and a spectrum called peptide mass fingerprint (PMF) is generated.

Uses:

- To identify gram-negative and gram-positive bacteria, aerobes, anaerobes, mycobacteria, Nocardia, yeast, filamentous fungi, and viruses.

- For antibiotic drug resistance.

- Used to identify bioterrorism organisms [22].

- Sensitivity: 76–80%; specificity: 96–100%.

Table 2.4 shows other PCR techniques.

Table 2.4   Other PCR Techniques

Methods	Technique	Advantages and Uses	Disadvantages
Lightcycler SeptiFast: The SeptiFast MGrade test (Roche Diagnostics, Mannheim, Germany)[23]	Multiplex PCR: Direct detection (from blood) – CE IVD approved.	Detects 25 causative agents of sepsis (19 bacterial and six fungal) directly from whole blood. Sensitivity: 68–75%; specificity: 86–99%.	Expensive High false-positive rates (up to 20% or higher) and false negatives (up to 14%)
T2 Candida assay and the T2Dx instrument (T2 Biosystems, Lexington, Massachusetts, USA)[22]	Combines nuclear magnetic resonance and PCR technology.	TAT: <3 hours. Accurate, sensitive (1–3 CFU/ml) Specific detection of five Candida spp. Strains (Candida albicans, Candida glabrata, Candida krusei, Candida parapsilo sis, and Candida tropicalis) in whole blood. Blood culture not necessary. Better analytical sensitivities (2.8–11.1 CFU/ml) and decreased time to positivity.	Expensive reagents and instrumentation.
Magicplex (Seegene, Seoul, South Korea)	Multiplex PCR	Detects 73 gram-positive and 12 gram-negative bacteria, six fungi, and three antibiotic resistance markers (vanA, vanB, and mecA). TAT of 4–5 h. Detection of clinically relevant pathogens from culture-negative material.	Low-to-moderate sensitivity and specificity (0.47 and 0.66, respectively).
Multiplexed-tandem PCR[22]	Nested real-time PCR • Uses two primer sets and two successive PCR reactions.	Detection of main bacterial pathogens in culture-negative samples (that were previously culture-positive). Higher sensitivity and specificity. Identifies candida spp. four days earlier than blood culture.	

(Continued)

Table 2.4 (Continued)

Methods	Technique	Advantages and Uses	Disadvantages
Verigene System (Nanosphere, now part of Luminex, Austin, TX, USA)[24]	Automated Multiplex PCR – Nucleic acid-based microarray Uses positive blood culture	Detects both gram-positive and gram-negative pathogens. Sensitivity: 92–96%. Panel of drug resistance markers (mecA for meticillin; vanA and vanB for vancomycin; and CTX-M for the detection of ESBLs, IMP, KPC, NDM, OXA, and VIM for carbapenemases) from positive blood cultures.	Occasional false-positive results.
The FilmArray Blood Culture Identification Panel (BCID; bioMérieux, Marcy l'Étoile, France, previously BioFire Diagnostics, Salt Lake City, Utah, USA)[22]	CE IVD approved and FDA-cleared multiplexed PCR system detection post-culture.	90% of causative agents of sepsis (19 bacterial and five Candida spp.) and three antibiotic resistance genes (mecA, vanA/B, and blaKPC). Hands-on time: 2 minutes. Provides results in 1 h. Sensitivity: gram-positive 97%, gram-negative 98%, fungal 99%. Specificity: gram-positive, gram-negative, and fungal pathogens – 99%, 99% and 99%, respectively.	False negatives and false positives – mecA detection in coagulase-negative staphylococci and Staphylococcus aureus, Pseudomonas aeruginosa, and Enterococcus spp. inhibited by prior antimicrobial therapy. Expensive.

Advanced Methods and Point-of-Care Tests
Biosensors and Detection of Biomarkers [9,26,27,28, 29]

- It quantifies pathogens, plasma proteins, and cell-surface proteins, and uses microfluidics, lateral flow, dipstick, and smartphone technologies.

- Helps stratify sepsis at the bedside.

- Low cost, easy to use, and rapid.

Electrochemical Sensors [26, 27]

- Utilizes ZnO nanomaterial or nanozymes for the detection of biomarkers along with bacterial species.

- Has been used in the detection of biomarkers in blood by citicoline-bovine serum albumin conjugates and aptamer-functionalized gold nanoparticles nanozymes with high sensitivity.

- Has also been used for the detection of procalcitonin (Au nanoparticles, CuMn CeO2 matrix), IL-1β and TNF-α (functionalized double-walled carbon nanotube modified dual screen printed carbon electrode (SPCE)), and IFN-γ.

Immunosensors

- Utilize specific antibodies (monoclonal, polyclonal, and recombinant antibodies), antigen reactions, and antibody detection.

- Nanobodies (Nbs) are single-domain antigen-binding fragments. These are utilized for developing biosensors and sepsis therapeutics.

- Utilized for detection of C-reactive protein (CRP), procalcitonin, and TNF-α.

- Drug-loaded nanoparticles are used for the management of sepsis.
- Has a low specificity for detecting microbes.
- Advantages: sensitivity, ease of functionalization with nanoparticles and biomolecules, reproducibility, and reliability [26, 27].

Microfluidic-based lab-on-chip devices and other integrated sensors

- They are miniature devices that integrate multiple functionalities of one or more sensing platforms on a single platform.
- Polymers polydimethylsiloxane (PDMS) and polymethylmethacrylate (PMMA) are biocompatible materials used to make microfluidic devices.
- Techniques include dielectrophoresis, inertial effects, surface acoustic waves, and centrifugal microfluidics to separate infectious agents from blood cells.
- Low cost.
- Quantifies sepsis-associated serum proteins like IL-6, IL-8, IL-10, TNF-α, S-100, PCT, E-Selectin, CRP, and Neopterin.
- IBS (integrated biosensor for sepsis) gives test results within 1 hour from native blood samples.

Optical biosensors: Used for detection of CRP, IL6, PCT, and TNF-α [26, 27].

Integrative omics [9, 28]: Genomics, transcriptomics, proteomics, and metabolomics (which is the systemic study of metabolite byproducts from enzymatic reactions) utilize high throughput techniques for the detection of sepsis biomarkers.

Artificial intelligence and machine learning/network algorithms along with "omics" can be facilitated to study protein–protein interactions, identify pathways and biological function hits, and map therapeutic responses.

Table 2.5 describes other molecular techniques including Surface-enhanced Raman spectroscopy (SERS), High-resolution melting analysis technology (HRM), Whole-genome sequencing (WGS) and DNA Microarray. Figure 2.5 shows the different types of biomarkers (in rectangle boxes); and methods of biosensors (in oval boxes) used for the detection of biomarkers or as point-of-care tests.

Table 2.6 shows the advantages and disadvantages of commonly used biomarkers. Table 2.7 shows advances in sepsis diagnostic modalities. Table 2.8 shows specialised diagnostic tests using blood cultures and whole Blood.

CLINICAL PEARLS

- The heterogeneity of sepsis pathophysiology complicates its early detection; irrespectively, appropriate antibiotics should be initiated.
- Bedside clinics together with laboratory tools are pertinent to diagnostic stewardship in cases of sepsis.
- Various methods of laboratory assessment of sepsis include conventional methods, and modern and advanced techniques.
- There is no ideal test for the detection of sepsis; all methods come with some form of limitation.
- Blood culture-positive sepsis is detected only in 50% of individuals; henceforth, other techniques including PCR, multiplex PCR, point-of-care testing, and biomarkers should be considered as better alternatives.
- Artificial intelligence may play a huge role in the early detection of sepsis using inbuilt scoring systems. Hence, further studies in this direction should be made in the future.

FAQS

1) How do you define sepsis according to the sepsis-3 guidelines?

   According to the Third International Consensus Task Force, sepsis can be defined as a "Life-threatening organ dysfunction caused by a dysregulated host response to infection." [1]

2) What are the different laboratory methods for sepsis diagnosis?

Table 2.5 Other Molecular Techniques [22]

Methods	Working Principles	Advantages and Uses	Disadvantages
Surface-enhanced Raman spectroscopy (SERS)	Amplifies the Raman dispersing of the objective particles on a superficial layer of graphene or other metal →	Identifies reference profile of microorganisms. Used for antibiotic susceptibilities.	Cannot withstand high sensitivity and specificity. Polymicrobial testing restricted → lower reproducibility of the SERS signal.
High-resolution melting analysis technology (HRM)	Uses differences in melting temperature (Tm) to produce melt curve profile of the pathogen.	New hereditary mutations and variations. AMR detection.	
Whole-genome sequencing (WGS)	Tracking of bacterial and AMR genes using automated bioinformatics examination methods. 16S rDNA and r18S DNA sequencing used.	Has a high negative predictive value. Species detection and strain typing. Can identify fastidious and uncultivable organisms. Predicts the recolonization of micro-biota post-antibiotic treatment. Identification of new resistance genes.	Expensive. Labor-intensive.
DNA Microarray[12]	Sequence-specific complementary hybridization technique used to collect and categorize DNA/RNA of microorganisms using surface-immobilized probes.	Large-scale screening for the diagnosis and detection of many pathogens. Independent of culture. AMR detection.	Powerful interpretation software is required. Expensive. Trained personnel required.

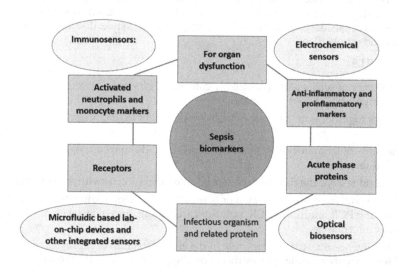

Figure 2.5 The different types of biomarkers (in rectangle boxes); and methods of biosensors (in oval boxes) used for the detection of biomarkers or as point-of-care tests.

Table 2.6 Advantages and Disadvantages of Commonly Used Biomarkers

Biomarker	Advantages	Disadvantages
Procalcitonin	Can accurately differentiate sepsis from SIRS. Sensitivity of 77% and specificity of 79%: Guides antibiotic de-escalation.	Non-specific. Single value does not give any interpretation.
Lactate	Has diagnostic and prognostic value. Higher levels co-relate with mortality 4.0 mmol/L–28.4% (21–36%).	Elevated lactate levels: cardiac arrest, trauma, seizure, or excessive muscle activity.
CRP (C-reactive protein)	Used as a diagnostic and prognostic marker. Correlates well with the severity of the infection. Cheap. Easy to perform. Widely available. As a marker for bacterial infections: sensitivity 68–92%, specificity 40–67%.	Non-specific marker. Unreliable in patients with a dysfunctional liver. Not as good as procalcitonin in discriminating infectious from non-infectious causes of fever.

Table 2.7 Advances in Sepsis Diagnostic Modalities

Automations in culture	BACTEC BacT/ALERT MGIT
Automations in ID and AST	VITEK2 Phoenix MicroScan WalkAway MALDI TOF-MS
Extended AST	Colistin microbroth dilution Carbapenem resistant gene Resistant markers in Biofire Direct susceptibility testing
Biomarkers	Procalcitonin Beta D Glucan Galactomannan
Point of Care (POC)	Latex agglutination test Immunochromatographic test
Molecular tests	GeneXpert(NAAT), Truenat RT-PCR

Table 2.8 Diagnostic Tests Using Blood Cultures and Whole Blood

Using blood cultures	PNA FISH Hyplex StaphPlex MALDI TOF Prove-it Sepsis Verigene Filmarray
Using whole blood	Xpert MRSA/SA SeptiFast VYOO SepsiTest

The different laboratory methods are leukocyte count, culture of different sources such as blood, urine, other body fluids, tissues, etc, and molecular diagnostic modalities.

3) Among the commercially available molecular tests, which ones use positive blood culture, and which ones use whole blood?

Commercial tests that use positive blood cultures include PNA FISH, Hyplex, StaphPlex, MALDI TOF, Prove-it Sepsis, Verigene and Filmarray, while those that use whole blood include Xpert MRSA/SA, SeptiFast, VYOO, SepsiTest.

4) What are the characteristics of an ideal sepsis biomarker?

The ideal sepsis biomarker would be affordable, feasible, objective, rapidly available, reproducible, with good sensitivity and specificity, dynamic, not dependent on the underlying pathology, not modified by any treatment or antibiotic, and able to correlate with clinical severity and mortality.

5) What is the working principle of PCR?

It comprises a three-step process of denaturation, annealing, and extension using DNA polymerase. It uses gene-specific primers or probes for amplification of the pathogen's target nucleic acid region.

6) What are the factors that interfere with molecular techniques, and how?

There are multiple factors that may impede the various molecular diagnostics, the most common of which is the cost of expensive reagents and instruments involved. Other factors include false-positive rates and low-to-moderate sensitivity and specificity for multiplex PCR. SERS is associated with a lower reproducibility of its signal. Whole genome sequencing is labor intensive. DNA Microarray requires powerful interpretation software and trained personnel.

Figure 2.6 shows the factors inhibiting nucleic acid amplification and their modes of action.

7) What is the best laboratory tool for the detection of infection?

An ideal diagnostic tool for sepsis is one that is cheap, easily available, has a low turnaround time to diagnose pathogens, can detect multiple organisms, is sensitive and specific, reliable and accurate, detects gene resistance, and has fast antimicrobial susceptibility. Diagnostic stewardship is individualistic and differs for different individuals. It is also dependent on comorbidities like immunocompromised state, burns, diabetes, older age, long-term hospital stay, undergoing dialysis, and whether the patient is on pre-existing antibiotics, steroids, or total parenteral nutrition. Some of the screening modalities include the Systemic Inflammatory Response Syndrome (SIRS) criteria, quick Sequential Organ Failure Score (qSOFA), SOFA

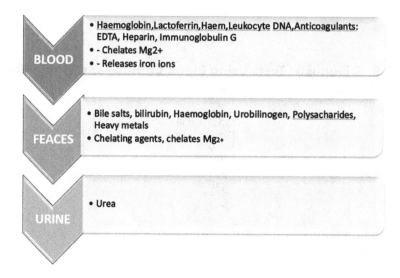

Figure 2.6 Factors inhibiting nucleic acid amplification and their modes of action.

criteria, National Early Warning Score (NEWS), and Modified Early Warning Score (MEWS) [2, 3]. The NEWS or SIRS score is preferred over qSOFA, as it has better sensitivity in predicting patient outcomes [3].

REFERENCES

1. Singer M., Deutschman C.S., Seymour C.W., Shankar-Hari M., Annane D., Bauer M., Bellomo R., Bernard G.R., Chiche J.-D., Coopersmith C.M., et al. The Third International consensus definitions for sepsis and septic shock (Sepsis-3). *JAMA* 2016;315:801–810. doi: 10.1001/jama.2016.0287.

2. Fulton II M.R., Zubair M., Taghavi S. Laboratory evaluation of sepsis. [Updated 2023 Aug 27]. In: *StatPearls* [Internet]. Treasure Island, FL: StatPearls Publishing; 2024.

3. Evans L., et al. Surviving sepsis campaign: International guidelines for management of sepsis and septic shock 2021. *Intensive Care Med*. 2021;47:1181–1247.

4. Rudd K.E., et al. Global, regional, and national sepsis incidence and mortality, 1990–2017: Analysis for the global burden of disease study. *The Lancet* 2020;395(10219):200–211.

5. Jeganathan, N. Burden of sepsis in India. *Chest* 2021;161(6):1438–1439.

6. Fleischmann-Struzek, C., Rudd, K. Challenges of assessing the burden of sepsis. *Med Klin Intensivmed Notfmed* 2023;118(Suppl 2):68–74.

7. Abe T., et al. Variations in infection sites and mortality rates among patients in intensive care units with severe sepsis and septic shock in Japan. *J. Intensive Care* 2019;7:28.

8. Coelho F.R., Martins J.O. (2012). Diagnostic methods in sepsis: The need of speed. *Revista Da Associacao Medica Brasileira* 58(4):498–504.

9. Pant A., Mackraj I., Govender T. Advances in sepsis diagnosis and management: A paradigm shift towards nanotechnology. *J Biomed Sci*. 2021;28:6.

10. Gupta E., et al. Fast track diagnostic tools for clinical management of sepsis: Paradigm shift from conventional to advanced methods. *Diagnostics* 2023;13(2):277.

11. Cockerill F.R. 3rd, Wilson J.W., Vetter E.A., Goodman K.M., Torgerson C.A., Harmsen W.S., Schleck C.D., Ilstrup D.M., Washington J.A. 2nd, Wilson W.R. Optimal testing parameters for blood cultures. *Clin Infect Dis*. 2004 Jun;38(12):1724–30.

12. Lamy B., Dargère S., Arendrup M.C., Parienti J.J., Tattevin P. How to optimize the use of blood cultures for the diagnosis of bloodstream infections? A state-of-the art. *Front Microbiol*. 2016 May;7:697.

13. Munson E.L., et al. Detection and treatment of bloodstream infection: Laboratory reporting and antimicrobial management. *J Clin Microbiol*. 2003;41(1):495–497.

14. Minassian A.M., Newnham R., Kalimeris E., Bejon P., Atkins B.L., Bowler I.C. Use of an automated blood culture system (BD BACTEC™) for diagnosis of prosthetic joint infections: easy and fast. *BMC Infect Dis*. 2014;14:233.

15. Ling T.K., Liu Z.K., Cheng A.F. Evaluation of the VITEK 2 system for rapid direct identification and susceptibility testing of gram-negative bacilli from positive blood cultures. *J Clin Microbiol*. 2003 Oct;41(10):4705–4707.

16. Ransom E.M., Alipour Z., Wallace M.A. Burnham C.A.D. Evaluation of optimal blood culture incubation time to maximize clinically relevant results from a contemporary blood culture instrument and media system. *J Clin Microbiol.* 2021;59:e02459-20.

17. Gonsalves W.I., Cornish N., Moore M., Chen A., Varman M. Effects of volume and site of blood draw on blood culture results. *J Clin Microbiol.* 2009;47:3482–3485.

18. Haselbeck A.H., Im J., Prifti K., Marks F., Holm M., Zellweger R.M. Serology as a tool to assess infectious disease landscapes and guide public health policy. *Pathogens* 2022 Jun;11(7):732.

19. Kozel T.R., Wickes B. Fungal diagnostics. *Cold Spring Harb Perspect Med.* 2014 Apr;4(4):a019299.

20. Singhal N, Kumar M, Kanaujia PK, Virdi JS. MALDI-TOF mass spectrometry: an emerging technology for microbial identification and diagnosis. Front Microbiol. 2015 Aug 5;6:791. doi: 10.3389/fmicb.2015.00791.

21. Liesenfeld O., Lehman L.H., Hunfeld K., Kost G.J. Molecular diagnosis of sepsis: New aspects and recent developments. *Eur J Microbiol Immunol.* 2014;4(1):1–25.

22. Ginn A.N., Halliday C., Douglas A., Chen S.C. PCR-based tests for the early diagnosis of sepsis. Where do we stand? *Curr Opin Infect Dis.* 2017;30(6):565–572.

23. Garibyan L., Avashia N. Polymerase chain reaction. *J Invest Dermatol.* 2013 Mar;133(3):1–4. doi: 10.1038/jid.2013.1.

24. Li Y., Xing Y., Zhao W. Emerging microtechnologies and automated systems for rapid bacterial identification and antibiotic susceptibility testing. *SLAS Technology* 2017;22(6):585–608. doi: 10.1177/2472630317727519.

25. Lukumbuzya M., Schmid M., Pjevac P., Daims H. A multicolor fluorescence in situ hybridization approach using an extended set of fluorophores to visualize microorganisms. *Front Microbiol.* 2019;10. doi: 10.3389/fmicb.2019.01383.

26. Kumar S., Tripathy S., Jyoti A., Singh S.G. Recent advances in biosensors for diagnosis and detection of sepsis: A comprehensive review. *Biosens. Bioelectron.* 2018. doi: 10.1016/j.bios.2018.10.034

27. Oeschger T., McCloskey D., Kopparthy V., Singh A., Erickson D. Point of care technologies for sepsis diagnosis and treatment. *Lab on a Chip* 2019;19(5): 728–737. doi: 10.1039/c8lc01102.

28. Langston J.C., Rossi M., Yang Q., Ohley W.J., Perez E., Kilpatrick L.E., Prabhakarpandian B., Kiani M.F. Omics of endothelial cell dysfunction in sepsis. *Vasc Biol.* 2022;4(1):R15–R34.

29. Ince J., McNally A. Development of rapid, automated diagnostics for infectious disease: Advances and challenges. *Expert Rev Med Devices* 2009;6(6):641–651. doi: 10.1586/erd.09.46.

3 Electrolyte and Acid-Base Disturbances in Intensive Care

Souvik Maitra

Electrolyte and acid-base disturbances are common in the intensive care unit (ICU) due to several pathophysiological reasons, such as organ dysfunction, activation of the sympathetic and renin-angiotensin-aldosterone system, and use of various medication and intravenous fluids, including resuscitation fluids. Common electrolyte and metabolic acid-base abnormalities encountered in critical care settings are discussed in this chapter.

ELECTROLYTE DISTURBANCES IN ICU

Disorders of Sodium Balance

Under physiological conditions, serum sodium concentration is maintained within a 135–145 mmol/l range. Sodium, urea, and glucose contribute to the serum osmolality, between 275 and 295 mOsm/kg. Serum osmolality can be estimated by the Smithline & Gardner formula (serum osmolality = 2*[Na]+[glucose]/18 + [blood urea nitrogen]/2.8) [1].

Serum sodium concentration is a function of total body water (TBW), and the following mechanisms regulate TBW:

1. Thirst mechanism. This is of limited significance in critically ill patients as they are often intubated, or oral water intake is not possible.

2. Hypothalamic osmoreceptors sense an increase in plasma osmolality and release vasopressin, which promotes free water absorption by activating V2 receptors in the collecting duct of the nephron, causing water retention [2].

3. Activation of the renin-angiotensin-aldosterone system causes renal sodium retention [3] and increased sodium uptake in the gastrointestinal tract.

Disorders of sodium balance are common in ICU and can both be a cause of ICU admission and can also be acquired subsequently. Both hypo- and hypernatremia in critically ill patients are associated with poor outcomes [4].

Hyponatremia

Hyponatremia (serum sodium < 130 mmol/L) is the most common electrolyte disorder in ICU, and nearly one-third of critically ill patients develop hyponatremia during an ICU stay [5, 6]. Traditionally, hypotonic hyponatremia is classified as hypovolemic (gastrointestinal tract loss, thiazide diuretics, hypoaldosteronism, cerebral salt wasting syndrome), euvolemic (syndrome of inappropriate anti-diuretic hormone secretion), or hypervolemic (heart failure, cirrhosis, nephrotic syndrome). However, in real-life situations, differentiation between hypovolemic and euvolemic patients is often less distinct. The following are the considerations when hyponatremia is encountered in the ICU:

A. Acute versus chronic hyponatremia: Traditionally, when hyponatremia develops over fewer than 48 hours, it is considered 'acute hyponatremia.' When hyponatremia is present for more than 48 hours, it is considered 'chronic hyponatremia.' The risk of neurological symptoms, including herniation, is higher in patients with acute hyponatremia; on the contrary, the risk of neurological injury from rapid sodium correction is higher in patients with 'chronic hyponatremia.'

B. Degree of hyponatremia: Serum sodium < 120 mmol/L is considered 'severe,' and a serum sodium ≥ 130 mmol/L but less than 135 mmol/L is considered 'mild' hyponatremia. Serum sodium values between 130 mmol/L and 120 mmol/L are considered 'moderate' hyponatremia.

C. Degree of symptoms: Hyponatremia may be asymptomatic or may cause significant neurological symptoms. Neurologic symptoms (such as seizure, coma, and obtundation) are the hallmarks of severe symptoms, and seizure is typically associated with acute hyponatremia. Mild to moderate symptoms are usually non-specific and include fatigue, headache, myalgia, nausea, and vomiting.

DOI: 10.1201/9781003449713-3

Management

The management plan depends upon the three above-mentioned clinical factors of hyponatremia. Hyponatremia with severe symptoms should be treated with 150 ml of 3% sodium chloride over 20 minutes and repeated serum sodium values after that [7].

Otherwise, the general rule for sodium correction is 8–10 mmol/L over 24 hours. However, in symptomatic patients with acute hyponatremia or severe symptoms, a target of 4–6 mmol/L should be achieved in 6 hours. If the initial serum sodium is < 120 mmol/L, along with other risk factors of osmotic demyelination, the target rate should be < 8 mmol/L over 24 hours.

Hypernatremia

The incidence of hypernatremia (serum sodium > 145 mmol/L) at the time of ICU admission is around 9% [8], and another nearly 4% of patients develop hypernatremia during the ICU stay [9]. Hypernatremia in critically ill patients is associated with an increased risk of mortality and prolonged ICU stay [9]. The primary mechanism of hypernatremia is loss of electrolyte-free water, but it may be contributed by sodium administration, particularly in critically ill patients. Hypernatremia causes hyperosmolality, and under physiological conditions, hyperosmolality activates thirst and free water retention by ADH [10]. In the ICU, the thirst mechanism is usually not practical because of several reasons, and hypernatremia cannot be corrected on its own. Loss of free water in critically ill patients may be both renal (diuretics, osmotic diuresis, renal failure causing hyposthenuria, diabetes insipidus) and extrarenal (insensible loss, lactulose therapy) and can be identified by electrolyte-free water clearance (EFWC). EFWC can be calculated by measuring urine sodium and potassium [$EWFC = $ Urine volume x $(1 - (Na_{urine} + K_{urine})/Na_{serum})$]—a positive EFWC, along with hypernatremia indicative of renal water loss.

Symptoms of hypernatremia are predominantly cardiac (ECG changes such as T wave flattening, QT prolongation, and poor myocardial contractility) and neurological (muscle weakness, confusion, coma).

Management

Assessment of intravascular volume and estimation of total body water deficit is the first step of management. Then, the rapidity of development of hypernatremia should be assessed. When hypernatremia develops within hours, it is prudent to correct sodium at a rate of 1 mmol/kg/h, as the risk of cerebral edema is minimal in these patients. When the duration of hypernatremia is longer or unknown, a slower rate of correction (0.5 mmol/L per kg per hour) is desirable to prevent cerebral edema and seizure. The expected decrease in serum sodium level depends upon the concentration of sodium and potassium in the infused fluid [change in serum sodium= [$(Na_{ifusate} + Ki_{nfusate} - Na_{serum})/$ (total body water+1)]] and proportion of the amount of fluid retained in the extracellular compartment [11]. Enteral-free water correction and parenteral 5% dextrose effectively correct hypernatremia; however, the parenteral route may be more efficacious [12].

Disorders of Potassium Balance

Potassium is a major intracellular ion; only a small portion of total body potassium is in the plasma. The incidence of abnormal serum potassium levels in critically ill patients may be more than 50% [13]. Both hypokalemia (< 3.5 mmol/L) and hyperkalemia (> 5.5 mmol/L) are associated with an increased incidence of arrhythmia and poor outcomes in critically ill patients [13] and in patients with acute myocardial infarction [14].

Hypokalemia

Hypokalemia (serum potassium < 3.5 mmol/L) in different critical care settings was found to be associated with poor outcomes [13–15]. Usually, mild hypokalemia (serum potassium between 3.0 and 3.5 mmol/L) is asymptomatic, and moderate hypokalemia (serum potassium between 2.5 and 3.0 mmol/L) can cause ileus and increase the risk of arrhythmia. Severe hypokalemia may be associated with muscle weakness, including respiratory paralysis, heart failure, ventricular arrhythmia, and rhabdomyolysis. Hypokalemia is associated with typical ECG changes such as prolonged PR interval, ST segment depression, shallow T wave, and prominent U wave. Causes of hypokalemia in critically ill patients are intracellular shift (insulin therapy, refeeding syndrome, beta-agonists), renal potassium loss (hypomagnesemia, diuretics, metabolic alkalosis, recovery phase of acute tubular necrosis, renal tubular acidosis I or II, mineralocorticoid excess), and extrarenal potassium loss (diarrhea, vomiting, etc.) [16].

Management

The usual goal of serum potassium is > 3.5 mmol/L except in patients with AMI (goal is 3.5– 4.5 mmol/L), renal insufficiency (> 3.0 mmol/L), and diabetic ketoacidosis with normal renal function (> 5.5 mmol/L). The enteral route is preferred for potassium supplementation unless enteral feeding is contraindicated or emergent treatment is required. Enteral potassium chloride is supplemented at a dose of 40 mmol three times a day in patients with normal renal function, and daily potassium monitoring is required. Intravenous potassium supplementation should be at 10 mmol/h (peripheral access) or up to 20 mmol/h (central venous access). Frequent serum potassium and continuous ECG monitoring are desirable for intravenous potassium supplementation. Concurrent magnesium deficiency should also be corrected.

Hyperkalemia

Hyperkalemia is defined as serum potassium > 5.5 mmol/L, and the European Resuscitation Council guideline classify hyperkalemia as mild (serum potassium 5.55.9 mmol/L), moderate (serum potassium 6.0--6.4 mmol/L), or severe (serum potassium ≥ 6.5 mmol/L) [17]. Causes of hyperkalemia in critically ill patients are several, such as decreased excretion (acute kidney injury, chronic kidney disease), transcellular shift (major trauma, rhabdomyolysis, burn, metabolic acidosis), and drugs (potassium-sparing diuretics, ACE inhibitors).

Hyperkalemia typically presents as neuromuscular weakness, characteristics of ECG changes (peaked T wave, flattened or absent P wave, increased PR interval, wide QRS and sine wave), and arrhythmia.

Management

Hyperkalemia, when present with typical ECG changes, requires immediate management by calcium gluconate (or chloride). The membrane stabilizing effect of calcium is fast (approximately 5 minutes) but short-lived (30–60 minutes). The recommended dose is 10–20 ml of 10% calcium gluconate or an equivalent dose of another salt [18]. The role of sodium bicarbonate in the management of hyperkalemia is less clear; some studies reported no change in serum potassium level, and on the other hand, a recent randomized trial reported a reduction in serum potassium level in patients with metabolic acidosis. Sodium bicarbonate is also associated with reduced serum calcium levels, which might contribute to poor myocardial contractility. Recent guidelines generally recommend 8.4% sodium bicarbonate at 100–250 ml doses in patients with metabolic acidemia or contraindication to calcium gluconate. Insulin-dextrose (10 U regular insulin with 25–50g of dextrose) and salbutamol (intravenous or nebulized) are probably equally efficacious in reducing serum potassium. However, insulin-dextrose has a faster onset of action. The use of diuretics for potassium lowering is of limited use, as potassium excretion is often limited and unpredictable in patients with acute kidney injury and heart failure [18]. Though potassium-binding resins are often used to increase gastrointestinal excretion of potassium, evidence is lacking.

Disorder of Magnesium Balance

Magnesium is a predominantly intracellular ion; serum magnesium represents only 0.03% of total body content [19]. Normal serum magnesium concentration is 1.8–2.3 mg/dL (0.7–1.0 mmol/L or 1.5–1.9 mEq/L) [20]. Approximately 70% of the serum magnesium is ionized, and the rest is protein-bound [21]. Around 95% of the filtered magnesium is reabsorbed in the nephron [22], and reabsorption of magnesium in the kidney is increased by calcitonin, parathyroid hormone, and acidemia.

Hypomagnesemia

The incidence of hypomagnesemia in ICU is around 40–65% and is often associated with hypokalemia, hypocalcemia, and metabolic alkalosis. Hypomagnesemia is associated with increased mortality, longer length of stay, and longer duration of mechanical ventilation in critically ill patients [23]. Deficient intake, gastrointestinal loss, renal loss, and transcellular shift all contribute to hypomagnesemia in critically ill patients. Clinical manifestations of hypomagnesemia are mainly cardiovascular (wide QRS complex, peaked T wave, prolonged PR interval) and neuromuscular hyperexcitability. Hypomagnesemia also increases the risk of atrial fibrillation in different clinical settings.

Management

The magnitude of the actual magnesium deficit is difficult to assess, as serum magnesium does not reflect total body magnesium. However, as a 'rule of thumb,' magnesium deficit is considered 1–2 mEq/kg body weight [24]. Mild hypomagnesemia (serum magnesium 1.5–2.0 mg/dL) may be managed by oral magnesium supplementation (magnesium oxide or hydroxide) [25]. Moderate (1.2–1.5 mg/dL) and severe (< 1.2 mg/dL) require parenteral magnesium supplementation. Moderate hypomagnesemia is usually treated with intermittent magnesium boluses of 2–4 gm. Severe hypomagnesemia is treated with 2–4 gm magnesium sulfate every 6–8 hours or continuous infusion of 4–8 gm over 24 hours. Nearly 50% of the infused magnesium is lost through the kidney.

Hypermagnesemia

Hypermagnesemia (serum magnesium > 5mg/dL) is typically present in clinical scenarios where there is renal failure and some other source of magnesium (rhabdomyolysis, hemolysis, tumor lysis syndrome, or magnesium therapy). Hypermagnesemia is typically associated with cardiac (hypotension, bradycardia) and neurologic symptoms (neuromuscular weakness, smooth muscle paralysis, delirium).

Management

Volume resuscitation, diuretics, and treatment of the underlying cause are the cornerstones for managing moderate hypermagnesemia. Severe hypermagnesemia requires intravenous calcium (2 gm of calcium gluconate) and renal replacement therapy when associated with renal failure.

Disorders of Calcium and Phosphorus Metabolism

Calcium and phosphorus homeostasis are interlinked, and a thorough understanding is required for bedside clinical management. The major regulators of calcium and phosphate metabolism are parathyroid hormone (PTH), fibroblast growth factor 23 (FGF 23), vitamin D3, and calcitonin [26]. The major target organs are the bone, kidney, and GI tract.

Calcium is the most abundant ion in the human body, and 99% is located as hydroxyapatite in the bone. Less than 1% of the total body calcium is in the extracellular fluid, and approximately 50% is in the ionized form. The remaining 40% is bound to the proteins (primarily albumin), and 10% is bound to the organic anions. Serum-ionized calcium is primarily regulated by PTH, which is secreted from the parathyroid gland and causes calcium reabsorption from the renal tubules and bone resorption by activating the osteoclasts. Prolonged elevation of the serum PTH increases intestinal calcium absorption through 1,25, $(OH)_2$- vitamin D. Calcitonin has a role in increasing calcium excretion by the kidney and decreasing bone resorption.

Approximately 1% of the total body phosphorus remains in the extracellular fluid, and around 75% of the phosphorus in the ECF is in free form. Phosphorus is absorbed from the intestine by passive pathways and 1,25, $(OH)_2$- vitamin D-dependent active pathways. Both PTH and FGF23 increase renal excretion of phosphorus and reduce serum levels.

Hypocalcemia

Incidence of hypocalcemia (ionized calcium < 1.5mmol/L) in critically ill patients is around 50–55% [27] and associated with poor outcomes [28], including longer length of stay and critical illness-related polyneuropathy/myopathy [27]. The classical signs and symptoms of hypocalcemia, such as increased neuromuscular excitability, are rarely seen in critically ill patients.

Management

In the case of mild hypocalcemia (serum calcium > 1.9 mmol/L), management of the underlying cause of hypocalcemia (such as vitamin D deficiency) along with oral calcium supplementation is the recommended management. In case of severe hypocalcemia, intravenous supplementation of 10% calcium gluconate at a dose of 10–20 ml diluted in 5% dextrose is recommended. Intravenous calcium gluconate infusion should be administered over 10–20 minutes and under ECG guidance. [29]

Hypercalcemia

Hypercalcemia (serum calcium > 2.6 mmol/L or > 10.5 mg/dL) in the ICU often results from malignancy (hematological or solid organ) or endocrinopathies, and AKI is associated with hypercalcemia in more than 80% of cases [30]. As hypercalcemia is a late manifestation of solid organ malignancy, the outcome in these patients is generally poor. Patients with a serum calcium level < 11.5 mg/dL are usually asymptomatic and do not require immediate therapy. Though there is no standard definition of severe hypercalcemia, a serum calcium level > 3.0 mmol/L (> 12 mg/dL) is considered 'severe' [30]. Symptoms of hypercalcemia include polyuria leading to volume depletion, AKI, drowsiness, obtundation, and characteristics of ECG changes.

Management

The initial management of hypercalcemia is volume resuscitation, and intravascular volume expansion causes around 1–2 mg/dL reduction in serum calcium level. Whether further intravascular volume loading increases renal calcium excretion or not is controversial. Though often used, furosemide is of uncertain benefit in reducing serum calcium levels [31]. Calcitonin (nasal spray or subcutaneous) is also effective in reducing serum calcium levels, and it works within a few hours to reduce serum calcium by 1–2 mg/dL [32]. Bisphosphonates are effective, but onset is slower, and evidence is largely in malignancy-associated hypercalcemia. Denosumab (monoclonal antibody against RANKL) is possibly more effective than bisphosphonates in preventing hypercalcemia in patients with skeletal metastasis.

Hypophosphatemia

The incidence of hypophosphatemia varies widely between 30–80% of critically ill patients, and it depends upon the definition used [33]. Mild (2–2.5 mg/dL) to moderate (1–2mg/dL) hypophosphatemia in critically ill patients is usually asymptomatic [34]. Hypophosphatemia may be due to transcellular shift or gastrointestinal or renal loss. Severe hyperphosphatemia (serum phosphate < 1.5 mg/dl) may be associated with muscular (proximal myopathy, poor diaphragmatic contractility), cardiovascular (reduced myocardial contractility), neurological (delirium, confusion, metabolic encephalopathy) symptoms. However, clinical symptoms do not correlate with the degree of hyperphosphatemia [35]. Whether hypophosphatemia is an independent predictor of mortality or other poor outcome in critically ill patients is debatable [33, 35].

Management

Intravenous phosphate supplementation is indicated when serum phosphate levels are < 1.0 mg/dL, when there are significant symptoms, or when the enteral route is not available. Either sodium or potassium phosphate can be used, and a dose of 15–30 mM over 4 hours, depending upon serum phosphate level, can be administered. Caution should be exercised when renal failure and/or abnormal serum calcium levels are present. For patients with milder symptoms, oral phosphate supplementation should be used. Serum calcium and magnesium should also be monitored during phosphate therapy.

Hyperphosphatemia

The incidence of hyperphosphatemia (serum phosphate > 4.5 mg/dL or 1.45 mmol/L) is around 30% in critically ill patients [36]. Critically ill patients with hyperphosphatemia have an increased risk of mortality, and the need for renal replacement therapy is also increased [36].

Hyperphosphatemia results from acute phosphate load (rhabdomyolysis, tumor lysis syndrome), transcellular shift (diabetic ketoacidosis, lactic acidosis), or reduced renal phosphate excretion. Hyperphosphatemia manifests as neurological (paresthesia, anxiety, confusion, seizure), cardiovascular (hypotension, ventricular arrhythmia), and muscle weakness.

Management

Along with restriction of enteral phosphate intake and avoidance of the offending agent, acute management of hyperphosphatemia requires volume loading and diuresis. In patients with acute kidney injury or chronic kidney diseases, renal replacement therapy is indicated. The role of oral phosphate binders (calcium acetate, sucralfate, sevelamer carbonate) is limited in acute care settings.

ACID AND BASE DISORDERS IN ICU

Human blood pH under physiological conditions is between 7.35 and 7.45. Any decrease in blood pH, along with a decrease in serum bicarbonate concentration, is known as metabolic acidosis. Nearly two-thirds of critically ill patients have metabolic acidosis [37], and alteration of blood pH in any direction is associated with poor outcomes.

Metabolic Acidosis

Metabolic acidosis (blood pH < 7.35) results from either overproduction and/or accumulation of acids or loss of bicarbonate. However, depending upon the presence of other acid-base disorders, pH may be normal or even elevated [38]. The calculation of the anion gap [AG, AG= (Na+ K)- (Cl+ HCO3)] is the first step in identifying the cause of metabolic acidosis. In critically ill patients, AG should be corrected (cAG) for the serum albumin [cAG= AG- 2.5x (4- serum albumin)]. AG is primarily constituted by serum albumin and, to some extent, by phosphate, and a value of 12 (±4) is considered normal. An increased AG metabolic acidosis is usually associated with ketoacidosis, lactic acidosis, poisoning (glycol, methanol, or salicylate), and uremia. Non-AG metabolic acidosis is usually associated with renal tubular acidosis (Type I, II, and IV), intestinal loss of bicarbonate, and chronic kidney disease with tubular dysfunction. Differentiation between renal and non-renal causes can be done by urine AG [Urine AG= Urine Na+ Urine K- Urine Cl]. A positive urine AG is indicative of the renal cause of normal AG metabolic acidosis.

Management

Primary management of metabolic acidosis is the management of the etiology of acidosis. The role of sodium bicarbonate is controversial in this setting and not routinely recommended. However, in critically ill patients with an acute kidney injury network score of 2 or 3, using 4.2% bicarbonate was associated with improved 28-day survival [39]. A French expert panel guideline [40] recommends only the use of sodium bicarbonate in patients with severe metabolic acidosis (pH ≤7.20, PaCO2 < 45 mmHg) and AKI. Bicarbonate therapy is generally not recommended in patients with diabetic ketoacidosis. Renal replacement therapy is recommended in patients with refractory acidosis (pH ≤7.15) without concomitant respiratory acidosis.

Metabolic Alkalosis

Metabolic alkalosis is a disorder where serum bicarbonate levels are higher than normal. Metabolic alkalosis requires an initiation and maintenance process [41]. The initiation phase of metabolic alkalosis is either loss of H+ ion (diuretics, nasogastric suction, vomiting) or gain of bicarbonate (sodium bicarbonate therapy, citrate from massive blood transfusion). Factors responsible for the maintenance of alkalosis are chloride depletion, reduced glomerular filtration rate, potassium depletion (mineralocorticoid excess), and volume contraction. Urine chloride < 20 mmol/L indicates volume depletion, and these patients usually respond to intravascular volume expansion [42, 43]. Metabolic alkalosis is usually associated with hypokalemia, hypocalcemia, and hypomagnesemia. Mild to moderate metabolic alkalosis (serum bicarbonate < 38 mmol/L) is usually asymptomatic. Clinical manifestations of metabolic alkalosis are cardiovascular (reduced myocardial contractility, arrhythmia), neurological (confusion, obtundation, seizure), and reduced tissue oxygen delivery.

Management

Management of the cause of alkalosis is critical. Also, maintenance factor management, such as intravascular volume loading with normal saline, is required when metabolic alkalosis is chloride sensitive. Management of the primary cause and potassium supplementation is indicated in chloride-resistant cases.

REFERENCES

1. Najem O, Shah MM, De Jesus O. Serum osmolality. 2022. In: *StatPearls* [Internet]. Treasure Island (FL): StatPearls Publishing, 2023.

2. Bichet DG. Physiopathology of hereditary polyuric states: a molecular view of renal function. *Swiss Med Wkly.* 2012;142:w13613.

3. Cano A, Miller RT, Alpern RJ, Preisig PA. Angiotensin II stimulation of Na-H antiporter activity is cAMP independent in OKP cells. *Am J Physiol.* 1994;266(6 Pt 1):C1603–C1608.

4. Funk GC, Lindner G, Druml W, Metnitz B, Schwarz C, Bauer P, Metnitz PG. Incidence and prognosis of dysnatremias present on ICU admission. *Intensive Care Med.* 2010;36(2):304–311.

5. DeVita MV, Gardenswartz MH, Konecky A, Zabetakis PM. Incidence and etiology of hyponatremia in an intensive care unit. *Clin Nephrol*. 1990;34(4):163–166.

6. Padhi R, Panda BN, Jagati S, Patra SC. Hyponatremia in critically ill patients. *Indian J Crit Care Med*. 2014;18(2):83–87.

7. Spasovski G, Vanholder R, Allolio B, Annane D, Ball S, Bichet D, Decaux G, Fenske W, Hoorn EJ, Ichai C, Joannidis M, Soupart A, Zietse R, Haller M, van der Veer S, Van Biesen W, Nagler E. Hyponatraemia Guideline Development Group. Clinical practice guideline on diagnosis and treatment of hyponatraemia. *Eur J Endocrinol*. 2014;170(3):G1–G47.

8. Polderman KH, Schreuder WO, Strack van Schijndel RJ, Thijs LG. Hypernatremia in the intensive care unit: an indicator of quality of care? *Crit Care Med*. 1999;27(6):1105–1108.

9. Waite MD, Fuhrman SA, Badawi O, Zuckerman IH, Franey CS. Intensive care unit-acquired hypernatremia is an independent predictor of increased mortality and length of stay. *J Crit Care*. 2013;28(4):405–412.

10. Chand R, Chand R, Goldfarb DS. Hypernatremia in the intensive care unit. *Curr Opin Nephrol Hypertens*. 2022;31(2):199–204.

11. Adrogué HJ, Madias NE. Hypernatremia. *N Engl J Med*. 2000;342(20):1493–1499.

12. Suzuki R, Uchino S, Sasabuchi Y, Kawarai Lefor A, Shiotsuka J, Sanui M. Enteral free water vs. parenteral dextrose 5% in water for the treatment of hypernatremia in the intensive care unit: a retrospective cohort study from a mixed ICU. *J Anesth*. 2023;37(6):868–879.

13. Tongyoo S, Viarasilpa T, Permpikul C. Serum potassium levels and outcomes in critically ill patients in the medical intensive care unit. *J Int Med Res*. 2018;46(3):1254–1262.

14. Goyal A, Spertus JA, Gosch K, Venkitachalam L, Jones PG, Van den Berghe G, Kosiborod M. Serum potassium levels and mortality in acute myocardial infarction. i2012;307(2):157–164.

15. Safavi M, Honarmand A, Mehrizi MK, Dastjerdi MS, Ardestani ME. Hypokalemia at the time of admission to the intensive care unit (ICU) increases the need for mechanical ventilation and time of ventilation in critically ill trauma patients. *Adv Biomed Res*. 2017;6:50.

16. Lee JW. Fluid and electrolyte disturbances in critically ill patients. *Electrolyte Blood Press*. 2010;8(2):72–81.

17. Truhlář A, Deakin CD, Soar J, Khalifa GEA, Alfonzo A, Bierens JJ, *et al*. European resuscitation council guidelines for resuscitation 2015. *Resuscitation*. 2015;95:148–201.

18. Dépret F, Peacock WF, Liu KD, Rafique Z, Rossignol P, Legrand M. Management of hyperkalemia in the acutely ill patient. *Ann Intensive Care*. 2019;9(1):32.

19. Elin RJ. Assessment of magnesium status. *Clin Chem*. 1987;33(11):1965–1970.

20. Jahnen-Dechent W, Ketteler M. Magnesium basics. *Clin Kidney J*. 2012;5(Suppl 1):i3–i14.

21. Hansen BA, Bruserud Ø. Hypomagnesemia in critically ill patients. *J Intensive Care*. 2018;6:21.

22. Sutton RA, Domrongkitchaiporn S. Abnormal renal magnesium handling. *Miner Electrolyte Metab*. 1993;19(4–5):232–240.

23. Jiang P, Lv Q, Lai T, Xu F. Does Hypomagnesemia impact on the outcome of patients admitted to the intensive care unit? A systematic review and meta-analysis. *Shock*. 2017;47(3):288–295.

24. Tong GM, Rude RK. Magnesium deficiency in critical illness. *J Intensive Care Med.* 2005;20(1):3–17.

25. Yamamoto M, Yamaguchi T. Causes and treatment of hypomagnesemia. *Clin Calcium.* 2007;17(8):1241–1248.

26. Shaker JL, Deftos L. Calcium and phosphate homeostasis. [Updated 2023 May 17]. In: Feingold KR, Anawalt B, Blackman MR, *et al.*, editors. *Endotext* [Internet]. South Dartmouth (MA): MDText.com, Inc., 2000. Available from: https://www.ncbi.nlm.nih.gov/books/NBK279023/

27. Melchers M, van Zanten ARH. Management of hypocalcaemia in the critically ill. *Curr Opin Crit Care.* 2023;29(4):330–338.

28. Zhang Z, Xu X, Ni H, Deng H. Predictive value of ionized calcium in critically ill patients: an analysis of a large clinical database MIMIC II. *PLoS One.* 2014;9(4):e95204.

29. Turner J, Gittoes N, Selby P, Society for Endocrinology Clinical Committee. Society for endocrinology endocrine emergency guidance: emergency management of acute hypocalcaemia in adult patients. *Endocr Connect.* 2016;5(5):G7–G8.

30. Mousseaux C, Dupont A, Rafat C, Ekpe K, Ghrenassia E, Kerhuel L, Ardisson F, Mariotte E, Lemiale V, Schlemmer B, Azoulay E, Zafrani L. Epidemiology, clinical features, and management of severe hypercalcemia in critically ill patients. *Ann Intensive Care.* 2019;9(1):133.

31. LeGrand SB, Leskuski D, Zama I. Narrative review: furosemide for hypercalcemia: an unproven yet common practice. *Ann Intern Med.* 2008;149(4):259–263.

32. Kammerman S, Canfield RE. Effect of porcine calcitonin on hypercalcemia in man. *J Clin Endocrinol Metab.* 1970;31(1):70–75.

33. Sin JCK, King L, Ballard E, Llewellyn S, Laupland KB, Tabah A. Hypophosphatemia and outcomes in ICU: a systematic review and meta-analysis. *J Intensive Care Med.* 2021;36(9):1025–1035.

34. Bsar AEME, El-Wakiel SA, El-Harrisi MA, Elshafei ASH. Frequency and risk factors of hypophosphatemia in patients admitted to emergency intensive care unit in Zagazig University hospitals. *Indian J Crit Care Med.* 2023;27(4):277–282.

35. Suzuki S, Egi M, Schneider AG, Bellomo R, Hart GK, Hegarty C. Hypophosphatemia in critically ill patients. *J Crit Care.* 2013;28(4):536.e9–19.

36. Zheng WH, Yao Y, Zhou H, Xu Y, Huang HB. Hyperphosphatemia and outcomes in critically Ill patients: a systematic review and meta-analysis. *Front Med (Lausanne).* 2022;9:870637.

37. Gunnerson KJ, Saul M, He S, Kellum JA. Lactate versus non-lactate metabolic acidosis: a retrospective outcome evaluation of critically ill patients. *Crit Care.* 2006;10(1):R22.

38. Achanti A, Szerlip HM. Acid-base disorders in the critically Ill patient. *Clin J Am Soc Nephrol.* 2023;18(1):102–112.

39. Jaber S, Paugam C, Futier E, Lefrant JY, Lasocki S, Lescot T, Pottecher J, Demoule A, Ferrandière M, Asehnoune K, Dellamonica J, Velly L, Abback PS, de Jong A, Brunot V, Belafia F, Roquilly A, Chanques G, Muller L, Constantin JM, Bertet H, Klouche K, Molinari N, Jung B, BICAR-ICU Study Group. Sodium bicarbonate therapy for patients with severe metabolic acidaemia in the intensive care unit (BICAR-ICU): a multicentre, open-label, randomised controlled, phase 3 trial. *Lancet.* 2018;392(10141):31–40.

40. Jung B, Martinez M, Claessens YE, Darmon M, Klouche K, Lautrette A, Levraut J, Maury E, Oberlin M, Terzi N, Viglino D, Yordanov Y, Claret PG, Bigé N, Société de Réanimation de Langue Française (SRLF), Société Française de Médecine d'Urgence (SFMU). Diagnosis and management of metabolic acidosis: guidelines from a French expert panel. *Ann Intensive Care.* 2019;9(1):92.

41. Seldin DW, Rector FC Jr. Symposium on acid-base homeostasis. The generation and maintenance of metabolic alkalosis. *Kidney Int.* 1972;1(5):306–321.

42. Tinawi M. Pathophysiology, evaluation, and management of metabolic alkalosis. *Cureus.* 2021;13(1):e12841.

43. Do C, Vasquez PC, Soleimani M. Metabolic alkalosis pathogenesis, diagnosis, and treatment: core curriculum 2022. *Am J Kidney Dis.* 2022;80(4):536–551.

4 Polytrauma and Multi-Organ Dysfunction

Rahul Chaurasia and Kapildev Soni

Laboratory investigations are integral to the management of polytrauma and multiple organ dysfunction syndrome (MODS), serving crucial roles in initial assessment, treatment guidance, complication detection, and patient outcome monitoring. The categorization of laboratory investigations for polytrauma and MODS is based on temporal considerations, distinguishing between basic and advanced tests. These assessments are pivotal for comprehensive patient care and optimization of therapeutic interventions in the context of complex trauma and multi-organ dysfunction scenarios.

BASIC LABORATORY TESTS

Fundamental laboratory analyses including hematological assessments, coagulation profiling, blood typing, crossmatching, serum electrolyte quantification, and arterial blood gas analysis are imperative for the initial evaluation of patients afflicted with polytrauma and MODS. The details of these investigations are given as follows:

i. **Blood counts**: Complete blood counts, encompassing measurements of hemoglobin, hematocrit, platelet counts, and leukocyte counts, serve as pivotal assessments to gauge the extent of anemia, thrombocytopenia, and inflammatory processes in patients with polytrauma and MODS. Although the absolute values obtained upon admission may not be immediately indicative in cases of acute bleeding, they establish a baseline for subsequent evaluations and aid in the ongoing monitoring of blood loss, transfusion requirements, and surgical interventions.

ii. **Coagulation testing:** Coagulopathy is a common occurrence reported in 25–30% of severely injured patients. The pathobiology of acute coagulopathy of trauma is multifactorial and related to the injury severity and nature of resuscitation. Hemostatic derangements encompass a spectrum of abnormalities including fibrinogen depletion, impaired thrombin generation, dysfunctional platelet activity, and dysregulated fibrinolysis. Thus timely identification of coagulopathy and its underlying etiology is imperative to facilitate prompt initiation of appropriate therapeutic interventions and transfusion strategies. Evaluation of trauma-associated coagulopathy typically involves assessment of prothrombin time (PT), activated partial thromboplastin time (aPTT), fibrinogen levels, and D-dimer/fibrin degradation product (FDP) assays.

iii. **Blood grouping and crossmatching:** Blood samples are expeditiously dispatched to the blood center to facilitate timely ABO and RhD typing of the patient. This critical step aids in the selection of compatible blood units tailored to the patient's specific blood group, ensuring availability for immediate issuance as needed during resuscitative efforts or operative interventions.

iv. **Blood gas analysis:** Arterial blood gas (ABG) analysis is performed to assess the partial pressures of gases in the blood and acid-base equilibrium. This diagnostic modality serves as an essential component of initial patient assessment, facilitating the identification of underlying etiologies contributing to respiratory and metabolic disturbances, thereby guiding the implementation of targeted therapeutic interventions. Additionally, ABG analysis plays a pivotal role in monitoring the efficacy of supplemental oxygen therapy and prognosticating outcomes in affected patients. The components of ABG include:

- PaO_2: Measures the partial pressure of oxygen in arterial blood. It reflects the adequacy of the blood oxygenation in the lungs and diagnosing respiratory failure.

- P_{50}: The determination of partial pressure of oxygen (pO2) at 50% oxygen saturation is a valuable metric for evaluating oxygen release to tissues.

- SaO_2: Arterial oxygen saturation reflects utilization of the currently available oxygen transport capacity and the oxygen delivery at the tissue levels.

- $PaCO_2$: Partial pressure of carbon dioxide in arterial blood reflects the "respiratory" contribution to acid-base status. Provides evidence of the adequacy of alveolar ventilation.

- pH: Assesses acid-base balance of the blood.

- HCO_3^-: The calculated concentration of bicarbonate (HCO_3^-) in arterial blood serves as an indicator of blood's buffering capacity. Together with pH and partial pressure of carbon

DOI: 10.1201/9781003449713-4

dioxide (pCO2), it is used for diagnosing and monitoring acid-base disturbances. It reflects the "non-respiratory" or "metabolic" component of acid-base status.

- Anion gap (AG) and base excess: AG is the difference between unmeasured anions and unmeasured cations. The clinical utility lies in the detection and analysis of acid-base imbalances, particularly metabolic acidosis. Furthermore, base excess levels aid in identifying the severity of hemorrhagic shock and serve as a prognostic indicator among severely bleeding trauma patients.

- In addition to these parameters of ABG analysis, there are equipments that can assess additional parameters such as electrolytes, lactate levels, and hemoglobin.

v. **Blood chemistry:** This comprehensive evaluation includes assessments of electrolyte concentrations, lactate levels, and baseline liver and kidney function tests. This includes assessment of:

- **Potassium (K⁺):** The concentration of K⁺ in the extracellular fluid is influenced by the acid-base equilibrium. Therefore, monitoring its levels aids in elucidating the anion gap and facilitates the assessment of any condition resulting in significant cellular destruction or lysis.

- **Sodium (Na⁺):** Assessment of Na⁺ helps in identifying disturbances of the sodium and water metabolism and calculating the anion gap.

- **Chloride (Cl⁻):** Monitoring Cl⁻ levels helps in the calculation of the anion gap and elucidates underlying etiology.

- **Calcium (Ca²⁺):** Evaluation of Ca²⁺ levels is essential for the initial assessment and guidance of calcium supplementation, given the frequent occurrence of calcium metabolism disturbances and abnormal Ca²⁺ levels among critically ill patients and those undergoing extensive blood transfusions. Blood units typically contain citrate as an anticoagulant.

- **Lactate:** Elevation in lactate levels serves as an early and sensitive indicator of an imbalance between tissue oxygen demand and oxygen supply. Serum lactate levels exceeding > 2.0 mmol/L are utilized for the prompt identification of hemorrhagic shock as well as monitoring response to resuscitation. Additionally, initial lactate levels are used for prognostication.

- **Glucose levels:** Hyperglycemia can be a significant problem in trauma patients and is associated with increased morbidity and mortality. It results from a hypermetabolic reaction to stress and appears to represent a distinct entity rather than merely a marker. It is highly sensitive in indicating cerebral cellular injury secondary to head trauma. While the exact pathophysiology of hyperglycemia's neuropathic impact remains incompletely understood, reports suggest it exacerbates ischemic acidosis, consequently aggravating brain edema.

vi. **Urine analysis:** Urine analysis is used for monitoring the water balance and hematuria, hemoglobinuria, or myoglobinuria. The presence of microscopic or macroscopic hematuria suggests genitourinary injuries. Thus, it serves as a screening tool for guiding further radiological investigations in blunt abdominal injuries. It also helps in identifying ketones and urinary tract infections in acutely ill trauma patients.

vii. **Pregnancy tests:** The monitoring of β-human chorionic gonadotropin (β-HCG) levels in urine provides a rapid and efficient means of detecting pregnancies in polytrauma patients.

ADVANCED LABORATORY TESTS

Advanced laboratory tests complement routine laboratory and imaging investigations by facilitating early identification of organ involvement, detection of infectious complications, and prognostication in affected patients. The details of the advanced tests are given as follows:

viii. **Viscoelastic assays (VEAs):** VEAs are comprehensive hemostatic assessments utilized to monitor the intricate dynamics of both coagulation and fibrinolysis processes. Initially described by Hartert in 1948 as thromboelastography, VEA enables the evaluation of the entire coagulation cascade in whole blood. By inducing clot formation under conditions simulating sluggish venous flow, VEA elucidates the kinetics of clot initiation, propagation, and stabilization, as well as the subsequent fibrinolysis process. This approach provides a holistic understanding of clot formation, strength, and breakdown within the physiological context of whole blood, incorporating contributions from platelets, fibrinogen, and coagulation factors. Based on Hartert's work, two technologies, i.e., Thrombelastograph® [TEG®] by Haemonetics, and Thromboelastometry (ROTEM®) by Werfen, are currently available. A brief description of both these assays are described as follows:

- **TEG:** as shown in Figure 4.1, TEG5000 uses a heated cup, which oscillates through a 4°45′ angle. A pin is suspended within the cup by a torsion wire, which monitors the shear stress during the process of clot formation and transfers the signal through an electromechanical transducer to produce a graphical representation, known as thromboelastography. The details of the parameters recorded with their clinical correlation are shown in Table 4.1. A newly developed TEG6s system uses a microfluidic system that monitors the clot resonance frequency to produce thromboelastography.

- **ROTEM:** The ROTEM delta device has a fixed cup within a heating block and a suspended rotating pin as shown in Figure 4.1. During clot formation, the rotation of the pin is detected optically, producing a graphical representation of the dynamic of the clot.

  Although both technologies assess clot kinetics, strength, and lysis, their results are not interchangeable due to variations in their operational characteristics. Discrepancies in parameter nomenclature are outlined in Table 4.2. Additionally, Table 4.2 provides a comprehensive overview of the assays and parameters employed within both systems.

ix. **Screening for bacterial infections:**

- **Culture and sensitivity:** Infections and sepsis represent prominent contributors to morbidity and delayed mortality among trauma patients. Microbiological cultures obtained from affected injury sites, coupled with sensitivity assays, play a pivotal role in identifying causative pathogens and guiding the selection of appropriate antibiotic therapy.

x. **Biomarkers:** While microbiologic cultures and clinical judgment serve as the gold standard for diagnosing infection/sepsis, early detection of infections using biomarkers is increasingly recognized as valuable. C-reactive protein (CRP) has been investigated as a marker for sepsis; however, its lack of specificity hinders its ability to differentiate systemic inflammatory response syndrome (SIRS) from sepsis following trauma. In contrast, procalcitonin (PCT)

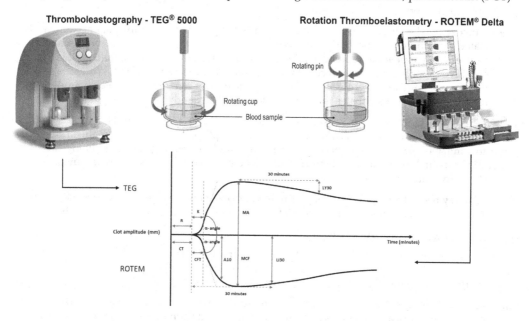

Figure 4.1 Principle and results of viscoelastic assays. TEG – R: Reaction time (min), K: Kinetics time (min), α: Angle (degrees), MA: Maximum amplitude (mm), LY 30: lysis 30 after MA (%); ROTEM – CT: Clotting time (s), CFT: Clot formation time (s), α: Angle (degrees), A10: Amplitude 10 min after CT, MCF - Maximum clot firmness (mm), LI30 – lysis index 30 min after CT (%).

Table 4.1   Viscoelastic Assays – TEG and ROTEM

	TEG® 5000	ROTEM® Delta	
Clot initiation	R – reaction time (min)	CT – clotting time (s)	Time to initial clot formation: represents activation of coagulation cascade, thrombin generation, and influence of anticoagulants.
Clot kinetics	α – angle (degrees) K – kinetics time (min)	α – angle (degrees) CFT – clot formation time (s)	Speed of clot propagation: represents fibrin activation and polymerization.
Clot strength	MA – maximum amplitude (mm)	A10 – amplitude 10 min after CT MCF – maximum clot firmness (mm)	Strength of clot: represents contribution of fibrinogen and platelet to the clot formed.
Clot stability	LY 30 – lysis 30 after MA (%)	LI30 – lysis index 30 min after CT (%)	Fibrinolysis: represents rate of fibrinolysis.

emerges as a specific marker for systemic bacterial infection and sepsis, with levels correlating with the bacterial burden and infection severity. It is noteworthy that PCT levels exhibit a rapid increase immediately after injury and remain elevated for approximately 48 hours post-trauma. Consequently, monitoring procalcitonin becomes particularly relevant beyond this timeframe. Compared to CRP, PCT boasts a shorter plasma elimination half-life, rendering it advantageous for regular monitoring purposes. Furthermore, PCT serves as a prognostic marker, as higher levels have been observed among non-survivors compared to survivors.

xi. **Serum amylase and lipase levels:** Persistently elevated or increasing levels of serum amylase and lipase serve as dependable indicators of pancreatic injury, with their diagnostic utility being time-dependent. Notably, these markers are nondiagnostic within the initial 6 hours following trauma. In resource-limited settings where computed tomography (CT) is unavailable, the combined estimation of serum amylase and lipase levels may provide supportive evidence for clinical suspicion of pancreatic injury.

Table 4.2   Available Assays on TEG® 5000 and ROTEM® Delta Analyzers

TEG® 5000	ROTEM® Delta	Clinical Significance
Standard TEG (Kaolin activator)	INTEM (Ellagic acid as activator)	Assessment of intrinsic pathway of coagulation and provides information similar to aPTT.
NA	EXTEM (contains tissue factor as activator)	Assessment of extrinsic pathway of coagulation and provides information similar to PT.
rTEG (contains tissue factor and kaolin as activator)	NA	Assessment of both extrinsic and intrinsic pathways of coagulation and provides information similar to PT and aPTT.
Heparinase TEG	HEPTEM	Used for assessment of heparin effect on intrinsic pathway of coagulation (for TEG, use standard TEG; for ROTEM use INTEM).
Functional fibrinogen TEG Reagent contains tissue factor and abciximab, a GPIIb/IIIa inhibitor, to block the platelet contribution to clot formation.	FIBTEM Reagent contains tissue factor and cytochalasin D, an actin polymerization inhibitor, to block the platelet contribution to clot formation	Used for qualitative assessment of the contribution of fibrinogen to clot strength by blocking platelets. Used and compared with standard TEG, whereas for ROTEM, used and compared with EXTEM assay.
NA	APTEM Reagent contains aprotinin (fibrinolysis inhibitor)	Helps in discriminating between fibrinolysis and platelet-mediated clot retraction.
TEG platelet mapping		Used for assessment of platelet function or the effect of antiplatelet agents.

xii. **Biomarkers for organ injuries:** Testing for organ-specific biomarkers can serve to obviate or assist in the interpretation of radiological investigations and invasive procedures for confirming diagnosis, guiding treatment decisions, and prognostication. The list of organ-specific biomarkers and their clinical relevance is delineated in Table 4.3.

xiii. **Toxicology and alcohol screening:** Self-harm incidents, poisonings, and toxicological disasters represent a substantial portion of patient cases encountered in emergency departments. Toxicological screening is routinely conducted for both medico-legal reasons and to exclude poisoning, which can significantly influence treatment decisions for affected individuals. This screening entails the analysis of blood and urine samples to detect common substances of abuse (such as alcohol, opioids, cannabinoids, and amphetamines) as well as therapeutic drugs (such as cholinesterase inhibitors, salicylates, and benzodiazepines) that may be employed as agents of self-harm.

xiv. **Serological tests:** Testing for infectious markers such as human immunodeficiency virus (HIV), hepatitis B virus (HBV), and hepatitis C virus (HCV) should be conducted in accordance with institutional policies. While not mandatory, screening for these infectious markers affords healthcare organizations the opportunity to identify and provide treatment to at-risk populations. Serological testing also facilitates the monitoring of transfusion-transmitted infections and enables timely organ procurement for transplantation from brain-dead donors.

Table 4.3 Different Markers for Organ Dysfunctions

Affected Organ	Markers	Remarks
Acute systemic inflammatory markers	Leucocyte number C-reactive protein (CRP) Erythrocyte sedimentation rate (ESR) Interleukin-6 (IL-6) Interleukin-8 (IL-8) Procalcitonin (PCT)	Used for monitoring of the acute systemic inflammatory response. Correlates with the severity and is thus also used for identifying risk groups. Identifying/differentiating SIRS from infection or sepsis.
Cardiac injury	Cardiac Troponin I or T (cTnI/cTnT) Myoglobin Creatine kinase-myoglobin binding (CK-MB) Heart fatty acid binding protein Brain natriuretic peptide (BNP) and N-terminal proBNP (NT-proBNP)	Earlier detection of myocardial damage. May indicate functional, subcellular damage of the cardiomyocytes, which is not detectable in advanced imaging. Heart failure, including diastolic dysfunction.
Kidney injury	Neutrophil gelatinase-associated lipocalin (NGAL), Kidney injury molecule-1 (KIM-1) Cystatin C IL-18 Liver fatty acid binding protein (L-FABP)	Often used as adjunct diagnostics to routine biochemistry, urine analysis, ultrasonography, and other radiological investigations to improve the early detection, differential diagnosis, and prognostic assessment of acute kidney injury.
Liver injury	Aspartate aminotransferase (AST) Alanine aminotransferase (ALT) Lactate dehydrogenase (LDH)	Markers of hepatocellular injury, assist imaging methods in identifying the extent of injuries and risk stratification.
Traumatic brain injury	Angiopoetin-2 Endothelin-1 (ET-1) Endocan-2 (EC-2) Neuron specific enolase, Ubiquitin-C terminal hydrolase-L1 (UCH-L1) Glial fibrillary acidic protein (GFAP), S100B protein Myelin basic protein (MBP) Osteopontin (OPN) High Mobility Group Box 1 Protein (HMGB1)	Markers for cell damage in the central nervous system, assist imaging techniques in risk stratification and predicting prognosis.
Lung injury	Surfactant protein D (SP-D) Angiopoietin -2 (AP-2)	Indicator for alveolar damage. Assists imaging methods and helps in early diagnosis and reduced radiation exposure.

Table 4.4 Available Point-of-Care Tests (POCT) for Trauma

1. Hematology analyzers
   a. Devices measuring single parameters
      - Hb, HemoCue 201 (Hb), HemoCue
      - HemoCue WBC system (WBC), HemoCue
   b. Devices measuring multiple parameters
      - pocH-100i™ Automated Hematology Analyzer, Sysmex
      - Yumizen 500, Horiba
      - DxH 500, Beckman Coulter

2. Coagulation analyzer
   a. Devices measuring single parameters
      - CoaguChek XS, Roche
      - INRatio system, Alere
      - Xprecia Stride, Siemens Healthcare Diagnostics
   b. Devices measuring multiple parameters
      - i-STAT, Abbott
      - Hemochron signature elite, Werfen
   c. Viscoelastic assays
      - TEG 5000 and TEG 6s, Haemonetics
      - ROTEM delta and ROTEM sigma, Werfen

3. Blood gas analysis
      - i-STAT-1 and i-STAT Alinity, Abbott
      - Cobas b221 system and Cobas b123 POC, Roche
      - RAPIÐPoint 500e and ePOC blood analysis system, Siemens Healthcare Diagnostics
      - GEM premier 500, Werfen

4. Blood chemistry
   a. Devices measuring single parameters
      - HemoCue glucose 201 system, HemoCue
      - AccuTrend Plus, Roche
   b. Devices measuring multiple parameters
      - i-STAT and Piccolo Xpress, Abbott
      - Cobas C111, Roche
      - RAPIDChem 744/754, Siemens Healthcare Diagnostics
      - GEM Premier Chemstat, Werfen
      - IEM Premier 3500, Instrumentation Laboratory
      - ABL800 FLEX, Radiometer

5. Urine analysis
      - URISYS 1100, Roche
      - CLINITEK Status + Analyzer, Siemens Healthcare Diagnostics
      - UC-1000 urine, Sysmex

6. Cardiac markers
   a. Devices measuring a single parameter
      - TROP T, Roche
   b. Devices measuring multiple parameters
      - Stratus CS acute care diagnostic system, Abbott

7. CRP
      - Cobas b101, Roche

8. Traumatic brain injury
      - i-STAT TBI Plasma test, Abbott

9. Antimicrobial susceptibility testing
      - PA-100 AST System, Sysmex

10. Pregnancy
      - Immunochromatographic card tests

11. Serology tests
      - Immunochromatographic card tests

12. Platelet function
      - PFA100/200, Siemens Healthcare Diagnostics
      - Multiplate, Roche
      - VerifyNow, Accumetrics

Point-of-care (POC) testing: Traditional laboratory testing typically involves multiple steps for sample collection (appropriate for the tests), transportation, and pre-processing of the test samples. The time delays between the steps involved result in a longer time to produce the results and delay the clinical decision-making. POC or bedside testing for such decision-making steps provides rapid turnaround of test results so that appropriate treatment can be implemented in a timely manner and affect the overall patient outcomes. The description of various point-of-care tests available for polytrauma patients is shown in Table 4.4. While POC testing is advantageous for decision-making during clinical management, there are several disadvantages compared to the test results from traditional laboratory testing. These include (1) lack of quality assurance quality control data to ensure that the test results are reliable and valid, (2) increased rate of errors such as sample handling errors, post-analytical errors, improper training of staff, etc., (3) poor analytical performance, (4) increased costs, (5) lack of adequate documentation, (6) limited number of tests, and (7) unauthorized testing in certain scenarios. Thus, prior to the implementation of POC testing, the advantages and disadvantages should be weighed appropriately, and the tests should be validated within the institution.

CLINICAL PEARLS

- Early coagulopathy identification: Assess PT, aPTT, and fibrinogen to detect coagulopathy promptly, reducing hemorrhagic risks.

- Organ dysfunction detection: Utilize liver and renal function tests, along with arterial blood gas analysis, for early organ dysfunction recognition and targeted interventions.

- Inflammatory response monitoring: Track CRP and PCT levels to gauge systemic inflammation severity, guiding timely interventions and prognosis assessment.

- Infectious complications screening: Regularly screen for infectious markers like blood and wound cultures to detect and treat infections promptly, minimizing sepsis risks.

- Metabolic status assessment: Monitor electrolytes, blood glucose, and lactate to optimize resuscitative efforts and prevent metabolic imbalances and associated complications.

5 Emergency and Intensive Care Management for Acute Poisonings and Toxicities

Uttam Garg and Michael Christian

INTRODUCTION

Acute poisoning and toxicity refer to the ingestion of a toxic substance that results in a rapid onset of symptoms and potentially life-threatening complications. It is a common medical emergency that requires prompt assessment, diagnosis, and appropriate management of a patient to minimize morbidity and mortality [1].

Initial medical assessment and management consist of a two-pronged approach to the patient. The practitioner is simultaneously treating any life-threatening emergencies as well as ordering any necessary diagnostic studies in order to further elucidate the cause(s) for the patient's presentation [2]. The mainstays of medical management consist of supporting the ABCs (airway, breathing, and circulation) as well as aggressive supportive care for immediate life threats caused by a particular toxin or a combination of toxins ingested [3]. While a comprehensive summary of supportive care is beyond the scope of this chapter, a few mainstays of treatment can be discussed. A wide variety of xenobiotics can cause airway failure due to a variety of mechanisms. This can be due to mental status depression (i.e., opioids, sedative-hypnotics, etc.), seizures (sympathomimetics, antidepressants, GABA inhibition, etc.), and/or pulmonary edema (salicylates, cholinergics, etc.). In many cases, intubation and mechanical ventilation will be necessary. In other cases, timely administration of an appropriate antidote (i.e., naloxone for an opioid overdose) may obviate the need for intubation and mechanical ventilation. In a similar fashion, the patient's circulation may be impaired by a variety of mechanisms resulting in shock. This may be due to a profound metabolic acidosis (i.e., toxic alcohols, metformin-associated lactic acidosis), uncoupling of oxidative phosphorylation (i.e., cyanide, salicylates, iron), direct cardiac and smooth muscle vasculature impairment (i.e., beta-blockers, calcium channel blockers), and/or dysrhythmias (i.e., tricyclic antidepressants, sodium channel blockers like flecainide, digoxin, etc.). In most cases of shock due to an ingested toxin, care is supportive with IV fluid administration and the use of vasopressor medications (i.e., epinephrine, norepinephrine, etc.). Antidotal therapy is available for some toxins (Digibind for digoxin, hydroxocobalamin for cyanide, etc.). Table 5.1 lists antidotes for certain drugs and toxins. Other toxins are amenable to enhanced elimination through a variety of treatment modalities. Drugs like salicylates and certain barbiturates can be treated with sodium bicarbonate drips in order to ion trap and enhance their elimination. Similarly, hemodialysis can be used to enhance the elimination of a wide variety of drugs including but not limited to salicylates, toxic alcohols, lithium, and metformin [4]. Drug-induced hyperthermia should be treated with active cooling measures.

As the practitioner is treating any life threats due to an ingested toxin, they are simultaneously trying to determine what substance(s) the patient was exposed to in order to cause their presentation. In many cases, patients will exhibit a particular toxidrome (specific signs and symptoms associated with a particular group of pharmacologically similar drugs or toxins). Common toxidromes can include opioid, sedative-hypnotic, sympathomimetic, anticholinergic (a.k.a., antimuscarinic), and cholinergic. Other described syndromes include serotonin syndrome, neuroleptic malignant syndrome, and malignant hyperthermia. Yet other drugs may cause a recognizable pattern of symptoms (bradycardia, hypotension, and hyperglycemia caused by calcium channel blockers). In some cases, the patient's signs and symptoms can lead an astute practitioner to a specific toxin or at least a pharmacologic group of toxins ingested. In other cases, laboratory examination is paramount. A wide variety of toxins cause vague symptoms at least initially (i.e., acetaminophen, salicylates, etc. resulting in nausea and vomiting) and can only be diagnosed based on the patient's history (which requires a cooperative, honest, and informed patient) or through laboratory examination.

The laboratory plays an important role in the diagnosis and management of an overdose patient. Common laboratory tests include blood gases, electrolytes, glucose, lactate, renal function tests, cardiac and muscle tests, liver function tests, complete blood count (CBC), coagulation profile, and drug screening. Most chemistry, hematology, and coagulation tests are available in a hospital laboratory. Some drug tests are also generally available in a hospital laboratory. However, comprehensive drug screening which involves screening for several hundred toxins is sent to a specialized laboratory.

DOI: 10.1201/9781003449713-5

Table 5.1 Drugs and Toxins and Their Antidotes

Drug/Toxin	Antidote
Acetaminophen (paracetamol)	N-acetylcysteine (NAC)
Anticholinergics (e.g., atropine, scopolamine)	Physostigmine
Benzodiazepine (e.g., diazepam, alprazolam)	Flumazenil (Romazicon)
Beta-blockers, calcium channel blockers	High-dose insulin and intravenous glucose
Cyanide	Hydroxocobalamin (Cyanokit) or sodium thiosulfate
Digoxin	Digoxin-specific antibody (Digibind)
Iron	Deferoxamine (Desferal)
Opioids (e.g., heroin, morphine, oxycodone, etc.)	Naloxone (Narcan)
Organophosphates, nerve agents	Atropine and pralidoxime (2-PAM)

CLASSIFICATION OF ACUTE POISONINGS AND TOXICITIES

Acute poisonings and toxicities can be broadly classified based on the type of exposure and type of toxins. Exposure to a toxin can occur due to accidental exposure, overdose, or intentional self-harm. Common toxicities encountered in emergency departments and intensive care units are due to an overdose of prescription or over-the-counter medications or the use of recreational or illicit drugs. Other poisonings include chemical or environmental exposures such as exposure to household chemicals, pesticides, heavy metals, and toxic gases. Less common poisonings are from toxic plants, and snake and spider bites.

TYPES OF TOXINS

Therapeutic Drugs and Over-the Counter Medications

These drugs can be broadly classified as analgesics, anticonvulsants, antihistamines, antidepressants, antimicrobials, antineoplastics, cardiac drugs, and immunosuppressants. Of these classes of drugs, analgesics-antipyretic, antidepressants, and cardiac drugs are commonly encountered drugs in acute poisoning.

Analgesics-Antipyretic Drugs

Acetaminophen (N-acetyl-p-aminophenol), also known as paracetamol, is a widely used analgesic-antipyretic drug particularly in pediatrics due to a possible link between salicylates and Reye's syndrome. When used as directed, acetaminophen is generally safe. However, unintentional ingestion or inappropriate dosing may lead to acetaminophen toxicity. In adolescents, intentional overdose is not uncommon. Acetaminophen doses of 7.5 g in adults or 200 mg/kg in children can cause severe hepatotoxicity. When administered orally, acetaminophen is rapidly and nearly completely absorbed from the gastrointestinal tract, with peak plasma concentration reached within 30–60 minutes. The drug is 20–50% bound to proteins and has a half-life of 2–5 hours. Over 90% of the drug is metabolized in the liver and excreted in the urine as glucuronide or sulfate conjugates. Additionally, 5–10% of acetaminophen is transformed by P450 enzymes into a highly reactive intermediate called N-acetyl-p-benzoquinoneimine (NAPQI). This metabolite is conjugated with glutathione to form non-toxic cysteine and mercapturic acid conjugates. In cases of acetaminophen overdose, glutathione is depleted, and NAPQI causes liver toxicity, potentially leading to fulminant liver necrosis in 3–5 days. This is generally the stage when a patient will present to an emergency department. Children are less prone to acetaminophen toxicity, mainly due to lower cytochrome P-450 mixed-function oxidase activity in neonates and infants. Additionally, children are more prone to vomiting.

The primary treatment for acetaminophen overdose is the antidote N-acetylcysteine (NAC). NAC stimulates glutathione production. Its effectiveness is the highest when administered within 10 hours of overdose, before the accumulation of toxic metabolites. Oral and intravenous administration protocols are employed for NAC treatment. In the United States, standard oral NAC therapy involves a 72-hour course comprising a 140 mg/kg loading dose followed by 17 doses of 70 mg/kg every 4 hours, totaling 1,330 mg/kg. Intravenous administration (300 mg/kg of NAC over 21 hours) is used for patients with intractable vomiting or medical conditions that prevent oral use of NAC. A nomogram (Figure 5.1) is available to predict the likelihood of hepatic injury based on acetaminophen blood concentrations and time since ingestion. Patients whose concentrations exceed the line indicating "possible or potential" liver toxicity are eligible for NAC treatment.

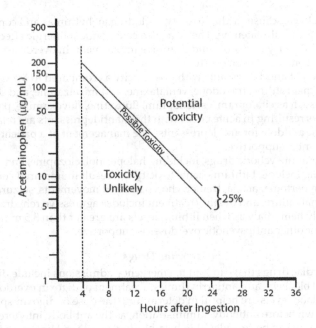

Figure 5.1 Nomogram for predicting acetaminophen toxicity. Figure adapted from [20]. Reproduced with permission from [9].

It is important to note that this nomogram is most applicable to acute ingestion cases involving immediate-release formulations and cannot be used for sustained-release preparations or patients with liver disease.

Another widely used analgesic-antipyretic drug is acetylsalicylic acid (aspirin). Acetylsalicylic acid is found in a number of prescription and over-the-counter preparations. When given orally, acetylsalicylic acid is almost completely absorbed, with a peak concentration in 1–2 hours. Once absorbed, acetylsalicylic acid is rapidly hydrolyzed to an active salicylic acid moiety. It is > 90% bound with a low volume of distribution of 0.20 L/kg and a half-life of 2–3 hours. The initial stage of salicylate overdose results in respiratory alkalosis due to hyperventilation from stimulation of the respiratory center. Respiratory alkalosis is followed by metabolic acidosis due to compensatory renal loss of bicarbonate. Salicylates also uncouple oxidative phosphorylation and inhibit the Krebs cycle, resulting in further metabolic acidosis. Treatment of salicylate overdose includes correction of electrolytes and acid-base imbalance and alkalization of urine to enhance the drug elimination. The Done nomogram was designed to assess the severity of salicylate intoxication; however, it has not been found to be clinically useful in predicting toxicity in the majority of salicylate exposures.

Antidepressants/Antipsychotics

Depression is a prevalent condition in both adults and children. Due to the instability of these patients, overdose with antidepressants is common. Antidepressants include monoamine oxidase inhibitors (MAOIs), tricyclic antidepressants (TCAs), selective serotonin reuptake inhibitors (SSRIs), serotonin-norepinephrine reuptake inhibitors (SNRIs), tetracyclic antidepressants and other atypical non-cyclic compounds, N-methyl D-aspartate (NMDA) antagonists, and neuroactive steroid gamma-aminobutyric acid (GABA)-A receptor positive modulators. Recently, in August 2022, the FDA approved Auvelity®, a fast-acting extended-release antidepressant [5].

Although an overdose of any antidepressant can cause serious toxicity, TCAs and MAOIs are the most concerning. Monoamine oxidase inhibitors (MAOIs) such as phenelzine and tranylcypromine inhibit monoamine oxidase, resulting in increased concentration of serotonin, norepinephrine, and dopamine. MAOIs overdose can lead to a hypertensive crisis. This potentially life-threatening condition is characterized by a sudden increase in blood pressure, severe headache, palpitations, chest pain, and confusion. Tricyclic antidepressants (TCAs), such as amitriptyline, doxepin, and imipramine, are an older class of antidepressants that have a high potential for significant toxicity. TCAs exert their therapeutic effects by blocking the reuptake of serotonin and norepinephrine. TCAs can cause cardiac toxicity, including arrhythmias and conduction abnormalities, which can be life-threatening. They can also cause anticholinergic effects, such as dry mouth, constipation, urinary retention, and cognitive impairment. In overdose situations, TCAs can lead to seizures, coma, and even death.

The next generation of antidepressants with less toxicity as compared to MAOIs and TCAs include amoxapine, maprotiline, trazodone, venlafaxine, and mirtazapine, and selective serotonin reuptake inhibitors such as citalopram, escitalopram, fluoxetine, fluvoxamine, paroxetine, and sertraline. Overdoses resulting in acute crises with these antidepressants are relatively small.

There is no specific antidote for antidepressants. The management of a patient who overdosed with an antidepressant is supportive.

Lithium and other antipsychotic drugs, including haloperidol, clozapine, and risperidone, can cause acute poisoning include. Lithium's acute toxicity can result in impaired consciousness, apathy, hyperreflexia, hypertonia, ataxia, tremor, choreoathetoid movements, seizures, cardiac dysrhythmias, acute renal failure, and death. Treatment includes aggressive rehydration with isotonic fluids and potentially hemodialysis when lithium levels are greater than 3.5 mmol/L in the acute setting. Treatment for other antipsychotic overdoses is supportive.

Cardiac Drugs

Commonly used cardiac drugs that can lead to emergency admissions include digoxin, beta-blockers, calcium channel blockers, and antiarrhythmics. Treatment of digoxin overdose is digoxin-antibody. Digoxin blood levels are helpful in determining the dose of digoxin-specific antibodies. Blood should be drawn before antibody administration, as the antibody interferes with digoxin measurement. Glucagon can be considered in beta-blocker overdose. High-dose insulin can be utilized in calcium channel blocker overdose. Central alpha-agonists like clonidine can sometimes show a response in treatment with naloxone. Otherwise, treatment is supportive.

Drugs of Abuse

Global use of drugs of abuse is increasing at an alarming rate [6]. Many drugs of abuse can lead to acute toxicity and emergency admissions [1]. Some examples of drugs of abuse are discussed below.

Opioids

Opioid abuse has become a global epidemic [7]. Common opioids that are abused include heroin, fentanyl, and oxycodone. Opioid overdose can cause respiratory depression and could be potentially fatal. Emergency admissions from opioid overdose are common. Naloxone is often administered as an antidote for opioid overdose.

Stimulants

Stimulant drugs include cocaine, amphetamines, cathinones, and methylenedioxymethamphetamine (MDMA, ecstasy). Abuse of these drugs is a common cause of emergency visits, as they can cause severe cardiovascular effects, including increased heart rate, blood pressure, and the risk of heart attack or stroke. Acute toxicity from these drugs may manifest as chest pain, palpitations, agitation, and seizures. Treatment for stimulant overdose is supportive as there is no specific antidote for these drugs.

Sedative-Hypnotics

Drugs in this category include benzodiazepines (e.g., diazepam, alprazolam), barbiturates, and gamma-hydroxybutyrate. These substances can lead to respiratory depression, sedation, and overdose. Emergency admission from sedative-hypnotic drugs is rare unless they are consumed with other substances like ethanol, which increases the risk of acute toxicity. Flumazenil is used as an antidote for benzodiazepine overdose.

Hallucinogens

Substances like cannabinoids, phencyclidine, LSD, psilocybin mushrooms, and synthetic cannabinoids (e.g., Spice, K2) can cause hallucinations, delusions, paranoia, and extreme agitation. These drugs rarely cause life-threatening issues. However, individuals may experience severe anxiety and panic attacks which may lead to self-harm leading to emergency admissions.

Inhalants

Inhalant abuse is generally seen in young adults and involves the intentional inhalation of volatile substances, such as solvents, aerosols, and gases found in common household products. These substances can cause acute symptoms such as central nervous system depression, cardiac arrhythmias, and seizures.

Alcohols

Ethanol is one of the most commonly abused drugs. Acute poisoning can lead to confusion, respiratory depression, coma, and in severe cases, death. Ethanol-related emergencies often involve auto-vehicular accidents. Other important alcohols are methanol and ethylene glycol. Methanol is widely found in paint thinners, gasoline additives, and windshield washer fluids. Consumption of adulterated alcoholic beverages, particularly in poor countries, is a common cause of methanol toxicity. Methanol toxicity is mostly from its metabolites formaldehyde and formic acid. Methanol overdose causes severe metabolic acidosis and increased anion gap, and can lead to respiratory depression, seizure, and coma. Blurred vision and blindness are caused by damage to the optic nerve by formic acid. Like methanol, ethylene glycol is relatively non-toxic. However, its metabolites glycolaldehyde, glycolic acid, and oxalic acid can cause severe metabolic acidosis and increased anion gap. Also, oxalic acid binds to calcium, leading to hypocalcemia, and the precipitation of calcium oxalate crystals in the kidneys leading to renal failure. Treatment of methanol and ethylene glycol poisoning involves the administration of ethanol or fomepizole. This treatment inhibits the formation of toxic metabolites by inhibiting the activity of alcohol dehydrogenase. Even after treatment with fomepizole, hemodialysis may be required if the patient has a significant metabolic acidosis.

Novel Psychoactive Substances (NPSs)

NPSs, also known as designer drugs, are marketed to deceive legal and drug detection systems. Common NPS are derivatives of amphetamines, opioids, and benzodiazepines. Generally, they are much more potent, mixed with other drugs, and have unpredictable action. Emergency admissions from these drugs are common [8].

Other Toxins

Other toxins that can result in emergency admission include metals (e.g., lead, arsenic, mercury, cadmium, iron), toxic gases (e.g., carbon monoxide and hydrogen sulfide), organophosphates, cyanide, and nitrites [9]. Measurement of cholinesterase is useful in the evaluation of organophosphate or carbamate exposure. In cases of cyanide toxicity, measurements of blood cyanide, thiosulphate, lactate, and blood gases can provide essential diagnostic information. To investigate suspected nitrite exposure, co-oximetry can be used to measure methemoglobin levels. Treatment for these toxins includes chelation therapy for metals, oxygen therapy for toxic gases, atropine and pralidoxime (2-PAM) for organophosphates, hydroxocobalamin or sodium thiosulfate treatment for cyanide, and methylene blue for nitrites poisoning.

MANAGEMENT OF A POISONED PATIENT

The management of the poisoned patient can be relatively straightforward or extraordinarily complex depending upon the xenobiotic(s) the patient was exposed to, the timing of exposure, the ability of the practitioner to obtain an accurate patient history, and the resources of the particular healthcare setting where the patient is being managed. As previously mentioned, aggressive supportive care with special attention to airway, breathing, and circulation is of paramount importance [10].

One unique aspect of managing a poisoned patient is the consideration of gastrointestinal (GI) decontamination. The most commonly used methods of GI decontamination are the administration of activated charcoal and whole bowel irrigation, which is typically performed with polyethylene glycol. An in-depth discussion of GI decontamination is beyond the scope of this chapter. Generally speaking, activated charcoal is considered when the patient has: 1) ingested a potentially life-threatening overdose, 2) presents within 1–2 hours of ingestion, 3) is awake, alert, and willing to swallow activated charcoal, 4) active bowel sounds and adequate perfusion for peristalsis of the charcoal by the gut, and 4) the ingested substance is not a liquid formulation (i.e., toxic alcohol) nor is it a metal (i.e., iron, lithium, lead, etc.) [11]. Whole bowel irrigation with polyethylene glycol is generally reserved for patients who ingest metals (again, examples include iron, lithium, lead, etc.), sustained-release medications, or body packers (intentionally ingested packets of illicit drugs for concealment and transportation). Other antiquated methods of GI decontamination like syrup of ipecac and gastric lavage have been supplanted by activated charcoal and whole bowel irrigation.

In addition to supportive care, there are many specific antidotal therapies for certain toxins (Table 5.1). Some antidotes are effective for specific symptoms that could be due to a heterogeneous toxin. As an example, sodium channel blockade of cardiac myocytes can be caused by a number of local anesthetics (bupivacaine), cardiac medications (flecainide), and antidepressants (amitriptyline). The use of IV sodium bicarbonate can be used for a prolonged QRS duration due to sodium channel blockade because of these pharmacologic classes as well as others. Similarly, intralipid rescue therapy has been utilized with varied success in a heterogeneous group of xenobiotics for patients in shock and/or cardiac arrest due to overdose [12]. Other antidotes are very toxin-specific (i.e., N-acetylcysteine for an acetaminophen overdose, hydroxocobalamin for a cyanide exposure, etc.). Lastly, the poisoned patient may require a myriad of antidotes and aggressive supportive care depending upon the substance(s) ingested.

ROLE OF LABORATORY IN THE MANAGEMENT OF ACUTE POISONINGS AND TOXICITIES

The laboratory plays an important role in the management of a poisoned patient. Laboratory tests can be categorized into the tests that are generally available in a hospital laboratory or on the bedside and tests that may not be available in a hospital laboratory and are sent out to a specialized laboratory [13].

Basic Laboratory and Point-of-Care Tests

Commonly used laboratory tests, for the management of a poisoned patient, include blood gases, electrolytes, glucose, lactate, renal function tests, liver function tests, complete blood count, coagulation profile, and drug screening (Tables 5.2 and 5.3). These tests, other than drug screening, are well standardized and are generally available in a hospital laboratory on an urgent basis. Point-of-care testing (POCT) devices are available for blood gases, glucose, electrolytes, and certain hematology and coagulation tests such as hemoglobin and prothrombin time. Turnaround time for these basic tests can be as short as 10 minutes for POCTs and 30 minutes for laboratory-based tests. POCTs are also available for drug testing, particularly for drugs of abuse. Most laboratories analyze certain drugs such as acetaminophen, salicylates, digoxin, common anticonvulsants (phenytoin, carbamazepine, valproate, and phenobarbital), lithium, and tricyclic antidepressants on automated chemistry analyzer by immunoassays. Certain drugs of abuse (individual and class) can also be assayed by immunoassays. These drugs include amphetamines, barbiturates, benzodiazepines, cocaine/metabolite, cannabinoid/metabolite, methadone, opioids, and phencyclidine. Due to cross-reactivity with other drugs and false positives, it is important to confirm drugs of abuse by more specific methods such as mass spectrometry [13, 14]. Drugs that can cause false positive results are listed in Table 5.4.

Table 5.2 Commonly Used and Available Non-Toxicology Laboratory Tests for the Management of a Poisoned Patient

Electrolytes: sodium, potassium, chloride, calcium, and magnesium

Renal function tests: creatinine, urea

Protein: albumin and total protein

Liver function tests: transaminases, bilirubin

Arterial blood gases: oxygen saturation (O_2Sat), partial pressure of oxygen (PaO_2), partial pressure of carbon dioxide ($PaCO_2$), pH, calculated bicarbonate, calculated base excess

Co-oximetry: oxyhemoglobin, carboxyhemoglobin, methemoglobin

Other chemistries: glucose, lactate, anion gap, creatinine kinase, osmolality, osmolal gap, urinalysis

Complete blood count (CBC) with hemoglobin

Coagulation tests: international normalized ratio (INR), prothrombin time (PT), activated partial thromboplastin time (aPTT)

Table 5.3   Commonly Used and Available Drugs and Toxins Testing for the Management of a Poisoned Patient

Acetaminophen
Carbamazepine
Digoxin
Ethanol
Iron with transferrin saturation
Lithium
Phenobarbital
Phenytoin
Salicylate
Theophylline
Tricyclic antidepressants (Qualitative)
Valproate
Drugs of abuse (Point-of-care device or automated chemistry analyzer): amphetamines, barbiturates, benzodiazepines, cannabinoid metabolite, cocaine/metabolite, opioids, phencyclidine

Table 5.4   Interferences in Drugs of Abuse Immunoassays [13]

Target Drug (s)	Interfering Drugs
Amphetamines	Pseudoephedrine, brompheniramine, phentermine, chlorpromazine, bupropion, fluoxetine, tricyclic antidepressants, methylphenidate, labetalol
Benzodiazepines	Oxaprozin, sertraline
Cocaine or metabolite (benzoylecgonine)	Procaine, lidocaine, levamisole
Opiates	Diphenhydramine, rifampin, dextromethorphan, verapamil, quinine
Phencyclidine	Dextromethorphan, diphenhydramine, ketamine, thioridazine, venlafaxine
Tetrahydrocannabinol (THC)	Non-steroidal anti-inflammatory drugs, pantoprazole
Methadone	Diphenhydramine

The potential for interference varies based on the specific immunoassay and the concentration of the interfering drugs.

Advanced Drug Testing

Drug screening varies significantly among laboratories. Some laboratories, as discussed above, screen for only a few drugs or toxins, while others may screen for hundreds of compounds. Comprehensive drug screening is generally not available in most hospital laboratories, but the samples are sent to a specialized laboratory. Urine is considered the best sample for drug screening, as most drugs are excreted in urine, and it is a standardized and simpler matrix to analyze [15]. For quantitative analyses, blood is the sample of choice. As described above, immunoassays are available for a limited number of therapeutic and illicit drugs. Chromatographic methods are used for comprehensive drug screening [16, 17]. These methods can screen for several hundreds of drugs. The methods include gas or liquid chromatography linked to various detectors. Mass spectrometry (MS) is a commonly employed technique for comprehensive drug screening. It is a fairly sensitive and very specific technique. MS should be used for the confirmation of drugs of abuse, particularly in children to avoid any legal issue. Gas chromatography-mass spectrometry (GC-MS) has been the gold standard for drug screening for several decades. The technology is well standardized, and the mass spectra produced in different laboratories are highly reproducible. Also, GC-MS mass spectral libraries containing hundreds of thousands of compounds are commercially available. In recent years, liquid chromatography linked to one or multiple mass spectrometers (LC-MS or LC-MS/MS) is gaining popularity [18, 19]. The advantages of LC-MS or LC-MS/MS include simpler sample preparation and a wider range of drug detection. The disadvantages include higher costs and less reproducible mass spectra among different laboratories. Other variations of MS include time-of-flight (TOF) and high-resolution mass spectrometry. Mass spectrometry is also commonly used for quantification of drugs. Turnaround time for comprehensive drug screening varies from a few hours if performed in-house to several days if the samples are sent out to a reference laboratory.

CONCLUSION

In conclusion, acute poisonings and toxicities can be complex medical emergencies that require rapid and comprehensive responses. Acute poisoning can result from diverse exposures surrounding therapeutic drugs and drugs of abuse. To effectively manage acute poisonings, it is imperative to conduct a careful patient history assessment, perform a comprehensive physical examination, and evaluate clinical symptoms. The treatment of acute poisoning includes a range of strategies, including decontamination, antidote administration, and supportive care, which depend on the toxin, dose, and patient's clinical condition.

Laboratory testing plays a pivotal role in evaluating acute poisonings. Basic tests that are generally available in a hospital laboratory include blood gases, electrolytes, glucose, lactate, renal function tests, liver function tests, complete blood count, and coagulation profiles. These tests can provide crucial insights into overall health and organ function. Toxicology screens are instrumental in identifying the specific toxin or drug involved, enabling tailored interventions. In some cases, measuring toxin levels or employing specialized methods can further enhance the accuracy of diagnosis and management.

CLINICAL PEARLS IN THE MANAGEMENT OF A POISONED PATIENT

1. For optimal outcomes, early intervention and recognition of the toxin(s) are important.

2. It is important to confirm the presence of drugs of abuse by definitive methods such as mass spectrometry.

3. Aggressive supportive care with special attention to airway, breathing, and circulation are the mainstays of therapy in the poisoned patient.

4. Be familiar with commonly used antidotal therapies for the poisoned patient.

5. Consider GI decontamination in the appropriate patient population.

FREQUENTLY ASKED QUESTIONS

1. What are the common signs and symptoms of drug overdose?

A wide variety of drugs can cause alterations in mental status, vital sign abnormalities, pupillary changes, skin manifestations, etc.

2. What are the common interferences in drug immunoassays?

Sympathomimetic amines in amphetamine assay, dextromethorphan in PCP assay.

3. What are common treatment modalities for drug overdose?

Most drug overdoses are treated with supportive care (i.e., intubation for impending airway compromise, IV fluids +/- vasopressors for hypotension, benzodiazepines for agitation, etc).

4. When should GI decontamination be considered?

In general, when the patient presents <1-2 hours after overdose, the patient's mental status is intact, the amount of drug ingested has the potential for harm, and the drug ingested is amenable to treatment to the specific modality of GI decontamination being considered (i.e., activated charcoal does not bind to heavy metals and liquids).

5. What are some specific antidotal therapies that are commonly used in the critical care setting?

N-acetylcysteine (NAC) for acetaminophen, naloxone for opioids, digoxin-specific antibody for digoxin, deferoxamine for iron.

6. When is hemodialysis considered in the poisoned patient?

When a life-threatening xenobiotic is relatively hydrophilic, has low protein binding, a molecular size <500 Daltons, and is not amenable to treatment with supportive care or a specific antidote.

REFERENCES

1. Thornton S. Management of an overdose patient. In: Ketha HK, Garg U, eds. *Toxicology Cases for the Clinical and Forensic Laboratory.* London: Academic Press, 2020, pp. 27–33.

2. Ornillo C, Harbord N. Fundaments of toxicology-approach to the poisoned patient. *Adv Chronic Kidney Dis.* 2020;27:5–10.

3. Skolnik A, Monas J. The crashing toxicology patient. *Emerg Med Clin North Am.* 2020;38:841–856.

4. Lavergne V, Nolin TD, Hoffman RS, Roberts D, Gosselin S, Goldfarb DS, *et al.* The EXTRIP (EXtracorporeal TReatments In Poisoning) workgroup: guideline methodology. *Clin Toxicol (Phila).* 2012;50:403–413.

5. Keam SJ. Dextromethorphan/Bupropion: First Approval. *CNS Drugs.* 2022;36:1229-1238.

6. United nations. Office of Drugs and Crime. *World Drug Report 2022.* 2022. https://www.unodc.org/unodc/en/data-and-analysis/world-drug-report-2022.html. Accessed July 18, 2023.

7. Robert M, Jouanjus E, Khouri C, Fouilhe Sam-Lai N, Revol B. The opioid epidemic: a worldwide exploratory study using the WHO pharmacovigilance database. *Addiction.* 2023;118:771–775.

8. Crulli B, Dines AM, Blanco G, Giraudon I, Eyer F, Liechti ME, *et al.* Novel psychoactive substances-related presentations to the emergency departments of the European drug emergencies network plus (Euro-DEN plus) over the six-year period 2014–2019. *Clin Toxicol (Phila).* 2022;60:1318–1327.

9. Garg U, Sandritter TL, Gaedigk A. Pediatric therapeutic drug monitoring, toxicology and pharmacogenomics. In: Dietzen D, Wong E, Bennett M, Haymond S, eds. *Biochemical and Molecular Basis of Pediatric Disease*, 5th ed. London: Academic Press, 2021, pp. 849–908.

10. Thompson TM, Theobald J, Lu J, Erickson TB. The general approach to the poisoned patient. *Dis Mon.* 2014;60:509–524.

11. Olson KR. Activated charcoal for acute poisoning: one toxicologist's journey. *J Med Toxicol.* 2010;6:190–198.

12. Cave G, Harvey M. Intravenous lipid emulsion as antidote beyond local anesthetic toxicity: a systematic review. *J Med Toxicol.* 2009;16:815–824.

13. Maharjan AS, Johnson-Davis KL. Issues of interferences with immunoassays used for screening of drugs of abuse in urine. In: Dasgupta A, ed. *Alcohol and Drugs of Abuse Testing.* London, UK: Academic Press, 2019, pp. 129–139.

14. Thompson JP, Watson ID, Thanacoody HK, Morley S, Thomas SH, Eddleston M, *et al.* Guidelines for laboratory analyses for poisoned patients in the United Kingdom. *Ann Clin Biochem.* 2014;51:312–325.

15. Moeller KE, Kissack JC, Atayee RS, Lee KC. Clinical interpretation of urine drug tests: what clinicians need to know about urine drug screens. *Mayo Clin Proc.* 2017;92:774–796.

16. Kyle PB. Laboratory medthods in toxicology. In: Ketha HK, Garg U, eds. *Toxicology Cases for the Clinical and Forensic Laboratory.* London: Academic Press, 2020, pp. 19–26.

17. Van Wijk XMR, Goodnough R, Colby JM. Mass spectrometry in emergency toxicology: current state and future applications. *Crit Rev Clin Lab Sci.* 2019;56:225–238.

18. Allen DR, McWhinney BC. Quadrupole time-of-flight mass spectrometry: a paradigm shift in toxicology screening applications. *Clin Biochem Rev.* 2019;40:135–146.

19. Su H, Huang MZ, Shiea J, Lee CW. Thermal desorption ambient ionization mass spectrometry for emergency toxicology. *Mass Spectrom Rev.* 2023;42:1828–1847.

20. Rumack BH, Matthew H. Acetaminophen poisoning and toxicity. *Pediatrics.* 1975;55:871–876.

6 Cardiac Arrest and Cardiopulmonary Resuscitation

Shaik Arif Pasha and Siva Prabodh Vuddandi

INTRODUCTION

Cardiac arrest is a critical medical emergency that requires swift intervention to restore blood circulation and prevent irreversible damage. Effective resuscitation is a multifaceted process that relies on accurate diagnostic information obtained through laboratory investigations. This article explores the essential laboratory tests involved in the management of cardiac arrest and resuscitation.

CLASSIFICATION OF DISEASE AND/-OR SEVERITY

Understanding the underlying cause and severity of cardiac arrest is crucial for tailoring the appropriate interventions. Laboratory investigations aid in classifying the condition, whether it is due to ischemic heart disease, arrhythmias, or other causes. Severity assessments may involve biomarkers like troponin levels, which are indicative of myocardial injury.

BASIC LABORATORY AND POINT-OF-CARE TESTS (WITH TIMELINES AND CLINICAL COURSE)

Blood Glucose

Glucose is a vital energy source for cells, particularly the heart and brain. Adequate blood glucose levels are necessary to support cellular metabolism and maintain cellular functions, including those critical for resuscitation.

a. **Hypoglycemia risk:**

- Prolonged cardiac arrest and stress of resuscitation efforts can deplete glucose stores, potentially leading to hypoglycemia which can adversely affect neurological function and compromise the effectiveness of resuscitation.

b. **Hyperglycemia concerns:**

- On the other hand, hyperglycemia can also occur during and after cardiac arrest. Stress-induced hyperglycemia is a common response to critical illness. Persistent hyperglycemia may be associated with worse outcomes and increased mortality in critically ill patients.

RELATIONSHIP WITH NEUROLOGICAL OUTCOMES:

Both hypoglycemia and severe hyperglycemia have been linked to poor neurological outcomes. Maintaining blood glucose within a targeted range (140–180 mg/dl) may be important for optimizing neurological recovery. The approach to blood glucose management during and after resuscitation is often individualized based on the patient's specific circumstances, underlying medical conditions, and the presence of comorbidities.

Arterial Blood Gas (ABG)

a. **Acid-base status:**

ABG helps in assessing the patient's acid-base balance, indicating whether the patient is in acidosis or alkalosis. During cardiac arrest, metabolic acidosis is common due to the accumulation of lactic acid. ABG can quantify the severity of acidosis and guide interventions such as sodium bicarbonate administration.

b. **Oxygenation status:**

ABG provides information about the partial pressure of oxygen (PaO_2) and oxygen saturation (SaO_2). In cardiac arrest, maintaining adequate oxygenation is critical for organ perfusion. ABG results help in adjusting ventilator settings and oxygen therapy to optimize oxygen delivery to tissues.

c. **Ventilation status:**

DOI: 10.1201/9781003449713-6

ABG provides data on the partial pressure of carbon dioxide ($PaCO_2$), which reflects the adequacy of ventilation. Hypercapnia may occur during cardiac arrest due to respiratory failure or inadequate ventilation. Monitoring $PaCO_2$ levels helps in adjusting ventilator settings to ensure proper ventilation.

d. **Guidance for advanced life support (ALS) interventions:**

ABG results can guide the administration of medications and interventions during advanced life support. For example, if the ABG shows severe acidosis, sodium bicarbonate may be considered. Additionally, it can help in titrating vasopressors and inotropic agents to optimize hemodynamics.

e. **Monitoring response to resuscitation:**

Serial ABG measurements can be used to monitor the patient's response to resuscitation efforts.

It is important to note that ABG results should be interpreted in conjunction with other clinical information, such as the patient's clinical status, ECG findings, and overall response to resuscitation efforts.

Lactate Levels

The normal range for lactate is 4.5 to 19.8 mg/L or 0.5 to 2.2 mmol/L.

a. **Indicators of tissue hypoperfusion:**

- Lactate is a by-product of anaerobic metabolism. Elevated serum lactate levels during cardiac arrest suggest inadequate tissue perfusion and oxygen delivery. The accumulation of lactate occurs when cells shift to anaerobic metabolism due to insufficient oxygenation, commonly seen in the setting of inadequate cardiac output.

b. **Prognostic indicator:**

- High initial lactate levels or a failure to decrease lactate levels during resuscitation may be associated with a poorer prognosis. Persistent elevation of lactate after resuscitation efforts may indicate ongoing tissue hypoperfusion and can be a predictor of mortality.

c. **Monitoring response to resuscitation:**

- A decreasing lactate trend is generally indicative of improved tissue perfusion and responsiveness to interventions.

d. **Differentiating types of lactic acidosis:**

- Lactic acidosis can be categorized into type A (due to inadequate tissue perfusion) or type B (related to underlying medical conditions). In the context of cardiac arrest, elevated lactate levels are typically associated with type A lactic acidosis, reflecting impaired tissue perfusion during the arrest.

e. **Post-resuscitation care:**

- In the post-resuscitation phase, persistently elevated lactate levels may guide ongoing management, including the need for advanced monitoring, consideration of targeted temperature management, and further investigations to identify and address the underlying causes.

It is important to note that while elevated lactate levels are informative, they should be interpreted in the context of the overall clinical picture and in conjunction with other markers and assessments.

Electrolyte Panel

Electrolyte abnormalities are among the most common reasons for patients to develop cardiac arrhythmias. Of all the electrolyte abnormalities, hyperkalemia is most rapidly fatal. A high degree of clinical suspicion and aggressive treatment of underlying electrolyte abnormalities can prevent many patients from progressing to cardiac arrest. Monitoring and managing serum electrolyte levels are important components of the comprehensive care provided during cardiac arrest and subsequent resuscitation efforts.

a. **Potassium (K+):** normal range 3.5–5.0 mEq/L

Hyperkalemia or hypokalemia can have significant effects on cardiac excitability and rhythm. During cardiac arrest, particularly if it is due to a primary cardiac cause, abnormalities in potassium levels may contribute to the dysrhythmia. Resuscitation efforts may involve interventions such as administering medications to stabilize potassium levels.

b. **Calcium (Ca2+):** normal range 8.5–10.5 mEq/L

Calcium is crucial for myocardial contraction and plays a role in the conduction of electrical impulses. Hypocalcemia can lead to impaired cardiac contractility and contribute to arrhythmias.

c. **Sodium (Na+):** normal range 135–145 mEq/L

Sodium is essential for maintaining cellular osmolarity and contributes to the regulation of water balance. Dysnatremia can affect neuronal function and contribute to neurological complications. Sodium levels are often monitored and corrected as part of post-resuscitation care.

d. **Magnesium (Mg2+):** normal range 1.3–2.2 mEq/L

Magnesium is involved in numerous cellular processes, including cardiac muscle contraction. Hypomagnesemia (low magnesium levels) can contribute to arrhythmias and affect the response to antiarrhythmic medications. Magnesium supplementation may be considered during resuscitation.

e. **Phosphate (PO4-):** normal range 3.4–4.5 mg/dl

Phosphate is important for cellular energy metabolism. During prolonged cardiac arrest and resuscitation efforts, changes in phosphate levels may occur. Monitoring and addressing severe imbalances may be necessary to prevent complications.

f. **Considerations of underlying causes:**

Identifying and addressing the underlying causes of electrolyte imbalances, such as renal dysfunction, medication effects, or metabolic disorders, are crucial for successful resuscitation and post-resuscitation care.

ADVANCED LABORATORY AND POINT-OF-CARE TESTS (WITH TIMELINES AND CLINICAL COURSE)

Complete Blood Count (CBC)

A CBC is a blood test that provides information about the cellular components of blood. A CBC can offer valuable insights into the patient's overall health and help guide management. Here are some aspects of the role of a complete blood count in the context of cardiac arrest and resuscitation.

a. **Hemoglobin levels:**

Hemoglobin is a crucial component of red blood cells that carries oxygen from the lungs to the rest of the body. Monitoring hemoglobin levels can provide information about the patient's oxygen-carrying capacity, helping healthcare providers assess the adequacy of oxygen delivery to tissues.

b. **Hematocrit:**

Hematocrit is the percentage of blood volume occupied by red blood cells. Changes in hematocrit can impact blood viscosity and oxygen-carrying capacity. Monitoring hematocrit levels may be relevant in assessing the patient's overall blood volume and potential need for fluid resuscitation.

c. **White blood cell count (WBC):**

White blood cells play a crucial role in the immune response. An elevated WBC count may indicate an inflammatory or infectious process, which can be important information for determining the underlying cause of the cardiac arrest or guiding post-resuscitation care.

d. **Platelet count:**

Platelets are involved in blood clotting. Monitoring platelet count is important, especially if there is concern about bleeding or if the patient has received anticoagulant medications during the resuscitation process.

e. **Monitoring for complications:**

Serial CBC measurements can be used to monitor for complications such as infections, bleeding disorders, or other hematological abnormalities that may arise during the post-resuscitation period.

While a CBC is not the primary diagnostic tool during cardiac arrest, it is part of the broader laboratory evaluation that healthcare providers use to gather information about the patient's condition.

Cardiac Biomarkers

Cardiac biomarkers are substances released into the bloodstream in response to cardiac injury or stress. Their measurement provides valuable information about myocardial damage, helps guide treatment decisions, and can assist in prognostication. Here are key aspects of the role of cardiac biomarkers in the context of cardiac arrest and resuscitation.

a. **Troponin:** normal range troponin I 0–0.4 ng/ml

- High-sensitivity troponin I ≤ 15 pg/ml for females and ≤ 20 pg/ml for males.
- Troponin is a sensitive and specific marker of myocardial injury.
- Elevated troponin levels suggest myocardial damage, which may occur during cardiac arrest due to ischemia or other cardiac events.
- Serial measurements of troponin may be useful to guide ongoing management.

b. **Creatine kinase-MB (CK-MB):** normal range 5–25 IU/L

- CK-MB is an enzyme that is released when there is damage to heart muscle cells.
- Although troponin is generally considered more specific for myocardial injury, CK-MB may also be measured in the context of assessing cardiac damage.
- Serial measurements of CK-MB may be performed to monitor the progression of myocardial injury.

c. **Myoglobin:** normal range 25–75 mcg/L

- Myoglobin is an early marker of myocardial injury but is less specific compared to troponin.
- Elevated myoglobin levels may be detected shortly after the onset of cardiac injury.

d. **Natriuretic peptides (BNP and NT-proBNP):** normal range < 125 pg/ml

- B-type natriuretic peptide (BNP) and its precursor, N-terminal pro-B-type natriuretic peptide (NT-proBNP), are released in response to cardiac stress and volume overload.
- Elevated levels of BNP or NT-proBNP may indicate heart failure, which can be a consequence of cardiac arrest or an underlying cause.
- Higher levels of troponin and natriuretic peptides have been associated with increased mortality and worse neurological outcomes.

Coronary Angiography Guidance:

Elevated cardiac biomarkers may prompt consideration of coronary angiography to assess and treat any underlying coronary artery disease. While elevated cardiac biomarkers are indicative of myocardial injury, they do not provide information about the cause of the arrest. Therefore, a comprehensive approach, including clinical assessment, imaging studies, and other laboratory tests, is crucial for optimal patient management during and after cardiac arrest.

Coagulation Profile

The coagulation system is essential for maintaining hemostasis, and disturbances in this system can have significant implications for patient outcomes. Here's the role of the coagulation profile in the context of cardiac arrest and resuscitation.

a. **Identification of bleeding risks:**

- The coagulation profile includes tests such as Prothrombin Time (PT), Partial Thromboplastin Time (PTT), International Normalized Ratio (INR), and D-dimer. These tests help identify bleeding risks that may arise during resuscitation efforts or as a complication of cardiac arrest.

b. **Management of anticoagulant-related complications:**

- Patients who experience cardiac arrest may have underlying conditions or medications that affect the coagulation system, such as anticoagulant therapy. Monitoring the coagulation profile is essential for managing anticoagulant-related complications and determining the need for reversal agents.

c. **Assessment for disseminated intravascular coagulation (DIC):**

- Disseminated intravascular coagulation is a serious condition characterized by widespread activation of the coagulation system, leading to both microvascular thrombosis and bleeding. Monitoring coagulation parameters, including fibrinogen levels, can help identify signs of DIC.

d. **Risk stratification for thromboembolic events:**

- While the focus is often on bleeding risks during resuscitation, an assessment of the coagulation profile can also help identify patients at risk for thromboembolic events. This is important for guiding interventions and post-resuscitation care.

e. **Guidance for blood product transfusion:**

- Abnormalities in the coagulation profile may prompt the administration of blood products, such as fresh frozen plasma (FFP), platelets, or clotting factor concentrates, to correct coagulation deficits and improve hemostasis.

f. **Prevention and management of hemorrhage:**

- In patients who have undergone successful resuscitation, coagulation monitoring remains important during the post-resuscitation phase to prevent or manage bleeding complications, particularly in those with ongoing critical illness.

The coagulation profile should be interpreted in conjunction with the patient's clinical presentation, underlying medical conditions, and other laboratory findings. Serial measurements of coagulation parameters provide information on the response to interventions.

Serum Creatinine and Blood Urea Nitrogen (BUN)

Serum creatinine and BUN are markers of kidney function. They play a role in the overall assessment and management of patients during and after resuscitation.

a. **Indicators of organ perfusion:**

- The levels of serum creatinine and BUN can be elevated as a result of reduced renal blood flow and impaired renal function during the period of inadequate perfusion due to cardiac arrest.

b. **Post-resuscitation care:**

- Post-resuscitation care involves addressing potential complications, and kidney function is a key consideration.

c. **Identification of renal complications:**

- Elevated serum creatinine and BUN levels may indicate acute kidney injury (AKI) or other renal complications following cardiac arrest.

Hemodynamic optimization: Abnormalities in serum creatinine and BUN may reflect inadequate hemodynamic status and compromised renal perfusion during the resuscitation process. Optimization of hemodynamics and perfusion is crucial for preventing further renal injury.

Fluid management: Serum creatinine and BUN levels can be influenced by fluid status. Close monitoring helps guide fluid management during resuscitation and post-resuscitation care, striking a balance between avoiding hypovolemia and preventing fluid overload.

In summary, while serum creatinine and BUN are not diagnostic markers for cardiac arrest, they play a crucial role in the ongoing assessment of renal function, fluid management, and the overall well-being of patients during and after resuscitation. The integration of these renal markers with other clinical and laboratory parameters is essential for providing comprehensive and individualized care to patients experiencing cardiac arrest.

Inflammatory Markers

Inflammatory markers play a role in the diagnosis and management of cardiac arrest and resuscitation by providing insights into the inflammatory response and potential complications. Monitoring these markers helps healthcare providers assess the severity of the incident, guide therapeutic interventions, and predict outcomes. Here are some key inflammatory markers and their roles in the context of cardiac arrest and resuscitation.

a. **C-reactive protein (CRP):** normal range 0.8–1.0 mg/dl

- CRP is an acute-phase protein produced by the liver in response to inflammation or tissue injury.
- Elevated CRP levels may indicate the presence and degree of systemic inflammation following cardiac arrest.
- Monitoring CRP can help assess the intensity of the inflammatory response and guide treatment decisions.

b. **Procalcitonin (PCT):** normal range < 0.05 ng/ml

- PCT is a precursor of calcitonin that is released in response to bacterial infections.
- Elevated PCT levels may suggest the presence of a bacterial infection, which can be a complication following cardiac arrest.
- PCT levels can aid in distinguishing between systemic inflammatory response syndrome (SIRS) and infection.

c. **Interleukins (IL-6, IL-10):** IL-6 normal range < 7 pg/ml IL-10 normal range 4.8–9.8 pg/ml

- IL-6 is a pro-inflammatory cytokine, while IL-10 is an anti-inflammatory cytokine.
- Monitoring these interleukins helps assess the balance between pro-inflammatory and anti-inflammatory responses.
- Elevated IL-6 levels are associated with the severity of inflammation, and increased IL-10 may indicate a compensatory anti-inflammatory response.

d. **Tumor necrosis factor – alpha (TNF-α):** normal range < 7.2 pg/ml

- TNF-α is a pro-inflammatory cytokine involved in the regulation of immune responses.
- Elevated levels of TNF-α may contribute to the inflammatory cascade and impact the post-resuscitation inflammatory state.
- Monitoring TNF-α levels provides insights into the inflammatory pathways activated during resuscitation.

It is important to note that while inflammatory markers provide valuable information, they should be interpreted in the context of the overall clinical presentation and other diagnostic findings. The management of patients during and after cardiac arrest involves a multidisciplinary approach, and the role of inflammatory markers is just one aspect of the comprehensive care provided to these patients.

Neurological Biomarkers

Neurological biomarkers play a crucial role in the diagnosis, prognosis, and management of patients during and after cardiac arrest and resuscitation. These biomarkers provide insights into the extent of neurological injury, guide treatment decisions, and help in predicting outcomes. Here are some key neurological biomarkers and their roles in the context of cardiac arrest and resuscitation.

a. **S100B:** normal range 0.02–0.15 μg/L

- S100B is a protein released from astrocytes and is considered a marker of glial cell damage.

- Elevated levels of S100B in blood or cerebrospinal fluid may indicate neurological injury and are associated with poor neurological outcomes after cardiac arrest.

b. **Neuro specific enolase (NSE):** normal range < 15 ng/ml

- NSE is an enzyme found predominantly in neurons, and its release into the bloodstream may indicate neuronal damage.

- Elevated NSE levels post-resuscitation have been correlated with poor neurological outcomes and may help in predicting the severity of brain injury.

c. **Glial fibrillary acidic protein (GFAP):** normal range 0.03–0.07 ng/ml

- GFAP is an astrocytic protein released in response to brain injury.

- Elevated levels of GFAP may indicate astrocytic damage and can be used as a marker of neurological injury in the context of cardiac arrest.

d. **Tau protein:** normal range < 300 pg/ml

- Tau is a protein found in neurons, and its abnormal accumulation is associated with neurodegenerative conditions.

- Measurements of Tau levels may provide insights into neuronal damage and be indicative of the severity of brain injury post-cardiac arrest.

Neurological biomarkers should be interpreted in conjunction with clinical neurological assessments, neuroimaging findings, and other diagnostic data.

- Elevated levels of these biomarkers, particularly in the early post-resuscitation period, are associated with poor neurological outcomes and increased mortality.

- This may include targeted temperature management and other strategies to mitigate secondary brain injury.

FREQUENTLY ASKED QUESTIONS

1. **What laboratory tests are crucial for diagnosing and managing cardiac arrest?**
   - Essential tests include troponin levels, blood glucose monitoring, arterial blood gas analysis, lactate levels, electrolyte panels, and a complete blood count.

2. **How does troponin aid in the diagnosis of cardiac arrest?**
   - Troponin is a biomarker of myocardial injury. Elevated levels help confirm cardiac involvement and assess the severity of damage during a cardiac event.

3. **Why is blood glucose monitoring important during resuscitation?**
   - Maintaining appropriate blood glucose levels is crucial for optimal cellular function, and abnormal levels (hypoglycemia or hyperglycemia) can impact neurological outcomes and resuscitation effectiveness.

4. **What information does an arterial blood gas (ABG) analysis provide during cardiac arrest?**
   - ABG assesses acid-base balance, oxygenation status, and ventilation adequacy, guiding interventions and monitoring the patient's response to resuscitation efforts.

5. **How does lactate contribute to the diagnosis and management of cardiac arrest?**

   - Lactate indicates tissue hypoperfusion, serves as a prognostic indicator, guides interventions, and monitors the patient's response to resuscitation efforts.

6. **What role does the electrolyte panel play in cardiac arrest diagnosis and management?**

   - Electrolyte imbalances, especially in potassium, calcium, sodium, magnesium, and phosphate, can affect cardiac rhythm and cellular function, necessitating close monitoring and targeted interventions.

7. **Why is a multidisciplinary approach important in interpreting laboratory results during cardiac arrest scenarios?**

   - A collaborative effort involving emergency medical services, physicians, and other healthcare providers ensures a comprehensive understanding of the patient's condition, leading to optimal patient care and outcomes.

8. **How does the laboratory diagnosis contribute to the ongoing management of patients in the post-resuscitation phase?**

   - Continuous monitoring of laboratory parameters helps to guide the ongoing interventions, prevent complications, and optimize recovery during the post-resuscitation period.

In conclusion, laboratory investigations play a pivotal role in managing cardiac arrest, guides the clinicians in making informed decisions, and improving the chances of successful resuscitation and patient outcomes.

REFERENCES

Rohan K, Vijay A, Daniel C, Pranitha PR and Mark SL, Diagnostic and prognostic utility of cardiac troponin in post-cardiac arrest care. *Circulation*. 2017;136:A17130.

Hou H, Pang L, Zhao L, *et al*. Hemoglobin as a prognostic marker for neurological outcomes in post-cardiac arrest patients: a meta-analysis. *Sci Rep*. 2023;13:18531.

Humaloja J, Ashton NJ, Skrifvars MB. Brain injury biomarkers for predicting outcome after cardiac arrest. *Crit Care*. 2022;26(1):81. doi: 10.1186/s13054-022-03913-5.

Hasper D, von Haehling S, Storm C, Jörres A, Schefold JC. Changes in serum creatinine in the first 24 hours after cardiac arrest indicate prognosis: an observational cohort study. *Crit Care*. 2009;13(5):R168.

Shin J, Lim YS, Kim K, *et al*. Initial blood pH during cardiopulmonary resuscitation in out-of-hospital cardiac arrest patients: a multicenter observational registry-based study. *Crit Care*. 2017;21:322.

Kim YJ, Lee YJ, Ryoo SM, Sohn CH, Ahn S, Seo DW, Lim KS, Kim WY. Role of blood gas analysis during cardiopulmonary resuscitation in out-of-hospital cardiac arrest patients. *Medicine*. 2016;95(25): e3960.

Gruebl T, Ploeger B, Wranze-Bielefeld E, *et al*. Point-of-care testing in out-of-hospital cardiac arrest: a retrospective analysis of relevance and consequences. *Scand J Trauma Resusc Emerg Med*. 2021;29:128.

Gruebl T, Ploeger B, Wranze-Bielefeld E *et al*. Point-of-care testing in out-of-hospital cardiac arrest: a retrospective analysis of relevance and consequences. *Scand J Trauma Resusc Emerg Med*. 2021:29:128.

7 Laboratory Diagnosis of Tropical Infections in the Intensive Care Unit

Tanu Singhal and Sweta Shah

INTRODUCTION

Tropical infections are those infections found in tropical and subtropical regions. Some of these infections are a common cause of hospitalization in the intensive care unit (ICU). While the list is exhaustive (Table 7.1), common illnesses in the Indian setting include dengue, malaria, leptospirosis, and rickettsial infections [1]. These infections generally present as fever with multi-organ dysfunction or acute febrile encephalopathy. They share several common clinical and laboratory features and mimic other infectious illnesses including bacterial sepsis. Hence, appropriate empiric therapy with a beta-lactam antibiotic and doxycycline is recommended in patients presenting with suspected severe tropical infection while waiting for the results of laboratory tests [2]. Laboratory tests are crucial to make an accurate diagnosis and institute targeted therapy. We discuss here the role of various laboratory tests in diagnosis of the common tropical infections, especially in the Indian setting. These include non-specific tests such as CBC, acute phase reactants, liver and renal functions, and imaging, and specific tests including cultures, serology, and molecular tests.

NON-SPECIFIC TESTS

Complete Blood Count

This is the first test and perhaps the most important. This test has the ability to triage various tropical infections, as depicted in Table 7.2 [3–5]. However, there is a significant overlap in the white cell count and platelet counts, making etiologic diagnosis challenging.

Acute Phase Reactants [6–8]

ESR is not a useful test in the ICU setting for the diagnosis of infections. C-reactive protein (CRP) is a commonly used test. Mild elevations of CRP can happen in both viral and bacterial infections, but very high levels are usually seen in bacterial infections. From the tropical infection perspective, dengue comes with normal or mildly elevated CRP while significant elevations can be seen in all other infections including leptospirosis, enteric fever, malaria, and rickettsia. Chikungunya, a viral infection, can sometimes be associated with a high CRP. Therefore the discriminatory value of CRP for making an etiologic diagnosis is limited. Procalcitonin is more specific than CRP, as it generally rises in bacterial but not viral infections. Hence like CRP, it will be elevated in leptospirosis, rickettsia, and malaria but not in dengue. However, it does not add significantly to the differential diagnosis of tropical infections beyond CRP.

Liver and Renal Function Tests [2]

Liver and renal function derangement is seen in most tropical infections once multi-organ dysfunction sets in. Leptospirosis is associated with the most remarkable changes. There is marked direct hyperbilirubinemia with only mild elevations of transaminases. There is a marked elevation of creatinine with non-oliguric renal failure. Direct hyperbilirubinemia and transaminitis can also be seen in malaria, dengue, and rickettsial infections.

Imaging [2]

CXR and USG of the abdomen and pelvis are important first-line investigations in patients admitted to ICU with sepsis. CT imaging of the chest and abdomen is a second-line imaging procedure

Table 7.1 Tropical Infections Associated with Severe Illness in the Indian Setting [1, 2]

Bacterial	Viral	Parasitic
Leptospirosis	Dengue	Malaria
Rickettsial infections	Chikungunya	Leishmaniasis
Enteric fever	Japanese encephalitis	
Melioidosis	Nipah virus disease	
Amoebic liver abscess	Crimean Congo hemorrhagic fever	
	Hantavirus	
	Rabies	

DOI: 10.1201/9781003449713-7

Table 7.2 Use of CBC in the Differential Diagnosis of Tropical Infections

Parameter	Significance
Hemoglobin	Low in malaria (may be low due to nutritional anemia)
	High in dengue (may also be high due to dehydration resulting from fever)
Total leucocyte count	Very low/low: Dengue, viral infections, malaria, overwhelming sepsis
	Normal: Enteric fever
	High: Leptospirosis, rickettsial infections
Differentials	Polymorph predominance: Enteric fever, leptospirosis, rickettsia
	Lymphocyte predominance: Dengue, malaria, chikungunya
	Eosinopenia: Any acute infection
Platelet count	Very low: Dengue, malaria, leptospirosis, rickettsial infections
	Low: Chikungunya, serious bacterial infections
Peripheral smear	Malaria, reactive lymphocytes in viral infections such as dengue

to localize the source of infection in patients with severe sepsis or septic shock. Imaging is however of limited value for differential diagnosis of tropical infections except for amoebic liver abscess, melioidosis (cavitary pneumonia/liver and splenic abscesses), or enteric fever (terminal ileal thickening, splenomegaly, and mesenteric adenopathy).

The role of CNS imaging especially MRI is particularly important in patients presenting with acute febrile encephalopathy [9]. Japanese encephalitis is associated with changes in basal ganglia and thalami, while the emerging Nipah virus encephalitis is characterized by multiple small discrete high-intensity lesions scattered throughout the deep and subcortical white matter [10]. Rabies is associated with rhombencephalitis.

SPECIFIC TESTS

These tests confirm the etiologic diagnosis and include microscopy, cultures, serology, and molecular tests. While the mainstay has been serologic tests, molecular tests are rapidly emerging as important diagnostic tools (For Summary of tests: See Table 7.4).

Bacterial Infections

Blood cultures should be sent for all patients with suspected sepsis admitted to the ICU irrespective of whether or not tropical infections are suspected. At least two sets of blood (each set has an aerobic and anaerobic bottle) or 40 ml of blood should be collected in adults. From the tropical infection perspective, enteric fever and melioidosis are two illnesses for which blood cultures are indispensable for diagnosis [11]. Infection due to *Burkholderia pseudomallei* can present with septicemia, septic shock, or necrotizing pneumonia in the ICU. The point to note is that the isolate may be misidentified as Pseudomonas species and dismissed as a contaminant. WIDAL and Typhidot IgM tests are not very sensitive and specific and are not recommended for diagnosis of enteric fever [12]. PCR has also not been found to be useful for the diagnosis of enteric fever. Conversely, diagnosis of melioidosis by PCR and antigen detection by lateral flow assay has been encouraging [13].

Malaria

Falciparum and Vivax can both cause severe malaria. The gold standard for diagnosis of malaria is a carefully examined thick smear, while a thin smear gives a species diagnosis [14]. Besides diagnosis, smear examination also gives an estimate of disease burden (parasite index which is the percentage of RBC that are parasitized), prognosis, and response to therapy. The presence of mature schizonts in the peripheral blood indicates poor prognosis. The smear should become negative no later than 72 hours after initiation of therapy. The main disadvantage of the smear is that it is observer-dependent. False positive results may occur due to stain deposits and false negative due to inexperience/cursory examination. The malarial rapid diagnostic tests (RDTs) are rapid point-of-care immune chromatographic tests that are based on the detection of parasite antigens, usually LDH/aldolase. The tests are not observer-dependent, and the sensitivity is comparable to smear microscopy However, the sensitivity varies widely with kit and storage conditions. Species diagnosis and diagnosis of mixed infection are possible with the current antigen tests. However, RDTs do not give an estimate of the disease burden, prognosis, or response to therapy. They may remain positive for 1–2 weeks after successful treatment. If malaria is strongly suspected and the initial thick smear and RDT are negative, then tests can be repeated every 6–8 hours. Performing the test at the height of fever does not enhance sensitivity.

Molecular diagnosis of malaria by PCR is now commercially available as a standalone test or as part of a multiplex fever panel. It has high sensitivity and can pick up 1–5 parasites per microliter as compared to 50–100 parasites detected by smear/RDTs. PCR has been used as the gold standard in drug efficacy trials. The sensitivity of PCR has been reported to be 98–100% as compared to 85–95% of smear/RDTs. In a study evaluating 2333 patients of fever from nine malaria-endemic states in India, PCR performed better than smear and RDT for diagnosis of malaria [15]. It is also superior to smear and RDT for the diagnosis of mixed infection and species identification. The specificity of PCR is however lower than smear/RDT (88–94% versus 95%). A malaria PCR may be requested if clinical suspicion is strong and the smear and RDT are negative.

Dengue

Dengue serology is the mainstay of diagnosis and includes testing for NS1 antigen, IgM, and IgG [16]. The NS1 antigen is a conserved non-structural protein specific to the dengue virus. It appears in the first two days of the illness and declines by days 5–7. In primary infection, NS1 antigen sensitivity in the first few days is close to 90%. The dengue IgM rises after 5–7 days and remains elevated for months. This prolonged persistence and cross-reactivity with other viruses lowers the specificity of IgM testing. The dengue IgG rises later and remains positive at low levels throughout a person's life. In secondary dengue infection, due to another serotype, the NS1 antigen declines rapidly due to mopping up by the antibodies. IgM also rises, but in 20% IgM may not rise at all. In secondary dengue, there is an exuberant IgG response with high titers of IgG. The test kits are designed to detect this high titer IgG, and hence a positive high titer IgG is suggestive of secondary dengue and not a past infection. Therefore IgG determination is of value in dengue, unlike other infections. The best sensitivity for dengue diagnosis is achieved by conducting NS1 antigen, IgM, and IgG tests together, irrespective of the time the patient presents to the hospital. Table 7.3 illustrates the interpretation of dengue serology.

Commercial tests are either rapid point-of-care immunochromatographic tests or ELISA-based tests. The ICT tests incorporate NS1 antigen, IgM, and IgG in a single card, have a quick turn-around time, are low-cost, and have good specificity but lower sensitivity than ELISA-based tests. They can be used as first-line tests. If negative, then ELISA testing can be requested.

The qRT-PCR for dengue is now commercially available. Studies evaluating the sensitivity of dengue diagnosis by NS1 antigen/RT-PCR compared to the gold standard by viral isolation have shown higher sensitivity of PCR as compared to the NS1 antigen (79% versus 73%) [17]. The sensitivity of PCR as compared to NS1 antigen is higher in patients with secondary dengue, severe dengue, and in the latter part of the illness [18].

Chikungunya [19]

Severe chikungunya and chikungunya encephalitis can lead to intensive care unit admissions. The chikungunya IgM antibodies are usually detectable in blood after 5–7 days of illness. The sensitivity of the commercial IgM ELISA assays was more than 90% after 1 week of infection but only 25% in the first week. Rapid immunochromatographic tests have poor performance with a sensitivity of only 46% beyond the first week. The chikungunya antigen tests have sensitivities of 90% in the first week but are not commercially available. Hence for diagnosis of chikungunya in the first week, chikungunya RT-PCR is recommended which has sensitivities greater than 90%. Chikungunya PCR is available as a standalone test or in combination with dengue or a part of the multiplex PCR panel (both are also available with TruNAT, Molbio platform apart from open real time PCR).

Rickettsia [20]

Rickettsial infections including scrub typhus and Indian spotted fever are an emerging cause of fever with multi-organ dysfunction and acute febrile encephalopathy in India [21]. The Weil-Felix

Table 7.3   Interpretation of Dengue Serology

NS1 antigen	IgM	IgG	Interpretation
Positive	Positive/Negative	Positive/Negative	Acute dengue infection
Negative	Positive	Negative	Acute primary dengue/other cause of fever
Negative	Negative	Positive	Acute secondary dengue
Negative	Negative	Negative	Serologically negative dengue/other diagnosis

Table 7.4   Recommended Diagnostic Tests in Tropical Infections in the Indian Setting

Indication	Tests
For all patients	CBC, CRP, blood culture, CXR, urine analysis, liver and renal function tests
Dengue	Dengue NS1, Dengue PCR, IgM and IgG rapid test/ELISA
Malaria	Smear/rapid diagnostic test
Chikungunya	PCR in first 5–7 days, IgM ELISA beyond 5–7 days
Leptospirosis	PCR in the first week, IgM ELISA beyond the first week
Rickettsial infections	Scrub typhus IgM/spotted fever IgM beyond day 5 If IgM ELISA is not available, then Weil-Felix test Rickettsia PCR in early disease if available

reaction is a heterophile antibody test based on the sharing of antigens between Rickettsia and Proteus. It demonstrates agglutinins to Proteus vulgaris OX19, OX2, and Proteus mirabilis OXK. Titers of more than 1:80 are considered significant (OX19 and OX2 for spotted fever and OXK for scrub typhus). The sensitivity and specificity of only 50% limits the diagnostic utility of this test. The indirect hemagglutination assay (IHA) and the indirect fluorescent assay (IFA) are the gold standard for diagnosis of rickettsial disease but are not available commercially. The commercially available IgM ELISA for scrub typhus and spotted fever are usually positive by the end of the first week. Rapid immunochromatographic tests are not recommended for diagnosis of rickettsial infections at this time. For diagnosis of rickettsial infections in the first week, PCR tests in blood or eschar tissue are recommended. But these tests are not readily available. Owing to the limitations of the currently available diagnostic tests in terms of availability, sensitivity, and specificity, empiric therapy with doxycycline is recommended in suspected cases [2, 21].

Leptospirosis

Traditionally the gold standard for diagnosis of leptospirosis is the microscopic agglutination test (MAT). The diagnosis is confirmed if there has been a fourfold rise in titer between the acute and convalescent sera or a single value of > 1:800. However the sensitivity of this test in a meta-analysis was reported to be 50%, although specificity was greater than 99% [22]. The limited sensitivity, need for live organisms, and availability only in reference laboratories make this an imperfect gold standard. The tests most commonly used in clinical practice are IgM and IgG ELISA. However, IgM test results can be false negative if done early in the illness, or false positive (50%) due to cross-reaction with other illnesses/exposure to leptospira in endemic areas [23]. Owing to the limitation of the serologic tests, molecular detection of leptospirosis has emerged as a promising modality. PCR tests for leptospira have a sensitivity ranging from 40 to 90% depending on the timing of collection, and specificities of greater than 95% [24]. Evaluation of TruNAT (chip-based NAAT) with RT-PCR as the gold standard showed that Truenat™ had a sensitivity of 97% and a specificity of 98%. The overall agreement with RT-PCR was 98% [25]. Widespread availability, low costs, and procedural ease make TruNAT a useful platform for molecular diagnosis of leptospirosis and other tropical illnesses.

Diagnosis of Emerging/Uncommon Infections

The last decade has seen the emergence of many severe and fatal viral infections in India, including Crimean Congo hemorrhagic fever and Nipah virus disease. The diagnosis of these illnesses is by RT-PCR in the first week of the illness from blood/body secretions and IgM ELISA after the first week [26, 27]. Samples have to be sent to reference laboratories for the same.

Role of Multiplex PCR in Blood for Diagnosis of Tropical Infections

Multiplex PCR-based panels have been introduced, which detect several tropical infections including dengue, malaria, chikungunya, rickettsia, leptospira, and enteric fever [28]. These are expensive panels with limited clinical studies on sensitivity and specificity. They are not recommended as first-line tests for tropical infections at this time.

CONCLUSION

The diagnosis of tropical infections should start with a good history with a focus on epidemiologic exposure and a thorough clinical examination for certain pathognomonic signs (e.g., eschar for scrub typhus). Important first-line investigations for suspected tropical infections include complete blood count with peripheral smear, CRP, blood cultures, smear or rapid antigen test for malarial parasites, CXR, liver and renal function tests, and urine analysis. If the initial evaluation is suggestive of a tropical infection, then further tests should be ordered. These include dengue serology, leptospira/chikungunya/rickettsia serology, and PCR. Empiric therapy with a beta-lactam antibiotic and doxycycline should be initiated while awaiting the results of investigations. The results of serologic tests should be interpreted carefully and correlated with the clinical presentation and results of other investigations, including complete blood count. Co-infections are the exception rather than the rule. Multiplex PCR panels should be used rationally. Intensivists should be aware of emerging infections and send investigations to referral labs in the appropriate setting.

REFERENCES

1. Karnad DR, Patil VP, Kulkarni AP. Tropical infections in the Indian intensive care units: the tip of the iceberg! *Indian J Crit Care Med.* 2021;25(Suppl 2):S115–S117.

2. Singhi S, Chaudhary D, Varghese GM, Bhalla A, Karthi N, Kalantri S, *et al.*, from The Indian Society of Critical Care Medicine Tropical fever Group. Tropical fevers: management guidelines. *Indian J Crit Care Med.* 2014;18(2):62–69.

3. Potts JA, Rothman AL. Clinical and laboratory features that distinguish dengue from other febrile illnesses in endemic populations. *Trop Med Int Health.* 2008;13(11):1328–1340.

4. Adiga DSA, Mittal S, Venugopal H, Mittal S. Serial changes in complete blood counts in patients with leptospirosis: our experience. *J Clin Diagn Res.* 2017;11(5):EC21–EC24.

5. Peter JV, Sudarsan TI, Prakash JA, Varghese GM. Severe scrub typhus infection: clinical features, diagnostic challenges and management. *World J Crit Care Med.* 2015;4(3):244–250.

6. Simon L, Gauvin F, Amre DK, Saint-Louis P, Lacroix J. Serum procalcitonin and C-reactive protein levels as markers of bacterial infection: a systematic review and meta-analysis. *Clin Infect Dis.* 2004;39(2):206–217.

7. Maillard O, Hirschinger D, Bénéteau S, *et al.* C-reactive protein: an easy marker for early differentiation between leptospirosis and dengue fever in endemic area. *PLoS One.* 2023;18(5):e0285900.

8. Otten T, de Mast Q, Koeneman B, Althaus T, Lubell Y, van der Ven A. Value of C-reactive protein in differentiating viral from bacterial aetiologies in patients with non-malaria acute undifferentiated fever in tropical areas: a meta-analysis and individual patient data study. *Trans R Soc Trop Med Hyg.* 2021;115(10):1130–1143.

9. Ramli NM, Bae YJ. Structured imaging approach for viral encephalitis. *Neuroimaging Clin N Am.* 2023;33(1):43–56.

10. Anam AM, Ahmad J, Huq SMR, Rabbani R. Nipah virus encephalitis: MRI findings. *J R Coll Physicians Edinb.* 2019;49(3):227–228.

11. Parry CM, Hien TT, Dougan G, White NJ, Farrar JJ. Typhoid fever. *N Engl J Med.* 2002;347(22):1770–1782.

12. Wijedoru L, Mallett S, Parry CM. Rapid diagnostic tests for typhoid and paratyphoid (enteric) fever. *Cochrane Database Syst Rev.* 2017;5(5):CD008892.

13. Shaw T, Tellapragada C, Ke V, AuCoin DP, Mukhopadhyay C. Performance evaluation of active melioidosis detect-lateral flow assay (AMD-LFA) for diagnosis of melioidosis in endemic settings with limited resources. *PLoS One.* 2018;13(3):e0194595.

14. Mbanefo A, Kumar N. Evaluation of malaria diagnostic methods as a key for successful control and elimination programs. *Trop Med Infect Dis*. 2020;5(2):102.

15. Siwal N, Singh US, Dash M, *et al.* Malaria diagnosis by PCR revealed differential distribution of mono and mixed species infections by *Plasmodium falciparum* and *P. vivax* in India. *PLoS One*. 2018;13(3):e0193046.

16. Muller DA, Depelsenaire AC, Young PR. Clinical and laboratory diagnosis of dengue virus infection. *J Infect Dis*. 2017;215 (Suppl_2):S89–S95.

17. Ahmed NH, Broor S. Comparison of NS1 antigen detection ELISA, real time RT-PCR and virus isolation for rapid diagnosis of dengue infection in acute phase. *J Vector Borne Dis*. 2014;51(3):194–199.

18. Balasubramanian S, Chandy S, Peter R, *et al.* Utility of a multiplex real-time polymerase chain reaction for combined detection and serotyping of dengue virus in paediatric patients hospitalised with severe dengue: a report from Chennai. *Indian J Med Microbiol*. 2020;38(3 & 4):288–292.

19. Johnson BW, Russell BJ, Goodman CH. Laboratory diagnosis of chikungunya virus infections and commercial sources for diagnostic assays. *J Infect Dis*. 2016;214(Suppl 5):S471–S474.

20. Devasagayam E, Dayanand D, Kundu D, Kamath MS, Kirubakaran R, Varghese GM. The burden of scrub typhus in India: a systematic review. *PLoS Negl Trop Dis*. 2021;15(7):e0009619.

21. Rahi M, Gupte MD, Bhargava A, Varghese GM, Arora R. DHR-ICMR guidelines for diagnosis & management of Rickettsial diseases in India. *Indian J Med Res*. 2015;141(4):417–422.

22. Limmathurotsakul D, Turner EL, Wuthiekanun V, *et al.* Fool's gold: why imperfect reference tests are undermining the evaluation of novel diagnostics: a reevaluation of 5 diagnostic tests for leptospirosis. *Clin Infect Dis*. 2012;55(3):322–331.

23. Desakorn V, Wuthiekanun V, Thanachartwet V, Sahassananda D, Chierakul W, Apiwattanaporn A, *et al.* Accuracy of a commercial IgM ELISA for the diagnosis of human leptospirosis in Thailand. *Am J Trop Med Hyg*. 2012;86(3):524–527.

24. Yang B, de Vries SG, Ahmed A, *et al.* Nucleic acid and antigen detection tests for leptospirosis. *Cochrane Database Syst Rev*. 2019;8(8):CD011871.

25. Rajamani M, Maile A, Sugunan AP, Vijayachari P. Truenat™: micro real-time-polymerase chain reaction for rapid diagnosis of leptospirosis at minimal resource settings. *Indian J Med Res*. 2021;154(1):115–120.

26. Vanhomwegen J, Alves MJ, Zupanc TA, *et al.* Diagnostic assays for Crimean-Congo hemorrhagic fever. *Emerg Infect Dis*. 2012;18(12):1958–1965.

27. Mazzola LT, Kelly-Cirino C. Diagnostics for Nipah virus: a zoonotic pathogen endemic to Southeast Asia. *BMJ Glob Health*. 2019;4(Suppl 2):e001118.

28. Manabe YC, Betz J, Jackson O, *et al.* Clinical evaluation of the BioFire Global Fever Panel for the identification of malaria, leptospirosis, chikungunya, and dengue from whole blood: a prospective, multicentre, cross-sectional diagnostic accuracy study. *Lancet Infect Dis*. 2022;22(9):1356–1364.

8 Organ-Support Devices

Sayan Nath and Shashikant Sharma

INTRODUCTION

A significant number of patients in intensive care units (ICU) require invasive or semi-invasive life modalities to support organ function. Monitoring patients on such devices requires an in-depth understanding of both the disease processes and the working principles of such devices. These patients are best monitored with a combination of clinical parameters, bedside point-of-care (POC) tests, and certain laboratory tests. Of course, there are additional on-device monitors necessary for smooth functionality like those for circuit pressures, flows, etc. that are integral to the working of such devices. This chapter primarily focuses on the point-of-care and laboratory parameters relevant to the monitoring of patients on continuous renal replacement therapy (CRRT), extra-corporeal membrane oxygenation (ECMO), and other temporary mechanical circulatory support (tMCS) devices.

CONTINUOUS RENAL REPLACEMENT THERAPY (CRRT)

There is wide variability in the literature regarding the incidence of RRT requirements in the ICU, with the range varying from 5 to 60%. Continuous forms of renal replacement therapies are often preferred in hemodynamically unstable patients. These modalities require complex machinery, circuits, and anticoagulation. Periodic evaluation of the functioning and safety of such devices is imperative. A detailed description of monitoring efficacy of CRRT is beyond the scope of this chapter. Instead, this chapter will provide an overview of monitoring the safety and most common concerns during CRRT.

Monitoring Anticoagulation

Circuit clotting is the most frequent cause of therapy interruption in CRRT. Additionally, many critically ill patients have higher bleeding risks owing to their underlying disease conditions. Hence, effective monitoring of anticoagulation is of prime importance. One has to choose from a wide number of available anticoagulants during CRRT, and the practice varies from institution to institution. Unfractionated heparin (UFH) is the most commonly used anticoagulant worldwide owing to rapid onset, lower costs, ease of monitoring, and reliable reversibility with protamine in case of overdose. However, low molecular weight heparin, direct thrombin inhibitors (DTI), factor Xa inhibitors, protease inhibitors, heparinoids, etc. are also used infrequently. The DTIs are useful in cases of heparin resistance and heparin-induced thrombocytopenia. Each of these anticoagulants has a unique chemistry and is monitored using different tests. A summary of the different tests used for monitoring systemic anticoagulation is given in Table 8.1). A strategy of no anticoagulation may be adopted for patients who have a platelet count < 50,000, an international normalized ratio > 2.0, an aPTT > 60 seconds, or who are actively bleeding or who have had a hemorrhagic event in the previous 24 hours.

Regional heparin–protamine anticoagulation may be used in patients with higher bleeding risk. It is administered by infusing pre-filter UFH into the extracorporeal circuit followed by post-filter infusion of protamine to bind excess UFH so that the blood returned to the patient is heparin-free. In these patients, the circuit aPTT should be maintained at therapeutic levels, while aPTT from the patient's blood should be normal. Laboratory-based aPTT measurements are commonly used. These are cheaper but have a delay depending on the individual lab's turnaround time. Nowadays, point-of-care cartridge-based aPTT measurement devices are available but have not seen wide acceptability owing to their higher cost and poor correlation with standard laboratory assays.

Citrate-based regional anticoagulation is achieved with pre-filter citrate and post-filter calcium infusion. When citrate is applied regionally, it binds calcium (a co-factor for multiple steps in coagulation) and thus prevents blood from clotting within the circuit. It has been seen that effective anticoagulation is achieved by reducing serum ionized calcium (iCa) to 0.25–0.4 mmol/L. This happens at a citrate concentration of 3–4 mmol/liter of blood. Citrate blood levels are not routinely measured, and instead indirect measurements like ionized calcium in the post-filter blood are obtained to determine the effectiveness of anticoagulation in the extracorporeal circuit. Due to the low molecular weight of citrate, its diffusion coefficient is quite high. However, calcium-bound citrate (which is slightly acidic in nature) passes through the filter at a rate of only 50–60%. Hence, it is necessary to apply calcium infusion into the systemic circulation (post-filter) in order to

DOI: 10.1201/9781003449713-8

Table 8.1 Systemic Anticoagulation During CRRT

Agent	Loading Dose	Maintenance Dose	Monitoring	Target	Frequency
Unfractionated heparin	5–15 IU/kg	5–10 units/kg/hour	Activated partial thromboplastin time (aPTT), anti-Xa activity	Target: aPTT in the circuit 45–60 anti-Xa activity 0.3–0.6 IU/mL	Initially every 6 hours until dose is stable, thereafter every 12 hours
Enoxaparin	0.15 mg/kg	0.05 mg/kg/hour	Anti-Xa activity	Anti-Xa 0.25–0.35 IU/mL	6–12 hourly
Dalteparin	15–25 IU/kg	5 IU/kg/hour	Anti-Xa activity	Anti-Xa 0.25–0.35 IU/mL	6–12 hourly
Nadroparin	15–25 IU/kg	5 IU/kg/hour	Anti-Xa activity	Anti-Xa 0.25–0.35 IU/mL	6–12 hourly
Danaparoid	750 U	1–2 U/kg/hour	Anti-Xa activity	Anti-Xa 0.25–0.35 IU/mL	6–12 hourly
Fondaparinux	–	2.5 mg/day	Anti-Xa activity	Anti-Xa 0.25–0.35 IU/mL	6–12 hourly
Argatroban	0.1 mg/kg	0.1–0.2 mg/kg/hour	aPTT	aPTT 1.5–2 times baseline (Some authors recommend 1–1.4 times in patients with higher bleeding risk)	Every 2–4 hours until aPTT target reached for two readings, then every 12 hourly
Bivalirudin	—	2 mg/hour	aPTT	aPTT 1.5–2 times baseline (Some authors recommend 1–1.4 times in patients with higher bleeding risk)	Every 2–4 hours until aPTT target reached for two readings, then every 12 hourly
Nafamostat mesylate	–	0.1–0.5 mg/kg/hour	aPTT	Pre-filter aPTT 2–2.5 times normal	Every 2–4 hours until aPTT target reached for two readings, then every 6–12 hourly
r-Hirudin	–	0.005–0.01 mg/kg/hour and after 1–2 days 0.005 mg/kg/hour or intermittent bolus 0.002 g/kg	Ecarin clotting time (ECT)	ECT 80–100 seconds	Not established. ECT is not a very good monitor during CRRT

replace the calcium loss due to the hemofiltration of bound Ca-citrate complexes. Citrate complexes that are returned to the patient are taken up by the liver (and to some extent muscle and kidneys) and metabolized by the Kreb's cycle to generate bicarbonate. In situations where citrate metabolism is impaired, citrate accumulates with its residual acidic effect. It further binds ionized calcium in the patient's blood and thus causes metabolic acidosis and hypocalcemia. Hence, for safety, normal ionized calcium in the patient's blood is generally targeted. An increased total serum calcium (tCa)/ iCa ratio above 2.5 is highly indicative of ongoing citrate accumulation.

The monitoring for regional anticoagulation is summarized in Table 8.2. Ionized calcium values may be obtained both from routine blood gas analyzers and laboratories.

Table 8.2   Monitoring Regional Anticoagulation

Agent	Loading Dose	Maintenance Dose	Monitoring	Target	Frequency
Regional heparin with protamine	–	Heparin pre-filter: 1000–1500 U/h Protamine post-filter: 10–12 mg/h	aPTT (both patient blood and circuit blood)	Patient aPTT < 45 s and circuit aPTT 50–80 s	4–15 min after dose and then every 2–8 h
Regional citrate anticoagulation	-	Variable, according to target	1. Post-filter ionized calcium (iCa) in blood gas from hemofilter circuit	Post-filter iCa < 0.35 mmol/lit	Hourly until target achieved and then 6 hourly
			2. Patient's systemic ionized blood calcium	1–1.3 mmol/lit	Hourly until normal and the 6 hourly
			3. Patient total calcium	2.2–2.5 mmol/lit	12 hourly
			4. Patient's total calcium ÷ Ionized calcium	< 2.5	12 hourly

Table 8.3   Metabolic Complications During RCA

	Citrate Accumulation	Insufficient Buffering	Net Citrate Overload
Mechanism	Decreased citrate metabolism	Insufficient buffer delivery	Excessive bicarbonate generation
pH	Metabolic acidosis	Metabolic acidosis	Metabolic alkalosis
HCO3	Low	Low	High
Lactate	High	Normal	Normal
iCa++	Low	Normal	Normal
Total calcium	High	Normal	Normal
Total Ca/iCa	High	Normal	Normal

For the reasons described above, citrate anticoagulation is often complicated by metabolic derangements. These are summarized in Table 8.3. Additionally, citrate anticoagulation may cause hypomagnesemia by chelation.

Monitoring Electrolytes
All forms of CRRT require protocolized electrolyte monitoring since these are often deranged. Monitoring of electrolytes and acid-base status should be done every 6 to 12 hours when starting CRRT. If stable after the first 24 to 48 hours, the interval can then be increased to 12 to 24 hours.

Dysnatremias
In hypernatremic patients who require RRT, the correction rate can be regulated by either hypertonic CRRT solutions (made by adding sodium chloride or sodium bicarbonate) or post-filter hypertonic saline infusions to prevent rapid correction of hypernatremia. The recommended sodium concentration for the initial CRRT solution is set to 5–10 mmol/lit lower than that of the patient. Change in sodium by more than 2 mmol/lit within the first 6 hours of CRRT requires modification of the dialysis solution or the prescribed dialysis dose. Hyponatremia, conversely, requires dilution of CRRT solutions with sterile water or concomitant post-filter administration of free water (5% or 10% dextrose water) in order to prevent rapid correction.

Dyskalemias
In hyperkalemic patients requiring CRRT, the dialysate potassium is usually low (0–2 mmol/lit). In patients with rhabdomyolysis, tumor lysis syndrome, hemolysis, etc., the ongoing potassium load should also be considered while prescribing the dose and solutions. On the other hand,

hypokalemia is a common complication of CRRT that can be treated or prevented with oral/intravenous potassium supplementation and/or potassium-containing CRRT solutions. Some centers use fixed protocols to prescribe the dialysate based on pre-RRT serum potassium and phosphate levels.

Dyscalcemias

In patients with hypercalcemia and concomitant renal insufficiency, RRT is the treatment of choice. Commercial CRRT solutions have iCa concentration of 1.25–1.75 mmol/L (2.5–3.5 mEq/L). When performing CRRT in AKI patients with significant hypercalcemia, calcium-free solutions can be used as dialysate and replacement fluid. Hypocalcemia, on the other hand, is generally a complication of RCA and is managed by intravenous calcium infusions or titrating the citrate anticoagulation as described before.

Dysphosphatemia

Severe hyperphosphatemia causing symptomatic hypocalcemia (for example in tumor lysis syndrome) is an indication of RRT. Conversely, hypophosphatemia is a frequent complication of CRRT with an incidence as high as 65%. Common CRRT solutions are phosphate-free. This can be avoided by newer phosphate-containing solutions or by supplementing intravenous/oral phosphate during CRRT. Some centers prescribe 15 mmol sodium phosphate intravenously two to three times per day during CRRT treatment.

Dysmagnesemia

Hypermagnesemia is most reliably treated by RRT if medical management fails. Not surprisingly, hypomagnesemia is a common complication of CRRT. In RCA protocols, a continuous MgS04 infusion of 2–4 g/day is generally recommended.

Hematological Parameters

CRRT may be frequently complicated by new onset thrombocytopenia and anemia, with etiology being multifactorial. This confounds the picture in patients with sepsis or other multi-organ dysfunctions where thrombocytopenia is generally common. Additionally, heparin-induced thrombocytopenia should be borne in mind. The latter needs laboratory confirmation with either immunoassays or functional assays. Immunoassays identify antibodies against heparin/platelet factor 4 (PF4) complexes. A functional assay that measures the platelet-activating capacity of PF4/heparin-antibody complexes is more specific, but it is time-consuming and not routinely available. Device-related consumption coagulopathy generally has associated elevation in D-dimer and a fall in fibrinogen levels. Hemolysis in the circuit can be identified by increasing plasma lactate dehydrogenase (LDH), rising indirect bilirubin, rising plasma free hemoglobin (pfHb), and reticulocyte count.

Other Parameters

Macro- and micronutrients are lost through CRRT circuits. Some authors recommend routine monitoring of nitrogen balance and micronutrients in patients having ongoing CRRT, though these assays are seldom cost-effective.

TEMPORARY MECHANICAL CIRCULATORY SUPPORT DEVICES

A large number of temporary mechanical circulatory support devices are used in patients with refractory cardiogenic shock. The type of these devices varies depending on the indications. The common devices in use are shown in Figure 8.1. The optimal functioning of these devices requires close hemodynamic monitoring, echocardiography, and monitoring for oxygenation and tissue perfusion, as well as controlling the on-device consoles. These are beyond the scope of this chapter. However, like other life support devices, these devices also require monitoring for certain complications and optimal anticoagulation.

Anticoagulation

The anticoagulation recommendations for the commonly used tMCS are summarized in Table 8.4.

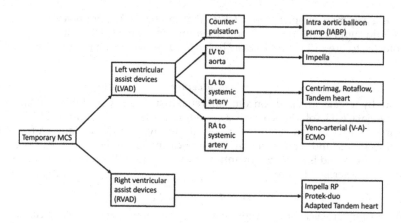

Figure 8.1 Temporary mechanical circulatory support devices.

Table 8.4 Anticoagulation in tMCS

Device	Comments	Anticoagulation
IABP	Not necessary in 1:1 support, use if 1:2 or 1:3 or if the device is in situ for more than 5 days or if the patient has high risk of thrombosis	Lower starting doses (10–12 U/kg/h of UFH) to start with aPTT goals of 50–70 seconds
Impella	Requires a heparin-based purge to prevent ingress of blood into the motor. Usual purge solution is 25,000 units of UFH in 1 L of intravenous dextrose 5% in water (D5W). The device automatically adjusts purge flow rates to target purge pressures, so additional systemic anticoagulation may be needed. When starting systemic anticoagulation, the amount of UFH from the purge solution should also be considered in initial dosing	25,000 units of UFH in 1 L of 5% D5W with or without systemic UFH to target anti-factor Xa 0.3–0.7U/ml Alternatively, sodium bicarbonate purge 25 mEq in 1 L of 5% D5W purge with or without systemic anticoagulation
Tandem heart	Uses heparin purge solution with or without systemic anticoagulation	UFH 9000 units in 1 L normal saline at 10 ml/h as purge solution
Centrimag	Generally used in post-cardiac surgery patients	Full anticoagulation (activated clotting time or ACT 300 sec) before device placement Start heparin infusion once chest tube output is less than 50 ml/hour targeting ACT 160–180 sec or aPTT 1.3–1.6 times normal, ACT 250–300 sec during low flow or weaning, antiplatelet on 4th post-operative day

Other Parameters

Like any other mechanical device, all the tMCS devices may cause hemolysis, consumption coagulopathy, thrombocytopenia, etc. The laboratory monitoring of these complications is similar to those in CRRT.

ECMO

Anticoagulation in ECMO

Like other life support devices, patients on ECMO are at increased risk of both thromboembolic and bleeding. Like CRRT, UFH is the most commonly used agent. However, others are also used, and the test for monitoring tests are of course similar, as mentioned previously in this chapter. Table 8.5 summarizes the three commonly used tests to monitor anticoagulation during ECMO. Apart from these, visco-elastic tests with or without platelet mapping are also used in some centers during ECMO. In contrast to techniques like ACT, aPTT, and PT/INR, which solely display the endpoint (the presence or absence of a thrombus), the viscoelastic tests provide information on several facets of the coagulation cascade, the dynamics of clot formation, clot strength and lysis, and fibrinolysis, and are often used. However, they do not offer information regarding the von

Table 8.5 Laboratory Assays to Monitor Anticoagulation and Targets in ECMO

Method	Purpose	Desired Target	Advantages	Disadvantages
aPTT	To monitor anticoagulant effect	25–90 s or 1.5–2.5 times baseline (depending on the device, anticoagulant, and utilized method)	• Widely available • Well-known method • Easy to interpret • Not affected by platelet count	• Nonspecific to heparin • Time-consuming and user-dependent • Can be affected by hematocrit, abnormalities in coagulation factors, fibrinogen, high C-reactive protein • Prolonged in the presence of lupus anticoagulant
ACT	To assess the anticoagulant effect	180–220 sec	• Point-of-care test • Low-cost and fast • Better correlation with high concentrations of heparin	• User- and instrument-dependent • Lacks specificity • Sensitive to (platelet dysfunction, temperature, hematocrit, anemia, hypothermia, hypofibrinogenemia, and activator type)
Anti-factor Xa assay	To monitor anticoagulant effect	0.3–0.7 IU/mL	• Sensitive to UFH • Independent of coagulopathy, thrombocytopenia, or dilution • Correlates better than ACT and aPTT with heparin concentration	• Affected by hyperlipidemia and hyperbilirubinemia • Not easily accessible • Costly • Time-consuming

Willebrand factor level (VWF). While the use of viscoelastic tests in ECMO has increased recently, most centers do not have routine access to them, limiting their widespread use.

ECMO and Infections

Infectious complications associated with the use of ECMO are common, and the reported incidence of hospital-acquired infections ranges from 10 to 12% with substantial mortality. Potential sources of sepsis in ECMO patients include ventilator-associated pneumonia, bloodstream infections, cannula infections, mediastinitis, catheter-associated urinary tract infections, infected pressure sores, and Clostridium difficile-associated diarrhea. The diagnosis requires routine tests including complete blood counts, liver and kidney function tests, urine analysis, and chest imaging. Samples such as blood, urine, and respiratory secretions should be sent for culture based on the suspected site of infection. Often pan-cultures are necessary. A high index of suspicion for fungal infections should be there, and unlike fungal cultures which come with significant delay, biomarkers such as beta-D-glucan and galactomannan may guide antifungal therapy. Newer rapid tests based on multiplex polymerase chain reaction (PCR), nucleic acid amplification, microarrays, etc. can provide a fast microbiological diagnosis. Empiric antimicrobial therapy is the same as for other critically ill patients; however, dosage should be appropriately adjusted with due consideration of the altered volume of distribution, protein binding, and organ dysfunction. Antimicrobial dosing in ECMO is beyond the scope of this chapter.

ECMO and Hypoxia

Blood gas analysis from different circuit sites in ECMO provides some idea about some causes of hypoxia in ECMO. Tissue level perfusion and microcirculatory function are checked by serial lactate and veno-arterial CO_2 gap. A decreased post-membrane oxygen ($PaO_2 < 200$ mm Hg in post-membrane blood despite maximal blood flow rate and FiO_2 at 1.0) suggests membrane dysfunction. A recirculation fraction (RF) of more than 30% contributes significantly to hypoxia in veno-venous ECMO. RF is given by the following formula:

$$\text{Recirculation fraction} = (SpreO_2 - SvO_2) / (SpostO_2 - SvO_2) \times 100$$

$SpreO_2$ = pre-membrane oxygen saturation; SvO_2 = Mixed venous oxygen saturation; $SpostO_2$ = Post-membrane oxygen saturation.

ECMO and Other Parameters

Like other life support therapies, patients on ECMO require close monitoring of electrolytes and signs of hemolysis, rhabdomyolysis, etc.

CONCLUSION

- Circuit clotting is a common cause of CRRT interruption, reducing the actual dose of CRRT delivered to the patient.

- Hemolysis and thrombocytopenia are complications common to all mechanical life support devices.

- Bloodstream infections on life support devices are difficult to treat since it is not possible to remove the invasive lines/foreign devices routinely in these patients.

- All point-of-care tests are theoretically advantageous, as they lessen the delay between assay and intervention. However, except for ACT, not all assays are standardized and hence not widely accepted for routine monitoring of patients on invasive life support devices.

BIBLIOGRAPHY

Baeg SI, Lee K, Jeon J, Jang HR. Management for electrolytes disturbances during continuous renal replacement therapy. *Electrolyte Blood Press*. 2022;20(2):64–75. https://doi.org/10.5049/EBP.2022.20.2.64.

Biffi S, Di Bella S, Scaravilli V, Peri AM, Grasselli G, Alagna L, Pesenti A, Gori A. Infections during extracorporeal membrane oxygenation: epidemiology, risk factors, pathogenesis and prevention. *Int J Antimicrob Agents*. 2017;50(1):9–16. https://doi.org/10.1016/j.ijantimicag.2017.02.025.

Boyaci Dundar N. Regional citrate anticoagulation: basic principles and clinical applications. *J Crit Intensive Care*. 2023;14:28–32.

Gautam SC, Lim J, Jaar BG. Complications associated with continuous RRT. *Kidney* 360 2022;3(11):1980–1990, https://doi.org/10.34067/KID.0000792022.

Gopalakrishnan R, Vashisht R. Sepsis and ECMO. *Indian J Thoracic Cardiovascular Surgery*. 2021;37:267–274.

Legrand M, Tolwani A. Anticoagulation strategies in continuous renal replacement therapy. *Semin Dial*. 2021;34(6):416–422. https://doi.org/10.1111/sdi.12959.

Levy JH, Staudinger T, Steiner ME. How to manage anticoagulation during extracorporeal membrane oxygenation. *Intensive Care Med*. 2022;48(8):1076–1079. https://doi.org/10.1007/s00134-022-06723-z.

MacLaren G, Brodie D, Lorusso R, Peek G, Thiagarajan R, Vercaemst L. *Extracorporeal life support: The ELSO Red Book*. 2022.

Makdisi G, Wang IW. Extra corporeal membrane oxygenation (ECMO) review of a lifesaving technology. *J Thorac Dis*. 2015;7(7):E166–E176. https://doi.org/10.3978/j.issn.2072-1439.2015.07.17.

Singh S. Anticoagulation during renal replacement therapy. *Indian J Crit Care Med*. 2020;24(Suppl 3):S112–S116. https://doi.org/10.5005/jp-journals-10071-23412.

Yin EB. Anticoagulation management in temporary mechanical circulatory support devices. *Texas Heart Instit J*. 2023;50(4): e238135.

Zakhary B, Vercaemst L, Mason P, Antonini MV, Lorusso R, Brodie D. How I approach membrane lung dysfunction in patients receiving ECMO. *Crit. Care*. 2020;24:1–4.

Zeibi Shirejini S, Carberry J, McQuilten ZK, Burrell AJ, Gregory SD, Hagemeyer CE. Current and future strategies to monitor and manage coagulation in ECMO patients. *Thrombosis J*. 2023;21(1):1–20.

9 Organ Retrieval and Transplant

Parshotam Lal Gautam

> *"While interpreting laboratory results and data, we must know whether we want to confirm or rule out disease. For quality interpretation of lab data, it is important to interpret data in the context of patient; knowing patient characteristics, disease pattern and laboratory limitation and patients purpose of investigation."*

INTRODUCTION

Investigational workup is the backbone of transplant services and plays a pivotal role in assessing the severity of disease, organ allocation, perioperative management, monitoring immunosuppression, and prognostication in the recipient. Laboratory workup plays an important role in the optimization of donors and inclusion of marginal donors. Many transplant service decisions are based on biochemical, radiological imaging, cytology, histopathology, and molecular genetics laboratory workups. Errors can happen at multiple levels, from the collection of samples to interpretation. The first consideration in each investigation should be rationale and purpose. Laboratory tests may be required to unmask subclinical or occult disease, differentiate and confirm the severity and activity, and guide the therapy in transplant services. Organ transplantation remains the best therapy for terminal and irreversible organ failure until we can find a magical and miraculous alternative to this modality.

Despite an upsurge in transplant facilities and the number of transplants, the number of recipients dying while waiting for a transplant is still high due to the paucity of donors. From multiple cohort studies, it can be estimated that 30–60% of potential donors are missed [1–3]. The solution is to convert these missed organ donors into the donor pool and prevent wastage. Novel *ex vivo* organ preservation and perfusion techniques such as hypothermic, normothermic, and subnormothermic machines may be useful to "resuscitate" marginal organs by reducing ischemia/reperfusion injury and prolonging preservation timings. These technologies may help in better assessment of marginal donors with serial laboratory tests. Determining that an organ is suitable for transplantation is based on a variety of factors, such as clinical and laboratory investigations that focus on the general health of the deceased donor, the cause of death, or the functional status of the potential donor organ. Appropriate use of investigations with clinical contexts and their interpretation play a pivotal role in improving the donor pool and the quality of organs, and making the right choices with accuracy and precision. The gained knowledge may improve organ function once administered to a deceased donor prior to organ recovery with a focus on a single specific organ such as a kidney (i.e., the target organ) or multiple organs and later other organs (i.e., non-target organs) [4]. Automated tools using artificial intelligence with machine learning may play a role in the future to alert physicians of these cases [5].

CLASSIFICATION OF DISEASE AND/OR SEVERITY

Allocation from the waiting list is done based on clinical status and investigations to make the distribution of organs fair, ethical, and equitable. Priority of different organs cannot be done with a single tool and is not simple. In end-stage renal disease, there are possibilities to extend life; however, this is more difficult in liver transplant patients. Furthermore, cardiac assist devices and extra-corporeal membrane oxygenation (ECMO) for lung transplant patients on waiting lists are invasive and costly. Disease severity and category of the patient determine priority. Interpretation of investigations on patients on waiting lists requires a thorough understanding of the disease in context to allow prognosis and a risk assessment of waiting time. In the time window between the declaration of the donor's death and the procurement of the donor's organs, donor management protocols are based on the patient's clinical parameters, lab values of electrolytes and hormones [6–8].

LABORATORY WORKUP

It is important to understand the laboratory tests and interpret the values in the context with clinical findings, reference range, timeline bias, sensitivity and specificity, accuracy, limitations of technology, etc. There are two types of laboratory tests: basic and point-of-care like biochemistry and imaging, and advanced investigations like genetics and molecular labs.

DOI: 10.1201/9781003449713-9

BASIC LABORATORY AND POINT-OF-CARE TESTS (WITH TIMELINES AND CLINICAL COURSE)

Most patients who are potential donors, are in an ICU. There may be investigations related to primary disease, death certification essentials, suitability as a donor, and organ preservation. Most of these investigations are either point-of-care biochemical testing such as blood gases and electrolytes, or radiological imaging such as chest X-ray, bedside ultrasonography, echocardiography, etc. Some of these are done in a central laboratory, but many others are done at the bedside at point-of-care. All tests need a diligent interpretation that considers the technology used to interpret the results and correlations with patient disease and characteristics, as investigations can have caveats and limitations because of technology, operation, and interpreter. Sampling technique and storage are a source of error. Thus, sound clinical decision-making must include the patient's status rather than focusing on investigation. However, in some conditions, laboratory values play a role more than clinics, for example in electrolyte imbalances. Sometimes you need to correlate multiple investigations to reach a conclusion on how to act. Interpretation has another major bias factor: human error. Medical errors are not uncommon. Not only human errors but laboratory test failures also qualify as errors. These may contribute to delayed or erroneous information resulting in error of omission or commission. Errors related to laboratory tests are more common than one might think. We must understand that these aren't always correct or incorrect, and they aren't always useful. However, that does not mean ignoring them. There are multiple ways and ample scope to improve the accuracy of any laboratory value and its interpretation. One should use the right test, with the correct standardized equipment, including calibration, and then use the proper collected sample and interpretation, keeping in mind the patient's characteristics. Common investigations are blood gases, clinical biochemistry, and hematological and infectious workups, including advanced microbiological workups.

Clinical Pearls in Laboratory Use in ICU

1 Using the right test is critical to obtaining the desired information.
2 One test may be performed by different devices with different technology, and results may not be the same; thus you should know the accuracy and limitations.
3 Proper sampling technique, transport, and storage of samples matter significantly in some investigations. These investigations can misguide you. We must be careful while collecting samples for sepsis.
4 Interpretation is another important step. Results must be put into context. Misinterpretation or misapplication of test results can lead to diagnostic errors. To best utilize lab testing, one must understand what the results mean in that particular scenario. When interpreting laboratory results, we must know whether we want to confirm or rule out disease. For quality interpretation of lab data, it is important to interpret data in the context of the patient: knowing patient characteristics, disease patterns, and laboratory limitations.
5 Lab errors happen despite a strong focus on quality operations.

ADVANCED LABORATORY AND POINT-OF-CARE TESTS (WITH TIMELINES AND CLINICAL COURSE)

The immune genetics laboratory in transplant medicine provides diagnostic testing of the disease, starting preoperatively in cross-matching to find the suitability of the donor and perioperatively to tailor immunotherapy. If the transplantation is genetically incompatible, then the allogeneic graft (allograft) is recognized as foreign and predominantly depends upon the differences between donor/recipient major histocompatibility complex (MHC) molecules, also known as the human leukocyte antigens (HLAs). Compatibility of HLA, a gene complex located in the short arm of chromosome 6 is the basic test for solid organ transplantation There are two major classes: class I (A, B, and C) and class II (DR, DQ, and DP). Both HLA classes are involved in maintaining the homeostasis of the immune system with their expression on CD8 and CD4 cells. In solid organ transplantation, a recipient receives a donor graft that usually carries different HLA antigens and triggers an alloimmune response, which could be humoral, cellular, or a mix. Some patients have pre-formed HLA antibodies due to previous sensitization events, which may react leading to graft rejection in the postoperative period. Thus, HLA matching is to assess and monitor the immunological risk of a donor-recipient pair. This HLA matching study can be done with different technologies such as PCR-targeted sequence-specific primer (SSP) or Luminex technology. These have variable turnaround times, accuracy, and precision in reporting. Thus, knowing the technique and its accuracy as well as the pitfalls are important while interpreting tests. Many international associations and country authorities set standards, regulations, and policies for uniform working, which are revised from time to time with updated knowledge. Antibody detection has to be performed by a solid phase method. One of the first used was ELISA, but it has been substituted by Luminex technology due to its versatility and accuracy. The other method is cross-matching, which is used to confirm compatibility between a patient/donor pair. Depending on the organ transplanted, this will be performed before the transplant or after, as there are differences in the immunogenicity of each organ. HLA laboratory testing for solid organ transplantation involves accurate typing for patients and donors and precise patients' HLA antibody profile determination for immunosuppression titration. For some organs, like the kidney, a physical XM pre-transplant is required. The purpose of the HLA testing is to provide an immunologic risk assessment for a given patient-donor pair.

HLA nomenclature—HLA typing data are reported at the antigen or allele level (version of DNA). Serologic typing has been replaced with molecular typing over time with advances in diagnostics. HLA allele names are reported with the gene (locus) designation, followed by an asterisk to denote that it was typed by molecular methods; colons separate the remaining fields. A high-resolution, "full" HLA typing can give a lot of information in advance regarding compatibility. There are multiple fields in HLA typing.

Serologic Methods

Serologic-based typing has been used for decades. This technique uses a panel of reference sera and lymphocytes from the donor or recipient. Following an initial incubation period, complement is added to wells, and a viability dye allows the detection of cell lysis. The presence of dead cells is a positive test. Major caveats in this testing include a large panel of sera required, and sera are seldom monospecific.

DNA-Based Molecular Methods

With the advent of the PCR technique, DNA-based molecular testing has evolved to more accurately determine an individual's HLA typing. There is further refinement in these which include sequence-specific primers (SSP) typing, sequence-specific oligonucleotide probes (SSOP) typing, and real-time PCR (RT-PCR)-based typing. SSP can be used for either low-resolution typing, by identifying allele groups of a particular antigen, or for high-resolution typing, which identifies a specific allele. A major advantage of the SSP method is its fast turnaround time of two hours. With SSOP typing, DNA is amplified using a set of primers that recognize a particular HLA locus. SSOP typing is well suited for typing large numbers of samples, with each assay capable of testing 80 to 180 samples, but it takes approximately two days to obtain results. The RT-PCR form of typing is based upon the use of allele-specific PCR similar to SSP methods. Automated data interpretation also simplifies the analysis significantly.

HLA Mismatches

The greater the disparity between the donor and recipient, the higher the likelihood of developing an all-immune response. All HLA components are not equally immunogenic. During kidney transplantation, only the *HLA-A*, *HLA-B*, and *HLA-DR* loci are compared between a donor and recipient. A zero-antigen mismatch refers to concordance at these loci but does not rule out disparities at the others (*HLA-C*, *HLA-DP*, or *HLA-DQ*). Since HLA genes are inherited as a set, related donor/recipient pairs are likely to also share the same antigens at the other loci, e.g., blood grouping. However, if the donor and recipient are unrelated, such derivations cannot be drawn [9]. The tests include histocompatibility testing, acceptable HLA mismatches, and tolerable donor-specific HLA antibodies (DSA). Substantial evidence suggests that not all HLA mismatches are detrimental to allograft survival. These days, incompatible donors are also accepted through close monitoring of the transplanted organ. In the post-transplant setting, the molecular profile of a biopsy picks up ongoing subclinical immune-mediated injury, as well as recognizes acute T cell-mediated rejection, even in samples without obvious histological evidence of inflammation. This may help to overcome the limitations of conventional biopsy diagnosis, which often relies typically on histopathology scores. Scores are often empirically derived, subjective, and opinion-based consensus. Using information from these investigations with appropriate relevance, we can design clinical decision pathways. Artificial intelligence and machine learning may prove to be successful tools.

DONOR FACTORS IMPACTING RECIPIENT OUTCOME

Donor characteristics are important. Some of these are associated with an adverse effect on graft function and/or graft survival, including "donation after circulatory death" (DCD), hemodynamic stability, advanced donor age, comorbidities, viral diseases, malignancies, and substance abuse. Initial work in donation aims at initial screening for suitability and excluding major contraindications. Common initial screening includes the age and sex of the patient, whether they are on a ventilator or have inotrope support, ruling out an active malignancy or a history of malignancy, infection workup, and specific organ function tests.

Marginal Liver Donors

Currently, with the use of marginal or extended criteria of liver grafts, many patients, who would have died on a liver transplant waiting list, survive. In an 18-year longitudinal study of over 2000 liver transplant recipients from a single center, authors found comparable and promising results. Short term outcomes following use of marginal allografts has been similar to nonmarginal allografts while reducing candidate wait time on the waiting list [10–13].

Hypernatremia

Worse outcomes have been reported in liver transplant grafts procured from donors with hypernatremia. Per se donor hypernatremia may be a surrogate marker for other factors affecting graft function, including prolonged ICU stay, secondary to diabetes insipidus with hypovolemia, catecholamine storm, excessive normal saline, negative water balance resulting from aggressive treatment of cerebral edema, and reduced antidiuretic hormone secretion after brain death. Most respondents to a survey of the South-Eastern Organ Procurement Foundation liver transplant centers indicated that the maximum donor serum sodium level that they would accept was 160 to 170 mEq/L [14, 15].

Hemodynamic Instability

Hepatic blood flow is dependent upon the portal system, which decreases during periods of shock and the use of high doses of vasopressors predisposing ischemic liver injury. Early graft dysfunction has been observed when donors experienced refractory shock. However, the use of high doses of dopamine was not associated with graft dysfunction when the donor's blood pressure was maintained above 90 mmHg [16].

Rejection vs Infection

Solid organ transplants are at risk of infection and rejection. Differentiation is a challenging task. Early detection of rejection and infection, and aggressive and timely management, have a remarkable impact on outcomes. Biopsy-based rejection monitoring is time-consuming as well as risky, particularly for organs like the heart and liver. There may be errors in the interpretation of biopsies due to a high degree of inter-observer variability in the grading of results. Also, the severity of rejection may not always coincide with the grading of the rejection according to the biopsy. It cannot be used to identify patients at risk of rejection, limiting the ability to initiate therapy early and in a presumptive approach to interrupt the development of rejection. Therefore, noninvasive methods of detecting cellular rejection have been explored. Noninvasive biochemical and molecular panels will assist in determining the appropriate approach for these patients to manage immunosuppression. The allograft rejection in heart transplant recipients produces oxidative stress which can be detected by breath markers (volatile organic compounds). Similarly, microfilm array technology for sepsis assessment permits the analysis of the gene expression of carbapenemaces, with a turnaround time of two hours. This helps not only to recognize the bug but also the enzymes. We need to understand the limitations that these can detect other forms of antimicrobial resistance. The panel is limited to certain bugs, and there remains the issue of other bugs not being included in the panel [17–19].

Renal Transplant Rejection

Allograft dysfunction is typically asymptomatic and remains often subclinical with wide differentials, including graft rejection. Surveillance of kidney function in recipients relies more on regular monitoring of serum creatinine, urine protein levels, and urinalysis. For immune suppression, there should be regular monitoring of calcineurin-inhibitor trough levels. Acute allograft dysfunction may also be demonstrated by a SIRS, a drop in urine output, or, rarely, as pain at the transplant site. With clinical suspicion of allograft rejection, bedside ultrasonography or radionu-clide imaging may be used. Renal biopsy allows definitive assessment of graft dysfunction and is typically a percutaneous procedure performed with ultrasonography or computed tomography guidance. Biopsy of a transplanted kidney is associated with fewer complications, as the allograft is placed superficially. Pathologic assessment of biopsies demonstrating acute rejection allows clinicians to further distinguish between acute cellular rejection (ACR) and antibody-mediated rejection (AMR), which are treated differently. There are other newer tests that measure the immune response of recipient lymphocytes to donor lymphocytes in cell culture, which predict the likelihood of acute cellular rejection after renal transplantation.[18–20] Risk assessment indices have been developed to evaluate marginal donors. A shortage of donor livers has led to the inclu-sion of these marginal donors judiciously and selectively to improve the survival of patients on waiting lists [20–23].

Identification of Potential Lung Donors

A good potential donor is younger than 55 years old, has a clear chest X-ray, $PaO_2/FiO_2 > 300$ mmHg at PEEP of 5, has not smoked within 20 years, has an absence of chest trauma, has no evidence of aspiration or sepsis, has had no prior cardiopulmonary surgery, and has an absence of purulent secretions or gastric contents on bronchoscopic visualization prior to procuring the lungs [24, 25].

The expanding role of artificial intelligence and machine learning in the healthcare delivery system will hopefully be integral in the allocation and management of patients [26].

We need to understand that accurate interpretation of laboratory workups is as important as getting it done.

REFERENCES

1. Krmpotic K, Payne C, Isenor C and Dhanani S. Delayed referral results in missed opportuni-ties for organ donation after circulatory death. *Crit Care Med.* 2017;45:989–992.

2. Kutsogiannis DJ, Asthana S, Townsend DR, Singh G, and Karvellas CJ. The incidence of potential missed organ donors in intensive care units and emergency rooms: a retrospective cohort. *Intensive Care Med.* 2013;39:1452–1459.

3. Sairanen T, *et al.* Lost potential of kidney and liver donors amongst deceased intracerebral hemorrhage patients. *Eur J Neurol.* 2014;21:153–159.

4. National Academies of Sciences, Engineering, and Medicine; Health and Medicine Division; Board on Health Sciences Policy; Committee on Issues in Organ Donor Intervention Research; Liverman CT, Domnitz S, Childress JF, editors. *Opportunities for Organ Donor Intervention Research: Saving Lives by Improving the Quality and Quantity of Organs for Transplantation.* Washington (DC): National Academies Press (US), 2017, p. 1.

5. Sauthier N, Bouchakri R, Carrier FM, *et al.* Automated screening of potential organ donors using a temporal machine learning model. *Sci Rep.* 2023;13:8459.

6. McKeown DW, Bonser RS, Kellum JA. Management of the heartbeating brain-dead organ donor. *Br J Anaesth.* 2012;108(Suppl 1):i96–i107.

7. Kotloff RM, Blosser S, Fulda GJ, *et al.* Management of the potential organ donor in the ICU: Society of Critical Care Medicine/American College of Chest Physicians/Association of Organ Procurement Organizations consensus statement. *Crit Care Med.* 2015;43(6):1291–1325.

8. Kumar L. Brain death and care of the organ donor. *J Anaesthesiol Clin Pharmacol.* 2016;32(2):146–152.

9. Vella, J. Kidney transplantation in adults: Risk factors for graft failure. https://www.uptodate .com/contents/kidney-transplantation-in-adults overview -of-hla-sensitization-and-cros smatch-testing. Accessed on August 24, 2023.

10. Gonzalez FX, Rimola A, Grande L, Antolin M, Garcia-Valdecasas JC, Fuster J, *et al.* Predictive factors of early postoperative graft function in human liver transplantation. *Hepatology.* 1994;20:565–573.

11. Figueras J, Busquets J, Grande L, Jaurrieta E, Perez-Ferreiroa J, Mir J, *et al.* The deleterious effect of donor high plasma sodium and extended preservation in liver transplantation. *Multivar Anal Transplantat.*1996;61:410–413.

12. Adam R, Reynes M, Johann M, Morino M, Astarcioglu I, Kafetzis I, *et al.* The outcome of steatotic grafts in liver transplantation. *Transpl Proc.* 1991;23:1538–1540.

13. Todo S, Demetris AJ, Makowka L, Teperman L, Podesta L, Shaver T, *et al.* Primary nonfunction of hepatic allografts with preexisting fatty infiltration. Transplantation. 1989;47:903–905.

14. Broughan TA, Douzdjian V. Donor liver selection. The South-Eastern organ procurement foundation liver committee. *Am Surg.* 1998;64:785.

15. Figueras J, Busquets J, Grande L, *et al.* The deleterious effect of donor high plasma sodium and extended preservation in liver transplantation. A multivariate analysis. *Transplantation.* 1996;61:410.

16. Mor E, Klintmalm GB, Gonwa TA, *et al.* The use of marginal donors for liver transplantation. A retrospective study of 365 liver donors. *Transplantation.* 1992;53:383.

17. Goldberg RJ, Weng FL, Kandula P. Acute and chronic allograft dysfunction in kidney transplant recipients. *Med Clin North Am.* 2016;100(3):487–503.

18. Solez K, Colvin RB, Racusen LC, *et al.* Banff 07 classification of renal allograft pathology: updates and future directions. *Am J Transplant.* 2008;8(4):753–760.

19. Haas. The Revised (2013) Banff classification for antibody-mediated rejection of renal allografts: update, difficulties, and future considerations. *Am J Transplant.* 2016;16(5):1352–1357.

20. Silberhumer GR, Rahmel A, Karam V, *et al.* The difficulty in defining extended donor criteria for liver grafts: the Eurotransplant experience. *Transpl Int.* 2013;26:990.

21. Croome KP, Mathur AK, Mao S, *et al.* Perioperative and long-term outcomes of utilizing donation after circulatory death liver grafts with macrosteatosis: a multicenter analysis. *Am J Transplant.* 2020;20:2449.

22. Giorgakis E, Khorsandi SE, Mathur AK, *et al.* Comparable graft survival is achievable with the usage of donation after circulatory death liver grafts from donors at or above 70 years of age: a long-term UK national analysis. *Am J Transplant.* 2021;21:2200.

23. Kotloff RM, Blosser S, Fulda GJ, *et al.* Management of the potential organ donor in the ICU: society of critical care medicine/american college of chest physicians/association of organ procurement organizations consensus statement. *Crit Care Med.* 2015;43:1291.

24. Heiden BT, Yang Z, Bai YZ, *et al.* Development and validation of the lung donor (LUNDON) acceptability score for pulmonary transplantation. *Am J Transplant.* 2023;23:540.

25. Duong Van Huyen JP, Tible M, Gay A, *et al.* MicroRNAs as non-invasive biomarkers of heart transplant rejection. *Eur Heart J.* 2014;35(45):3194–3202.

26. Sauthier N, Bouchakri R, Carrier FM, *et al.* Automated screening of potential organ donors using a temporal machine learning model. *Sci Rep.* 2023;13:8459.

10 Malnutrition and Related Complications

Sanjith Saseedharan, Surendra Shingnapurkar and Jayram Navade

INTRODUCTION

Malnutrition refers to a condition when there is an imbalance in energy and nutrient intake, either excesses or deficiency in any person. Insufficient intake of calories, protein, or various nutrients can lead to malnutrition. It is an effect of "not enough" as well as "too much" food, the wrong types of food, or the inability to use nutrients properly to maintain one's health.

Malnutrition is a considerable public health concern and is associated with an increased risk of disease and early death. WHO defines malnutrition as "the cellular imbalance between supply of nutrients and energy and body's demand for them to ensure growth, maintenance and specific functions".

Globally in 2020, 149 million children under 5 were estimated to be stunted (too short for age), 45 million were estimated to be wasted (too thin for height), and 38.9 million were overweight or obese.

1.9 billion adults are overweight or obese, while 462 million are underweight.

Around 45% of deaths of children under 5 years of age are linked to undernutrition. These mostly occur in low- and middle-income countries. At the same time, in these same countries, rates of childhood overweight and obesity are rising.

Complications arising from malnutrition can have significant and sometimes severe consequences on physical and mental health.

CLASSIFICATION OF MALNUTRITION

Typically, malnutrition can be classed as either undernutrition or overnutrition.

1. Undernutrition

    This includes both macronutrient (underweight) and micronutrient deficiencies due to a lack of energy, proteins, vitamins, and minerals. Undernutrition is most common in developing countries and is associated with poverty and limited access to nutritious food.

2. Overnutrition

    This is a result of excessive consumption of calories, unhealthy fats, sugar, and salt. It results in weight gain and related health problems. The global rise in obesity rate is an indicator and is commonly associated with high-income countries.

Malnutrition can be further classified into specific nutrient deficiencies such as protein-energy malnutrition, iron deficiency anemia, vitamin A deficiency, and iodine deficiency disorders.

(A) Protein-energy malnutrition (PEM):

1. Marasmus: This is chronic energy deficiency resulting in severe wasting and loss of muscle mass. It is often characterized by emaciation and a "skin and bones" appearance.

2. Kwashiorkor: This is a protein deficiency leading to edema (fluid retention), enlarged liver, and changes in skin and hair. Kwashiorkor can occur even when caloric intake is adequate.

(B) Micronutrient deficiencies:

This results from insufficient intake of vitamins and minerals. The most common are

1. Vitamin A deficiency: This can lead to night blindness, dry skin, and increased susceptibility to infections.

2. Iron deficiency anemia: This is insufficient iron, leading to reduced hemoglobin levels and anemia.

3. Iodine deficiency disorders (IDD): This can result in goiter, mental retardation, and developmental issues.

(C) Undernutrition:

1. Stunting: This is chronic malnutrition causing impaired growth and development in children.

DOI: 10.1201/9781003449713-10

2. Underweight: This is insufficient weight for a given age, indicating a general lack of nutritional adequacy.

3. Wasting: This is rapid weight loss or failure to gain weight, often associated with acute malnutrition.

(D) Overnutrition:

1. Obesity: This is excessive accumulation of body fat, often associated with a diet high in calories and low in nutritional value.

However, in view of the lack of consensus in defining and classifying the severity of malnutrition in clinical settings, the Global Leadership Initiative on Malnutrition (GLIM) criteria was suggested in 2018 by a core leadership committee with representatives of several of the global clinical nutrition societies like ASPEN (www. nutritioncare.org), ESPEN (www.espen.org), FELANPE (www. felanpeweb.org), and PENSA (www.pensal-online.org). As per the GLIM criteria, the diagnosis of malnutrition would involve at least one phenotypic criterion and at least one etiologic criterion from the list below.

The phenotypic criteria would be satisfied by one or both of the following criteria:

1. Weight loss in percentage: > 5% in last 6 months, or > 10% in more than 6 months. Low body mass index (BMI) (kg/m2): < 20 if < 70 years, or < 22 if > 70 years. Asia: < 18.5 if < 70 years, or < 20 if > 70 years.

2. Reduced muscle mass as diagnosed by validated body composition measuring techniques like DEXA, bio-electrical impedance analysis (BIA), ultrasound, CT, or MRI. Alternatively calf or arm circumference or a thorough physical exam along with calibrated hand-grip strength using a validated hand-grip dynamometer can be used to correlate to muscle mass.

The etiologic criteria would be satisfied by any one or both of the following two criteria:

1. History of a reduction of intake of more than 50% of the requirement for more than a week 1 week, any reduction of intake for more than 2 weeks, or any chronic GI disorders with adverse nutrition impact.

2. An acute disease or injury with severe systemic inflammation, or socioeconomic or environmental starvation.

Malnutrition is further classified into stage 1 (moderate) and stage 2 (severe) (see Table 10.1) [1].

COMPLICATIONS OF MALNUTRITION

1. Poor overall intellectual development and learning abilities due to impaired cognitive development.

2. More susceptibility to infections due to impaired immune function.

3. Muscle wasting.

4. Poor response during tissue repair, leading to delayed wound healing.

5. Increased mortality because of higher vulnerability to diseases.

LABORATORY INVESTIGATIONS IN MALNUTRITION

1. CBC, iron, B12, folic acid.

Table 10.1   Severity of malnutrition by the Glim criteria

	Stage 1	Stage 2
Wt loss %	5%–10% in last 6 months, > 10%–15% more than 6 months	> 10% < 6 months, or > 20% > 6 months
BMI	< 20 if < 70 yrs, or < 22 if > 70 yrs	< 18.5 if < 70 yrs, or < 20 if > 70 yrs
Red muscle mass	Mild to moderate	Severe deficit

CBC helps in identifying common nutritional deficiencies of iron, vitamin B12 (a water-soluble vitamin), or folate.

B12 deficiency (< 200 pg/ml) would show up as low hemoglobin, low hematocrit, and a mean corpuscular volume of more than 100. A peripheral blood smear will show hypersegmented neutrophils having greater than or equal to five lobes. However, in order to confirm this deficiency, it is important to demonstrate increased levels of homocysteine and methylmalonic acid (MMA). In folic acid deficiency (< 2 ng/ml), there are increased levels of homocysteine without an increase in methylmalonic acid. The easiest option to differentiate between B12 deficiency and folic acid deficiency would be to find the levels of both. Severe folic acid deficiency may also lead to pancytopenia [2].

Anemia associated with hypochromic and microcytic erythrocyte morphology is common with iron deficiency. In the absence of inflammation, low ferritin is the best indicator of iron deficiency. Apart from ferritin, a low serum iron, high transferrin or total iron binding capacity (TIBC), and a low transferrin saturation indicate iron deficiency anemia.

Some investigators have shown that transferrin could be used as a marker of nutritional status [3, 4]. Since this functions as an acute phase reactant, some investigators have advised against its use as a nutrition marker [5].

2. Blood glucose, insulin levels, HbA1c

Prediabetes is known to be an increased risk for sarcopenia. Malnutrition is among the leading factors causing sarcopenia, and nutritional interventions as well as other interventions like physical rehabilitation have been used to mitigate sarcopenia. Prediabetes is characterized by impaired fasting glucose and impaired glucose tolerance and thus may be harbingers of malnutrition. Recent studies have linked HbA1c as an independent risk factor for loss of appendicular skeletal muscle mass and sarcopenia when HbA1c is greater than 5.2% in the male non-T2DM population [6].

A distinct entity referred to as malnutrition-related diabetes mellitus is defined by blood glucose > 200 mg/dl, onset before 30 years of age, BMI < 19, absence of ketosis on insulin withdrawal, insulin requirement more than 2 u/kg/day, and history of childhood malnutrition. The glucose intolerance of protein-energy malnutrition is known to be associated with structural changes in the beta cell, and in a significant proportion of undernourished subjects, it is irreversible despite prolonged and vigorous nutritional rehabilitation [7].

3. Liver function test – serum proteins, prealbumin, albumin, globulin

Albumin (half-life of approximately 20 days) has been used as an indicator of malnutrition for decades in clinically stable patients. Prealbumin and transthyretin, which have half-lives of less than 2 days, are considered more sensitive markers of malnutrition.

However it is important to note that both albumin and prealbumin cannot be used to define malnutrition, nor are they markers of muscle mass or total body protein. Even in instances of anorexia nervosa, albumin and prealbumin levels were maintained and lowered only when there was extreme starvation (BMI < 11 kg/m²) [8]. In fact, albumin and prealbumin both function broadly as acute phase reactants and are known to reduce in the presence of inflammation. Serum albumin concentrations not only decrease during decreased synthesis due to inflammatory cytokines like IL-6 and TNF-alpha leading to tissue catabolism or hepatic insufficiency, but they may also decrease following renal losses in nephrotic syndrome and losses via the GI tract in protein-losing enteropathies. However, low albumin and prealbumin can be used to indicate that a patient is at risk of malnutrition and poor outcomes if not supplemented adequately.

Prealbumin (transthyretin) is a transport protein for thyroid hormone and is synthesized by the liver and partly catabolized by the kidneys. Serum prealbumin concentrations less than 10 mg/dL are associated with malnutrition.

The use of prealbumin has been advocated as a nutritional marker, particularly during refeeding and in the elderly. The main advantage of prealbumin compared to albumin is its shorter half-life (two to three days), making it a more favorable marker of acute changes in the nutritional state. In addition, prealbumin was not influenced by intestinal protein losses in patients with protein-losing enteropathy.

4. Renal function test

Serum creatinine, BUN, and electrolyte levels are used to assess overall clinical and fluid volume status and need to be obtained if parenteral (intravenous) nutrition is a possibility. Plasma calcium, magnesium, and phosphorous concentrations should also be assessed periodically, particularly in the setting of poor oral intake or diarrhea. They are monitored regularly in patients receiving parenteral nutrition.

5. Urinary creatinine

Nutritional status will determine the amount of creatine and thus creatinine (as creatinine is the metabolic product of creatine) in the body. This is completely excreted in the urine. Hence, the amount of creatinine excreted in urine will be a direct estimate of the amount of skeletal muscle mass in the body. There are issues in measuring urinary creatinine, such as a cumbersome 24-hour urine collection period, errors in values due to the interference of ketones and other chromogens, almost 5 to 10% day-to-day variation even after accurate collection, and variations during impaired renal functions, fever, menstrual cycle, etc. Therefore, this measurement is not used regularly. Moreover, significant reduction is found only when more than 10% of skeletal muscle is lost. Urinary methylhistidine, another very similar protein from skeletal muscle like creatinine, continues to be used for research purposes, but the same issues are faced as those by urinary creatinine. Hence, urinary methylhistidine is not used in clinical practice [9].

6. Nitrogen balance

Nitrogen balance is the difference between nitrogen intake and nitrogen loss. It thus helps in assessing malnutrition, as nitrogen is an essential part of protein. Assessment is done by finding the nitrogen lost by measuring the urine urea nitrogen from a 24-hour urine sample. Then 4 is added to account for non-urinary urea nitrogen loss. The intake is found by dividing the protein by 6.25 (the average nitrogen content of proteins is about 16%, hence, to convert nitrogen into protein content N x 1/16, i.e., 6.25). The intake is subtracted from the nitrogen lost, and then nitrogen balance can be established (normal equilibrium is −4 or −5 g/day to +4 or +5 g/day) [10].

7. Serum cholesterol

Low serum cholesterol mirrors low lipoprotein and thus low visceral protein. Hence, cholesterol levels < 160 mg/dl are closely associated with protein-energy malnutrition.

The sensitivity and specificity of cholesterol as a marker to diagnose and monitor nutrition are very poor. Nevertheless, this marker has been incorporated into screening tools like the Elderly Nutritional Indicators for Geriatric Malnutrition Assessment (ENIGMA), Controlling Nutritional Status (CONUT), and the Mini Nutritional Assessment [11–13].

8. Serum zinc level

Zinc is extensively involved in protein, lipid, nucleic acid metabolism, and gene transcription. Individuals at high risk for malnutrition are found to have zinc deficiency. This abundant trace element is however bound to albumin, and hence assessment of zinc status is difficult. It is highly possible that zinc deficiency is thus under-recognized in malnourished individuals [14].

9. Immunity markers

Malnourished patients do not respond well to skin antigen tests and hence may demonstrate delayed hypersensitivity. In addition, they may also have reduced circulating lymphocytes (< 1500/mm^3) due to reduced maturation. Both these immunity markers would also point toward a malnourished state.

10. Tests for malabsorption

There is a close relationship between malabsorption and malnutrition, where malabsorption can be a cause as well as an effect of malnutrition. The laboratory plays a very important role in the diagnosis of malnutrition and a significant role in treatment.

Breath tests:
These tests are generally done for diagnosing carbohydrate malabsorption. In this test, the quantity of hydrogen exhaled is measured with the help of a gas chromatograph. Hydrogen is

generally produced by bacteria in the colon with the help of carbohydrates and transported to the lungs from where it is exhaled. Therefore, the more unabsorbed carbohydrate that reaches the colon, the more hydrogen. Similarly, the more small intestinal bacterial overgrowth, the more hydrogen in the breath.

A glucose hydrogen breath test will help in the diagnosis of small intestinal bacterial overgrowth. A lactulose hydrogen breath test will help in the diagnosis of SIBO as well as orocecal transit time. Lactose and fructose hydrogen breath tests will help in the diagnosis of lactose and fructose malabsorption, respectively [15].

Blood and urine tests for malabsorption:

This test is used to diagnose malabsorption. D-xylose is a pentose sugar that is not normally found in the blood. It can be easily absorbed by healthy intestinal cells without the aid of pancreatic enzymes and is poorly metabolized, where at least 50% of the dose is excreted in the urine within 24 hours. Adults (usually given an oral dose of 25 grams of D-xylose) should excrete at least 25% of the dose in a five-hour urine sample and have a two-hour blood level of at least 25 mg/dL [16].

Pancreatic elastase test:

This helps to detect pancreatic insufficiency. Pancreatic elastase 1 (PE1) is a proteolytic enzyme secreted exclusively by the human pancreas, and as such, it reflects overall pancreatic exocrine function. It is an extremely stable, reliable, and specific marker useful in differentiating pancreatic from nonpancreatic steatorrhea or diarrhea.

Fecal fat studies:

These help to diagnose steatorrhea (fat malabsorption).

a. Qualitative – The stool sample is examined under a microscope to check the number of fat globules or droplets.

b. Quantitative – A stool sample is collected over a period of 72 hours to measure the total amount of fat.

11. Other markers

Serum leptin, insulin-like growth factor-1, serum Nesfatin-1, and retinol-binding protein are other laboratory markers that hold promise in the assessment of malnutrition [17].

CONCLUSION

None of the existing biomarkers seem to be ideal for diagnosing malnutrition. Clearly, there is a dire need for biomarkers in the diagnosis of malnutrition. The ideal laboratory biomarker would have ease of measurement, be simple, highly sensitive, and specific to nutritional status, not be altered by inflammatory state, be available as point-of-care, and should be cheap. Until the ideal laboratory biomarker can be established, other biomarkers should be supplemental to a good nutrition-focused history and physical examination of the patient and taking advantage of screening tools such as SGA, standardized equipment like the bio-electrical impedance analyzer, DEXA scan, Ct, MRIm, and reasonably standardized measurements like hand-grip dynamometry and muscle mass estimation.

CLINICAL PEARLS

1. Judicious use of the laboratory supplemented with a thorough physical examination along with screening tools can help in the assessment of malnutrition.

2. All laboratory biomarkers to diagnose malnutrition are neither sensitive nor specific.

3. Most serum biomarkers tested for assessing malnutrition have a relationship with clinical outcomes.

REFERENCES

1. Jensen GL, Cederholm T, Correia MITD, Gonzalez MC, Fukushima R, Higashiguchi T,et al. GLIM criteria for the diagnosis of malnutrition: a consensus report from the global clinical nutrition community. *JPEN J Parenter Enteral Nutr.* 2019;43(1):32–40. doi: 10.1002/jpen.1440.

2. Bouri S, Martin J. Investigation of iron deficiency anaemia. *Clin Med (Lond).* 2018;18(3):242–244. doi: 10.7861/clinmedicine.18-3-242.

3. Shetty PS, Jung RT, Watrasiewicz KE, James WP Rapid-turnover transport proteins: AN index of subclinical protein-energy malnutrition. *Lancet.* 1979;314:230–232. doi: 10.1016/S0140-6736(79)90241-1.

4. Fletcher JP, Little JM, Guest PK A comparison of serum transferrin and serum prealbumin as nutritional parameters. *J Parenter Enter Nutr.* 1987;11:144–147.

5. Roza AM, Tuitt D, Shizgal HM. Transferrin—a poor measure of nutritional status. *J Parenter Enter Nutr.* 1984;8:523–528.

6. Li S, Mao J, Zhou W. Prediabetes is associated with loss of appendicular skeletal muscle mass and sarcopenia. *Front Nutr.* 2023;10:1109824.

7. Partha Sarathi C, Sanjib KG, Rita C, Prabir KK, Rabindranath C; Malnutrition-related diabetes mellitus (MRDM), not diabetes-related malnutrition: a report on genuine MRDM. *Diabetes Care* 1995;18(2):276–277.

8. Lee JL, Oh ES, Lee RW, Finucane TE. Serum albumin and prealbumin in calorically restricted, nondiseased individuals: a systematic review. *Am J Med.* 2015;128:1203.

9. Shenkin A, Cederblad G, Elia M, Isaksson B. Laboratory assessment of protein-energy status. *Clin Chim Acta.* 1996;253:S5–S9. doi: 10.1016/0009-8981(96)06289-4.

10. Rand WM, Pellett PL, Young VR. Meta-analysis of nitrogen balance studies for estimating protein requirements in health adults. *Am J Nutr* 2003;77:109–127.

11. Ng TP, Nyunt MSZ, Gao Q, Wee SL, Yap P, Yap KB. Elderly nutritional indicators for geriatric malnutrition assessment (ENIGMA): development and validation of a nutritional prognostic index. *Clin Nutr ESPEN.* 2017;22:54–63.

12. De Ulíbarri JI, González-Madroño A, De Villar N, González P, González B, Mancha A, Rodriguez F, Fernández G. CONUT: a tool for controlling nutritional status. First validation in a hospital population. *Nutr Hosp.* 2005;20:38–45.

13. Vellas B, Guigoz Y, Garry PJ, Nourhashemi F, Bennahum D, Lauque S, Albarede JL. The mini nutritional assessment (MNA) and its use in grading the nutritional state of elderly patients. *Nutrition.* 1999;15:116–122.

14. Yokokawa H, Fukuda H, Saita M, Miyagami T, Takahashi Y, Hisaoka T, Naito T. Serum zinc concentrations and characteristics of zinc deficiency/marginal deficiency among Japanese subjects. *J Gen Fam Med.* 2020;21(6):248-255.

15. Ghoshal UC. How to interpret hydrogen breath tests. *J Neurogastroenterol Motil.* 2011;17(3):312–317.

16. Craig RM, Ehrenpreis ED. D-xylose testing. *J Clin Gastroenterol.* 1999;29(2):143–150.

17. Atamer Y, Şahbaz T, Aşık HK, Saraç S, Atamer A. The relationship between serum leptin, insulin-like growth factor-1, and insulin-like growth factor binding protein-3 levels and clinical parameters in primary fibromyalgia patients. *Rev Assoc Med Bras (1992).* 2023;69(10):e20230240.

11 Reporting Critical Laboratory Values

Sridevi Devaraj and Anil K. Chokkalla

INTRODUCTION

Communication of critical laboratory results needs to be timely and accurate, and this is the basic requirement of critical alert reporting as required by Clinical Laboratory Improvement Amendments (CLIA). It is also codified in the International Organization for Standardization's standards for medical laboratories. Laboratory medicine professionals are often belabored by the need to establish relevant cutoffs for critical values in different populations and having to differentiate between alerts that are urgent but not critical. What is a critical value or critical alert? How does the lab establish criteria for reporting critical laboratory values, and how does effective reporting of laboratory critical values improve patient outcomes? This review will address the tenets of critical alert reporting and implementation strategies for the reporting of critical laboratory values.

WHAT IS A CRITICAL LAB VALUE?

A critical value is defined as "a laboratory test result that represents a pathophysiologic state at such variance with normal as to be life-threatening unless something is done promptly and for which some corrective action could be taken." This concept was first implemented by Dr. George D. Lundberg at Los Angeles County/University of Southern California Medical Center in 1972 [1].

Table 11.1   Sample Critical Value Formulary

Laboratory Division	Analyte	Critical Values
Blood Gas	Calcium ionized	< 3.2 or > 6.2 mg/dL
	Hemoglobin	< 6.5 g/dL
	PCO_2 (arterial, venous)	< 20 or > 75 mmHg
	pH (arterial, venous)	< 7.10 or > 7.59
	PO_2 (arterial)	< 40 mmHg
Chemistry	Bilirubin, total	> 15 mg/dL (0–3 months); > 20 mg/dL (4–6 months)
	Calcium	< 6.5 or > 14.0 mg/dL
	Carbon dioxide (total)	< 11 or > 40 mmol/L
	Glucose, CSF	< 40 mg/dL
	Glucose, Plasma	< 40 or > 500 mg/dL
	Lactate	> 4 mmol/L
	Lithium	> 1.8 mmol/L
	Magnesium	< 0.5 or > 2.4 mmol/L
	Osmolality, plasma, or serum	< 250 or > 335 mOsm/kg water
	Phosphorus	< 1.1 mg/dL
	Potassium	< 2.8 or > 6.0 mmol/L
	Sodium	< 120 or > 160 mmol/L
Hematology	Initial hematocrit	> 56% within 30 days
	Differential	Presence of blasts on initial smear within 30 days
	Initial hematocrit	≤ 20% within 30 days
	Initial platelet count	< 40 × 10^3/µL or > 999 × 10^3/µL within 30 days
	Initial WBC	< 1.5 or > 50 × 10^3/µL within 30 days
	INR	≥ 5.0
	Partial thromboplastin time	> 100 seconds
	Platelets	Patients < 20 years old with a platelet count of < 20 × 10^3/µL
Immunology	Viscosity	> 3 relative viscosity units

(Continued)

DOI: 10.1201/9781003449713-11

Table 11.1 *(Continued)*

Laboratory Division	Analyte	Critical Values
Microbiology	Blood and CSF cultures	Positive cultures
Toxicology/Therapeutic Drug Monitoring	Acetaminophen	> 50 mg/L
	Carbamazepine	> 20 µg/mL
	Digoxin	> 2.5 ng/mL
	Gentamicin	Peak/unknown: > 9.9 µg/mL; Trough: > 2.9 µg/mL
	Isopropanol	> 100 mg/L
	Methanol	> 100 mg/L
	Phenobarbital	> 70 µg/mL
	Phenytoin	> 30 µg/mL
	Tobramycin	Peak: > 9.9 µg/mL; Trough: > 2.9 µg/mL
	Vancomycin	Trough: > 39.9 µg/mL

Because of the critical nature of these laboratory results, immediate notification to the healthcare provider is necessary. They have alternatively been called panic values, but since the term carries some emotional stress with it, it is strongly dissuaded from future use.

STANDARD LIST OF CRITICAL VALUES

Currently, there is no standardized list and limits for critical values. Hospitals autonomously establish their critical value formulary based on the patient population and clinical setting. Clinical Laboratory Standards Institute guidance document (CLSI GP47-ED1), however, highlighted the benchmarks for critical values based on the College of American Pathologists (CAP) Q-Probe survey data from 163 laboratories across the US [2]. Table 11.1 shows a sample critical value formulary (adapted from CLSI GP47-ED1) [3].

REGULATIONS SURROUNDING CRITICAL VALUES

Critical value reporting is regulated and is part of many accreditation programs. In the United States, the Clinical Laboratory Improvement Amendments of 1988 (CLIA 88) regulations for critical lab value reporting specify that the laboratory manual must address critical values and have appropriate protocols for reporting critical value results [see §493.1251 (b; 11 and 13); and §493.1291 (g)] [4]. The Joint Commission National Patient Safety Goals also address critical value reporting and indicate that improving the effectiveness of communication among caregivers will be performed by timely reporting of critical test results and diagnostic procedures, and readback of such results is imperative, especially if the critical results are reported verbally [5]. This is imperative since several reports have been documented by erroneous telephone communications [6]. If there is an electronic way of seeing results in real-time while calling criticals, such readback after looking at results electronically needs to be documented and does not require readback. The CAP Laboratory Accreditation Program has critical lab value result reporting as part of their required standards in several checklist components (College of American Pathologists. *Laboratory General Checklist [components GEN.41320, GEN.41330, and GEN.41340])* and includes standards for documenting the procedure for critical lab value reporting, readback, or appropriate acknowledgment of the communicated critical lab results. In addition, the CAP also has a critical values list that can guide practitioners in understanding some tests that may require immediate attention and that laboratory directors can use at their discretion for their individual facilities [7]. Furthermore, the International Organization for Standardization (ISO 15189) also includes critical value reporting in its clinical laboratory standard [8].

The first step in communicating critical values is the appropriate identification of the critical value by the laboratory technologist. In most of the automated analyzers, either the middleware, such as data innovations or the laboratory information system, is equipped to flag critical results. In many instances, laboratory policies must indicate clearly whether the assay needs to be repeated and/or verified before reporting the critical. However, the policies should indicate the timeframe for repeating or verifying the test results since these need immediate medical attention and/or intervention [9]. Laboratory policies also need to indicate who reports the critical lab results and to whom. In several hospitals as well as outside clinics, there are several people who

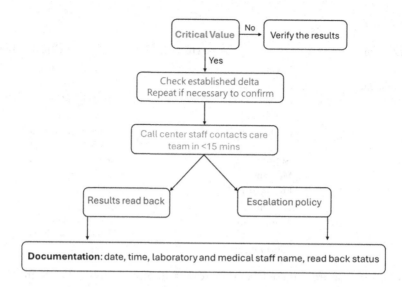

Figure 11.1 Key events in critical value reporting.

may be given the responsibilities of receiving and acting upon critical values and may include the ordering physician, on-call physician, trainee, or other appropriate caregiver who should acknowledge and document it. The CAP specifies that required information for a critical laboratory value are date, time, person notified, and responsible laboratory specialist, as well as who it was read to and whether it was read back, and all of the above needs accurate documentation during the process. Also, CAP requires the establishment of an escalation policy when the automated processes do not work or if the ordering provider cannot be found in a timely fashion, such as contacting the in-charge or pathology resident/fellow or medical director [2]. A typical workflow for reporting critical values is shown in Figure 11.1.

WHAT INTERVENTIONS IMPROVE CRITICAL LAB VALUE REPORTING?

In a rapidly evolving information technology infrastructure, laboratories need to use automated notification systems or best practice alerts or pathways such as secure chat on hospital information systems such as Epic to alert the care team/health provider of critical laboratory test results. This would enable the provider to acknowledge and confirm receipt of the alert electronically. In cases where automated notification systems do not exist, then laboratories should resort to manual critical alert notification systems.

With regard to critical alert notification systems, one strategy that improves critical result reporting is the use of laboratory technologists in call centers who are able to reach the healthcare provider in a reasonable timeframe and can ensure receipt and readback of critical lab values. It is also mandatory to document these calls for regulatory purposes. The advantage of the manual critical alert notification is that if the primary health provider is not able to be contacted, they can reach out to the alternate healthcare provider team [10]. Studies have contrasted the timeliness of call centers' critical test result reporting with manual (typically, laboratory personnel) notification systems [11–13]. Reviews have reported that by utilizing such call centers, the time to report randomly selected critical results is most often faster than using just the laboratory technologist to call a critical lab value.

Automated notification systems also provide an electronic audit trail that can be utilized for performance monitoring and evaluation. However, one drawback of the automated critical alert notification system is that there is a possibility of risks for patient privacy violations, especially if mobile phones are used and inappropriate security policies exist. Furthermore, with automated electronic notification systems, staff should always be competent concerning manual procedures, and downtime policies should be published when there is a disruption in power or electronic services.

CLINICAL PEARLS

Critical values should be interpreted in a given clinical context by factoring in the patient's condition and preanalytical factors. Using two case studies, this section exemplifies the importance of appropriately interpreting the critical values for effective patient care. The first case is based on a true critical value for glucose by point-of-care testing in a pediatric patient presenting with diabetic ketoacidosis. The second case highlights the preanalytical factors influencing critical value reporting for potassium by the central lab and point-of-care testing.

Case 1: A three-year-old female presents to the emergency room with sudden onset abdominal pain, nausea, and vomiting. Clinical history also includes polydipsia, fatigue, and appetite change. The glucose tested using the glucometer by the medical staff read a critically high value of 563 mg/dL. Other significant lab results include a pH of 6.86 and a beta-hydroxybutyrate of 8.4 mmol/L. Instead of waiting for glucose results from central laboratory testing, the care team administered insulin immediately, after which the patient's condition improved significantly. Clearly, the patient presented with diabetic ketoacidosis, and prompt management based on the critical glucose levels yielded optimal outcomes. Although the team performing the testing and managing this patient is the same, it is important to document these critical values for regulatory purposes.

Case 2: A 26-year-old male with a history of a complex congenital heart disease status post-heart transplant presents with central line-associated fungemia due to *Candida glabrata* infection. The patient is critically ill and on continuous renal replacement therapy. The potassium tested using the laboratory analyzer gave continuous critical potassium levels from 8.4 to 8.7 mmol/L. The lab noticed a delta flag and retested the sample. Additionally, the astute laboratory staff noticed that the complete blood count showed a marked leukocytosis of $54 \times 10^3/\mu L$. The medical director was informed, and point-of-care whole blood potassium was tested from the patient in the unit. The actual potassium result was 5.7 mmol/L, which is within the normal limits. Clearly, the critical potassium levels noticed by the laboratory team are spurious due to intracellular potassium release from the fragile white blood cells. Upon discussing with the medical director, a disclaimer saying false elevation due to leukocytosis was added to the laboratory potassium result, and the medical staff was informed of future testing of this patient. The care team thus did not go for inappropriate intravenous potassium administration, and furthermore, ECG was normal for this patient. Therefore, closed-loop communication is crucial for the appropriate utilization of critical values in patient care.

CONCLUSION

In conclusion, there needs to be effective and timely communication of critical laboratory results to the healthcare team. It is the responsibility of laboratory professionals to ensure that there is an appropriate list of critical values, and that there are defined policies and regular audits to ensure appropriate utilization of such policies. It should also be mentioned that one option to take is to limit the critical laboratory value list to only those that are indeed life-threatening and also include a list of medically urgent values that need not be as timely as the critical lab values. Furthermore, we, as laboratory professionals, need to partner with the emerging technology improvements in our laboratory information systems and health information systems and those that could utilize artificial intelligence to streamline the process of critical laboratory value reporting and employ state-of-the-art strategies to ensure patient safety and better outcomes.

REFERENCES

1. Lundberg GD. Critical (panic) value notification: an established laboratory practice policy (parameter). *JAMA*. 1990;263(5):709.

2. Wagar EA, Friedberg RC, Souers R, Stankovic AK. Critical values comparison: a College of American Pathologists Q-Probes survey of 163 clinical laboratories. *Arch Pathol Lab Med*. 2007;131(12):1769–1775. doi: 10.5858/2007-131-1769-CVCACO.

3. CLSI. *Management of Critical- and Significant-Risk Results*. 1st ed. CLSI guideline GP47. Wayne (PA): Clinical and Laboratory Standards Institute, 2015.

4. Medicare, Medicaid, and CLIA Programs: laboratory requirements relating to quality systems and certain personnel qualifications. *Fed Regist.* 2003;68:3639–3714. Codified at 42 CFR §493.

5. The Joint Commission. *Accreditation Program: Laboratory, National Patient Safety Goals (NPSG.02.03.01).* http://www.jointcommission.org/. Accessed on July 12, 2010.

6. Rensburg MA, Nutt L, Zemlin AE, Erasmus RT. An audit on the reporting of critical results in a tertiary institute. *Ann Clin Biochem.* 2009;46(Pt 2):162–164. doi: 10.1258/acb.2008.008182.

7. AlSadah K, S El-Masry O, Alzahrani F, Alomar A, Ghany MA. Reporting clinical laboratory critical values: a focus on the recommendations of the American College of Pathologists. *J Ayub Med Coll Abbottabad.* 2019;31(4):612–618.

8. ISO15189:2007: Medical laboratories: particular requirements for quality and competence [items 5.5.3n, 5.8.7, and 5.8.8].

9. Hanna D, Griswold P, Leape LL, Bates DW. Communicating critical test results: safe practice recommendations. *Jt Comm J Qual Patient Saf.* 2005;31(2):68-80. doi: 10.1016/s1553-7250(05)31011-7.

10. Liebow EB, Derzon JH, Fontanesi J, Favoretto AM, Baetz RA, Shaw C, Thompson P, Mass D, Christenson R, Epner P, Snyder SR. Effectiveness of automated notification and customer service call centers for timely and accurate reporting of critical values: a laboratory medicine best practices systematic review and meta-analysis. *Clin Biochem.* 2012;45(13–14):979–987. doi: 10.1016/j.clinbiochem.2012.06.023.

11. Valenstein PN, Wagar EA, Stankovic AK, Walsh MK, Schneider F. Notification of critical results: a College of American Pathologists Q-Probes study of 121 institutions. *Arch Pathol Lab Med.* 2008;132(12):1862–1867. doi: 10.5858/132.12.1862.

12. Etchells E, Adhikari NK, Cheung C, Fowler R, Kiss A, Quan S, Sibbald W, Wong B. Real-time clinical alerting: effect of an automated paging system on response time to critical laboratory values: a randomised controlled trial. *Qual Saf Health Care.* 2010;19(2):99–102. doi: 10.1136/qshc.2008.028407.

13. Kuperman GJ, Teich JM, Tanasijevic MJ, Ma'Luf N, Rittenberg E, Jha A, Fiskio J, Winkelman J, Bates DW. Improving response to critical laboratory results with automation: results of a randomized controlled trial. *J Am Med Inform Assoc.* 1999;6(6):512–522. doi: 10.1136/jamia.1999.0060512.

12 Respiratory Disorders

Manoj Goel and Aditi Singh

INTRODUCTION

Laboratory applications are revolutionizing the diagnosis and therapeutic course of all illnesses. Respiratory medicine is no exception, with the diverse tests and biomarkers raising expectations about better management of pulmonary diseases in the intensive care unit. The tests are diverse, their implications are also diverse, and their interpretation is cumbersome with individual-to-individual variation. When it comes to biomarkers, our knowledge is even less. The combined use of laboratory tests and biomarkers has a considerable bearing on treatment decisions. As respiratory diseases are heterogeneous due to different pathophysiological processes, their clinical manifestations, course, and drug responses are also variable. Thus, appropriate and judicious use of diagnostic tests and biomarkers is helpful for identifying the underlying pathogenetic mechanism, detecting definitive factors for specific diseases, expediting diagnosis, monitoring progression, and assessing treatment response.

CLASSIFICATION OF RESPIRATORY DISEASES

The major respiratory diseases can be classified into tumors, infections, airway diseases, e.g., chronic obstructive pulmonary disease (COPD) and bronchial asthma, pulmonary vascular diseases, e.g., pulmonary embolism, and interstitial lung diseases, e.g., sarcoidosis and pneumoconiosis. In this section, we shall discuss the biomarkers related to pneumonia due to bacterial and fungal infections, COPD exacerbation, pulmonary embolism, and pleural diseases.

BIOMARKERS FOR PNEUMONIA

The search for the ideal biomarker for pneumonia is ongoing, and multiple molecules are undergoing rigorous investigation. C-reactive protein (CRP) and procalcitonin (PCT) remain the most robust and widely used biomarkers, while interleukin 6 (IL-6) has been of particular interest research-wise.

BIOMARKERS FOR BACTERIAL INFECTION

Procalcitonin

For patients with lower respiratory tract infections, procalcitonin can help distinguish bacterial infections from other kinds of infections or inflammation. The rise of PCT occurs early and is identifiable within 2–3 hours, with a peak at 6 hours [1]. Rodriguez et al. [2] conducted a prospective, multicenter study in an intensive care unit (ICU) patients with H1N1 influenza. They found that procalcitonin had a 94% negative predictive value for excluding bacterial co-infection. For community-acquired pneumonia (CAP), serial examinations of procalcitonin can help to stop antibiotics. Ito et al. [3] demonstrated that procalcitonin can reduce the antibiotic duration in CAP from 12.6 days to 8.6 days. Both the European Respiratory Society (ERS) and American Thoracic Society suggested using the clinical criteria alone to determine when to start antibiotics, and utilizing clinical criteria together with procalcitonin to determine when to stop [4]. However, PCT has a number of limitations. It is elevated in a variety of inflammatory and non-infectious conditions, such as cirrhosis, pancreatitis, mesenteric infarction, burns, and aspiration pneumonitis.

C-Reactive Protein (CRP)

CRP secretion begins in 4–6 hours and peaks at 36–50 hours, potentially limiting its efficacy in predicting early treatment failure [5, 6]. CRP has poor specificity, as it is elevated in a variety of pathologies, such as trauma, surgery, burns, and immunological-mediated inflammatory diseases. However, CRP is an independent predictor for the absence of severe complications in CAP[7].

BIOMARKERS OF FUNGAL INFECTIONS

While pulmonary candidiasis is an extremely rare entity in ICU, the most common invasive fungal infection in the lungs is aspergillosis. The Aspergillus cell wall contains galactomannan (GM) and (1→3)-β-D-Glucan (BDG) which may be utilized for detection in blood and bronchoalveolar lavage (BAL).

DOI: 10.1201/9781003449713-12

Table 12.1 Sensitivity and Specificity of Serum Galactomannan

Population	Sensitivity, %	Specificity, %
Hematologic malignancy	58	95
Hematopoietic stem cell transplantation	65	65
Solid organ transplant	41	85

Galactomannan

GM is a useful diagnostic test for clinically suggestive invasive aspergillosis. The Optical Density Index (ODI) cut-off of serum GM is > 0.5 and BAL GM is > 1.0. The GM result can be false positive if the patient is receiving Beta-lactam antibiotics such as amoxicillin-clavulanate, piperacillin-tazobactam, cefepime, and cefoperazone-sulbactam, or carbapenems, colistin nebulization, or due to fungal colonization in BAL.

Serum galactomannan has a higher sensitivity and specificity in patients with hematological malignancies and allogeneic hematopoietic stem cell transplant recipients who have a higher burden of disease [8]. On the other hand, the serum GM has a relatively lower sensitivity and specificity in solid organ transplant patients, who typically have a lower burden of disease (Table 12.1) [9, 10].

ISDA guidelines recommend the use of serial serum galactomannan only in patients with hematologic malignancies and hematopoietic stem cell transplant recipients who have an elevated galactomannan at baseline to monitor disease progression, therapeutic response, and prediction of patient outcomes with IA [11].

(1→3)-β-D-Glucan (BDG) in IA

The utility of BDG testing in the therapeutic monitoring of patients with IA has been poorly characterized. Pazos et al.[12] evaluated BDG compared with galactomannan testing in a retrospective cohort of 40 high-risk neutropenic patients. The sensitivity, specificity, and positive and negative predictive values of galactomannan and BDG testing were almost identical. Serial BDG testing is not recommended because BDG kinetics are slow and may require > 4–6 weeks after treatment initiation to appreciably change. There is also intra-patient variability of BDG testing [13, 14].

BIOMARKERS FOR COPD

CRP

The most commonly studied biomarker in COPD exacerbation is CRP, followed by IL-6 and TNF-α. Elevated CRP levels in the presence of a major exacerbation symptom are useful in confirming the COPD exacerbation. The use of CRP as a biomarker was investigated in 28 studies, in which 26 of these reported a statistically significant increase in concentration during AECOPD versus stable COPD and/or healthy controls [15]. However, CRP levels were not helpful in predicting survival and mortality in the acute COPD exacerbation event [16].

Blood Eosinophil Levels

A large number of patients with COPD have high blood eosinophil counts exceeding 300. These patients had more severe disease and a better response to glucocorticoids than patients with normal eosinophil levels.

BIOMARKERS FOR PULMONARY EMBOLISM

D-Dimer

D-dimer levels are elevated in the presence of acute thrombosis because of the simultaneous activation of coagulation and fibrinolysis. The negative predictive value of D-dimer testing is high, and a normal D-dimer level renders acute pulmonary embolism (PE) or deep vein thrombosis (DVT) unlikely. On the other hand, the positive predictive value of elevated D-dimer levels is low, and D-dimer testing is not useful for confirmation of PE. D-dimer is also more frequently elevated in patients with cancer, severe infection, or inflammatory disease, and during pregnancy.

A multinational prospective management study evaluated a previously validated age-adjusted cut-off (age x10 µg/L, for patients aged > 50 years). Use of the age-adjusted (instead of the "standard" 500 µg/L) D-dimer cut-off increased the number of patients, in whom PE could be excluded, from 6.4 to 30%, without additional false-negative findings [17].

Biomarkers of Myocardial Injury

Elevated plasma troponin concentrations may be associated with a worse prognosis in the acute phase of PE. A meta-analysis showed that elevated troponin concentrations were associated with an increased risk of mortality, both in unselected patients (OR 5.2, 95% CI 3.3–8.4) and in those who were hemodynamically stable at presentation (OR 5.9, 95% CI 2.7–13.0) [18].

At the other end of the severity spectrum, the high-sensitivity troponin assays possess a high negative predictive value in the setting of acute PE. In a prospective multicenter cohort of 526 normotensive patients, high-sensitivity troponin T concentrations < 14 pg/mL had a negative predictive value of 98% for excluding an adverse in-hospital clinical outcome [19].

Biomarkers of Right Ventricular Dysfunction

RV pressure overload due to acute PE is associated with increased myocardial stretch, which leads to the release of B-type natriuretic peptide (BNP) and N-terminal (NT)-proBNP. Thus, the plasma levels of natriuretic peptides reflect the severity of RV dysfunction and hemodynamic compromise in acute PE. A meta-analysis found that 51% of 1132 unselected patients with acute PE had elevated BNP or NT-proBNP concentrations on admission; these patients had a 10% risk of early death (95% CI 8.0–13%) and a 23% (95% CI 20–26%) risk of an adverse clinical outcome [20].

PLEURAL EFFUSION

Pleural effusion may result from a variety of diseases, including malignant, inflammatory, infectious, and cardiovascular illnesses. Pleural fluid aspiration facilitates the measurement of various disease biomarkers. The pleural fluid biomarkers may obviate the need for pleural biopsy or other investigations and facilitate early treatment initiation, including early intercostal chest tube drainage (ICD) in patients with complex PPE or empyema.

Pleural Fluid pH

If pleural fluid pH is ≤ 7.2, there is a high risk of complicated parapneumonic pleural effusion (CPPE) or pleural infection, and an ICD should be done if the volume of accessible pleural fluid on ultrasound makes it safe to do so. If pleural fluid pH is ≥ 7.4, this implies a low risk of CPPE or pleural infection and no indication for immediate drainage. If pleural fluid pH is > 7.2 If pH and <7.4, this implies an intermediate risk of CPPE or pleural infection. Pleural fluid LDH should be measured and if >99IU/L. Chest tube drainage (ICD) should be considered, especially if other clinical parameters support CPPE (such as ongoing fever, low pleural fluid glucose <40mg/dL, contrast enhancement of the pleural membranes on CT imaging, or septations in the pleural space on ultrasound examination of chest [21].

Pleural Fluid Glucose

A low pleural fluid glucose level (< 3.4 mmol/l) may be found in complicated parapneumonic effusions, empyema, rheumatoid pleuritis, and pleural effusions associated with TB, malignancy, and esophageal rupture. The most common causes of a very low pleural fluid glucose level (< 1.6 mmol/l) are rheumatoid arthritis and empyema. Although glucose is usually low in pleural infection and correlates with pleural fluid pH values, it is a significantly less accurate indicator for chest tube drainage than pH [22]. However, in the absence of readily available immediate pleural fluid pH measurement, initial pleural fluid glucose < 3.3 mmol/L may be used as an indicator of a high probability of CPPE/pleural infection and can be used to inform the decision to insert ICD in the appropriate clinical context [23].

Pleural Fluid Adenosine Deaminase (ADA)

This is an enzyme produced by lymphocytes, and an elevated level of ADA in pleural fluid is a useful marker for the diagnosis of tuberculous pleurisy. The most widely accepted cut-off value for ADA in pleural fluid for the diagnosis of tuberculous pleurisy is 40 U/L, with a sensitivity and specificity of 92% and 90%, respectively. Pleural fluid ADA and IFN-gamma provide high sensitivity and specificity for diagnosing tuberculous pleural effusion [23].

Pleural Fluid N-Terminal Pro-Brain Natriuretic Peptide (NT-proBNP)

This provides high sensitivity and specificity for diagnosing heart failure in patients with unilateral pleural effusion. NT-proBNP is a sensitive marker of both systolic and diastolic cardiac failure.

Levels in blood and pleural fluid correlate closely, and measurements of both have been shown to be effective, hence, applying the NT-proBNP test to blood alone is sufficient.

The cut-off value NT-proBNP varies widely from 600 to 4000 pg/ml, with 1500 pg/ml being the most commonly used.

Pleural Fluid Amylase

Pleural fluid amylase levels are elevated if they are higher than the upper limit of normal for serum or if the pleural fluid/serum ratio is > 1.0. This suggests acute pancreatitis, pancreatic pseudocyst, rupture of the esophagus, ruptured ectopic pregnancy, or pleural malignancy (especially adenocarcinoma).

CHYLOTHORAX AND PSEUDOCHYLOTHORAX

Chylothorax and pseudochylothorax can be discriminated by lipid analysis of the fluid. Demonstration of chylomicrons confirms chylothorax, whereas the presence of cholesterol crystals diagnoses pseudochylothorax. A true chylothorax will usually have a high triglyceride level, usually > 1.24 mmol/l (110 mg/dl), and can usually be excluded if the triglyceride level is < 0.56 mmol/l (50 mg/dl). In pseudochylothorax, a cholesterol level > 5.18 mmol/l (200 mg/dl) or the presence of cholesterol crystals is diagnostic irrespective of triglyceride levels [24].

CONCLUSION

Current respiratory disease treatment relies on traditional evaluation based on clinical assessment, imaging, pulmonary physiology, and biochemical biomarkers. While some of the biomarkers especially in pulmonary embolism and pleural fluid have a definitive role, others are evolving. This will greatly improve the accuracy and efficiency of diagnosis, prognosis prediction, and tailored treatment for respiratory diseases.

Q&A

Q: Is high serum procalcitonin diagnostic of bacterial infection?
A: No, PCT is primarily used for de-escalation and stoppage of antibiotics in CAP.
Q: What is the role of CRP in respiratory infection?
A: CRP has a poor specificity for respiratory infections, but low CRP is an independent predictor for the absence of severe complications in CAP.
Q: What is the role of galactomannan in invasive aspergillosis?
A: Serial serum galactomannan is recommended only in patients with hematologic malignancies and hematopoietic stem cell transplant recipients who have an elevated galactomannan at baseline to monitor disease progression, therapeutic response, and prediction of patient outcomes with invasive aspergillosis.
Q: Should D-dimer be used for the screening of pulmonary embolism in the ICU?
A: A negative D-dimer in an OPD setting rules out the possibility of pulmonary embolism. However in an ICU setting, if there is a high clinical probability, the patient should be investigated for PE irrespective of D-dimer results.
Q: Which pleural fluid biomarker should be used for chest tube drainage in complicated parapneumonic effusion?
A: Pleural fluid pH < 7.2 is the most definitive indication for chest tube drainage. However, if pleural fluid pH measurement is not feasible, pleural fluid glucose < 3.3 mmol/L in the presence of appropriate clinical and imaging criteria is another biomarker.

REFERENCES

1. Matthaiou DK, Ntani G, Kontogiorgi M, *et al.* An ESICM systematic review and meta-analysis of procalcitonin-guided antibiotic therapy algorithms in adult critically ill patients. *Intensive Care Med.* 2012;38:940–949.

2. Rodriguez AH, Aviles-Jurado FX, Diaz E, *et al.* Procalcitonin (PCT) levels for ruling-out bacterial coinfection in ICU patients with influenza: a CHAID decision-tree analysis. *J Infect.* 2016;72:143–151.

3. Ito A, Ishida T, Tokumasu H, I Impact of procalcitoninguided therapy for hospitalized community-acquired pneumonia on reducing antibiotic consumption and costs in Japan. *J Infect Chemother*. 2017;23:142–147.

4. Zheng N, Zhu D, Han Y. Procalcitonin and C-reactive protein perform better than the neutrophil/lymphocyte count ratio in evaluating hospital acquired pneumonia. *BMC Pulm Med*. 2020;20:166.

5. Shepherd KE, Lynch KE, Wain JC, *et al.* Elastin fibers and the diagnosis of bacterial pneumonia in the adult respiratory distress syndrome. *Crit Care Med*. 1995;23:1829–1834.

6. Bloos F, Hinder F, Becker K, *et al.* A multicenter trial to compare blood culture with polymerase chain reaction in severe human sepsis. *Intensive Care Med*. 2010;36:241-247.

7. O'Dwyer MJ, Starczewska MH, Schrenzel J, *et al.* The detection of microbial DNA but not cultured bacteria is associated with increased mortality in patients with suspected sepsis-a prospective multi-centre European observational study. *Clin Microbiol Infect*. 2017;23:208.e1-208.e6.

8. Maertens J. Buve´ K, Theunissen K, Meersseman W, Verbeken E, Verhoef G, Van Eldere J, Lagrou K. Galactomannan serves as a surrogate endpoint for outcome of pulmonary invasive aspergillosis in neutropenic hematology patients. *Cancer*. 2009; 115:355–362.

9. Ledoux MP, Guffroy B, Nivoix Y, Simand C, Herbrecht R. Invasive pulmonary aspergillosis. Semin Respir Crit Care Med. 2020;41:80–98.

10. Miceli MH, Maertens J. Role of non-culture-based tests, with an emphasis on galactomannan testing for the diagnosis of invasive aspergillosis. *Semin Respir Crit Care Med*. 2015;36:650–661.

11. Patterson TF, Thompson GR, 3rd, Denning DW, *et al.* Practice guidelines for the diagnosis and management of aspergillosis: 2016 update by the infectious diseases society of America. *Clin Infect Dis*. 2016;63:e1–e60.

12. Pazos C, Ponton J, Del Palacio A. Contribution of (1→3)-Beta-D-glucan chromogenic assay to diagnosis and therapeutic monitoring of invasive aspergillosis in neutropenic adult patients: a comparison with serial screening for circulating galactomannan. *J Clin Microbiol*.2005;43:299–305.

13. Neofytos D, Railkar R, Mullane KM, Fredricks DN, Granwehr B, Marr KA, *et al.* Correlation between circulating fungal biomarkers and clinical outcome in invasive aspergillosis. *PLoS ONE*. 2015;10(6):e0129022.

14. Ellis M, Al-Ramadi B, Finkelman M, *et al.* Assessment of the clinical utility of serial beta-D-glucan concentrations in patients with persistent neutropenic fever. *J Med Microbiol*. 2008;57:287–295.

15. Chen Y-WR, Leung JM, Sin DD (2016) A systematic review of diagnostic biomarkers of COPD exacerbation. *PLoS ONE*. 2016;11(7):e0158843.

16. Stolz D, Christ–Crain M, Morgenthaler NG, Leuppi J, Miedinger D, Bingisser R, Tamm M Copeptin, C-reactive protein, and procalcitonin as prognostic biomarkers in acute exacerbation of COPD. *Chest*. 2007;131(4):1058–1067.

17. Righini M, Van Es J, Den Exter PL, *et al.* Age-adjusted D-dimer cutoff levels to rule out pulmonary embolism: the ADJUST-PE study. *JAMA*. 2014;311:1117–1124.

18. Becattini C, Vedovati MC, Agnelli G. Prognostic value of troponins in acute pulmonary embolism: a meta-analysis. *Circulation*. 2007;116:427–433.

19. Lankeit M, Jiménez D, Kostrubiec M, *et al.* Predictive value of the high-sensitivity troponin T assay and the simplified Pulmonary Embolism Severity Index in hemodynamically stable patients with acute pulmonary embolism: a prospective validation study. *Circulation.* 2011;124:2716–2724.

20. Klok FA, Mos IC, Huisman MV. Brain-type natriuretic peptide levels in the prediction of adverse outcome in patients with pulmonary embolism: a systematic review and meta-analysis. *Am J Respir Crit Care Med.* 2008;178:425–430.

21. Roberts ME, Rahman NM, Maskell NA, Bibby AC, Blyth KG, Corcoran JP, *et al.* British Thoracic Society Guideline for pleural disease. *Thorax* 2023;0:1–34.

22. Heffner JE, Brown LK, Barbieri C, *et al.* Pleural fluid chemical analysis. parapneumonic effusions. A meta-analysis. *Am J Respir Crit Care Med.* 1995;151:1700e8.

23. Liang QL, Shi HZ, Wang K, Qin SM, Qin XJ. Diagnostic accuracy of adenosine deaminase in tuberculous pleurisy: a meta-analysis. *Respir Med.* 2008;102(5):744–754.

24. Hooper C, Gary Lee YC, Maskell N. Investigation of a unilateral pleural effusion in adults: British Thoracic Society pleural disease guideline 2010. *Thorax.* 2010;65(Suppl 2):ii4–ii17.

13 Interpreting Laboratory Diagnosis for the Cardiovascular System in Intensive Care

David C. Gaze and Paul O. Collinson

INTRODUCTION

Patients requiring critical care in the intensive care unit (ICU) present with complex system disorders due to combined acute and chronic pathologies or following trauma, or require system support in the post-surgical phase. Central to the intensive support of patients is the maintenance of adequate cardiovascular physiology. Practitioners in the ICU have an armamentarium of diagnostic tests to assist in the diagnosis and prognosis of cardiovascular pathophysiology. This chapter reviews these diagnostic tests with emphasis on appropriate test utilisation in assessing the cardiovascular (CV) system in the intensive care setting. Laboratory tests are considered to contribute to 70% of clinical decisions about ICU patient management.

Although there has been a decline in cardiovascular mortality in the last 30 years, cardiac disease remains prevalent in the population. In patients over 65 years, acute heart failure (AHF) is responsible for 5% of all acute admissions with a corresponding mortality of approximately 10%. Of admissions to the ICU, 20% of patients present with heart failure (Adams *et al.*, 2005) and 32% with cardiogenic shock due to acute myocardial infarction (AMI) (Vallabhajosyula *et al.*, 2020), further complicated by multi-organ failure. Modern ICU practice requires intensive expert management of a variety of complex cardiovascular conditions either as the primary cause for admission or as comorbidity (Walker *et al.*, 2012).

Classification and severity of cardiovascular disease (CVD) are paramount in targeting appropriate management in the ICU. Laboratory-derived measurements are invaluable in differentiating between the aetiology of many cardiac pathologies including AMI, atrial fibrillation (AF) and chronic heart failure (CHF), cardio-renal syndrome, myopathies, cardiac inflammatory diseases or cardiac rhythm disorders. The Acute Physiology and Chronic Health Evaluation (APACHE) score and Sequential Organ Failure Assessment (SOFA) score require data from laboratory tests to assess CV dysfunction in the critically ill.

Appropriate front-line testing includes blood gas analysis, electrolytes, renal function, inflammatory markers, full (complete) blood count, assessment of coagulation, cardiac markers and secondary testing of glucose, lipid profiling and thyroid function (Tooth *et al.*, 2018). Such testing could be performed in the point-of-care/near-patient setting or provided by a centralised laboratory service. Assay performance (analytical sensitivity and specificity), methodological variation and appropriateness of reference intervals along with turnaround times to obtain results may play a role in the choice of testing requirements.

ARTERIAL BLOOD GAS ANALYSIS

Arterial blood gas (ABG) analysis of electrolytes, pO_2, pCO_2, blood pH, from which are calculated HCO_3^-, and standard bicarbonate and base excess provide valuable information on acid-base balance, oxygenation and ventilation. Continuous intra-arterial real-time monitoring of ABG is possible and useful in adjusting ventilator settings or during resuscitation, allowing precise adjustment of therapy. This is beneficial in the preservation of blood volume compared to intermittent arterial blood draws. Limitations to ABG analysis in the ICU involve patients with a hypercoagulable state causing clotting in the heparinised syringe, erroneous results due to the presence of air bubbles, or a delay between sample collection and measurement which should be done immediately.

ELECTROLYTES AND RENAL FUNCTION

Serum and plasma samples are both adequate matrices for the determination of electrolyte and renal function tests. The determination of sodium (Na^+) is dependent on sodium and fluid balance and is useful in determining hyponatraemia caused by excess fluid. Serum and urine plasma osmolality and Na^+ should be interpreted together. Serum osmolarity is decreased in true hyponatraemia. The osmolarity ratio in urine/plasma indicates net water loss (<1) or retention (>1). Urine sodium <10 mmol/L is indicative of sodium retention due to low circulating blood volume and is seen in patients with HF.

Potassium (K^+) is stored mainly in intracellular fluid and regulated by renal excretion via the hormonal action of aldosterone along with urine flow and sodium in the distal tubule of the nephron. The reference interval is tight due to the limited amount of potassium in circulation.

DOI: 10.1201/9781003449713-13

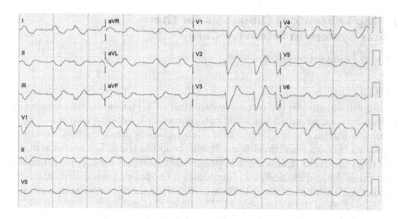

Figure 13.1 Sine-wave ECG pattern due to hyperkalaemia, demonstrating loss of P-waves, widening of QRS and fusion with T waves.

Acute disturbance to potassium balance is observed with changes in blood pH as a result of H^+ ion exchange in the extracellular compartment for K^+ ions in the intracellular compartment. Serum K^+ is elevated in acidosis and reduced in alkalosis. Hypokalaemia arises from many causes including renal or gastrointestinal loss but rarely due to an increase in aldosterone. Concomitant changes observed in electrocardiography include flattening and inversion of T waves in mild hypokalaemia, followed by prolonged QT interval, prominent U wave and mild ST-segment depression in severe hypokalaemia. Other arrhythmic patterns due to hypokalaemia include premature ventricular complexes, atrial fibrillation or flutter, supraventricular tachycardia and, in severe cases, torsade de pointes, ventricular tachycardia and ventricular fibrillation. Hyperkalaemia is normally a result of impaired renal function or as a result of pharmacological agents or over infusion of potassium. It is a common clinical observation that can induce catastrophic cardiac arrhythmias. Non-specific repolarisation abnormalities are observed with mild elevations of serum potassium to the classic sine-wave rhythm (QRS complex widens and blends with the T wave, Figure 13.1), which occurs in severe hyperkalaemia (Loubser *et al.*, 2023). It is important to remember that rapid changes in serum potassium are more likely to cause dysrhythmia than slow changes and this is most marked when patients have not previously been exposed to potassium fluctuations as seen in renal dialysis patients.

Renal function is assessed through the measurement of serum or plasma urea and creatinine along with the calculation of the estimated glomerular filtration rate (eGFR). There is a synergy between worsening renal and cardiac function potentiating each other into the cardio-renal syndromes with a cycle of worsening pathophysiology and prognosis. There are five types of cardio-renal syndrome (Figure 13.2). Types one to four involve acute chronic cardiovascular diseases causing renal dysfunction. Type 5 is due to acute or chronic renal disease, causing cardiovascular dysfunction (Loftus *et al.*, 2021).

INFLAMMATORY MARKERS

Markers of inflammatory processes can be measured as an indicator of cardiovascular disease severity and aetiology. Following AMI, wound healing occurs following the death of cardiomyocytes. Cardiac cell death can result within 3 to 6 hours of initial injury and can continue for 4 days. An inflammatory response begins approximately 12 hours from ischaemia. The next phase in wound healing is granulation tissue formation at the border zone of the infarcted area. The final phase in the healing process is cardiac remodelling and repair, which occurs two to three weeks after injury and can persist for one year. Several biomarkers of inflammation including the interleukins (IL-1a, IL-6, IL-8, IL-33), tumour necrosis factor alpha (TNF-a), myosin/tropomyosin autoantibodies, c-reactive protein (CRP), fibrinogen, pentraxins and matrix metalloproteinases have all demonstrated clinical promise. However, their diagnostic and clinical significance has yet to be determined in assessing cardiovascular function in critically ill patients (Pearson *et al.*, 2003). Nevertheless, readily available assays for CRP and fibrinogen are extremely reliable and offer diagnostic information to the ICU physician, however as coexisting infection is common in ICU

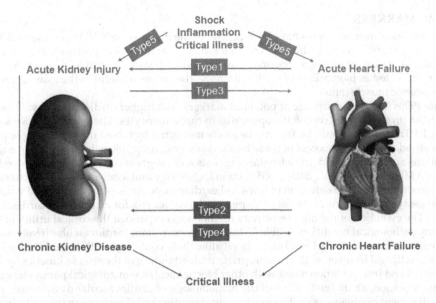

Figure 13.2 Development of the cardio-renal syndromes in critical illness. Acute illness results in acute cardiac disease and acute renal injury which can progress to chronic cardiac and kidney disease. Acute heart failure can precede acute kidney injury (type 1); chronic heart failure precedes chronic kidney disease (type 2); acute kidney injury proceeds acute heart failure (type 3); chronic heart failure precedes chronic kidney disease which precedes chronic heart failure (type 4); shock, inflammation and critical illness precede acute heart failure or acute kidney injury (type 5). [Adapted from (Loftus *et al.*, 2021)].

patients, interpretation of CRP and fibrinogen is influenced by factors other than acute cardiac injury.

FULL (COMPLETE) BLOOD COUNT

The full/complete blood count (FBC/CBC) is a useful and inexpensive laboratory test for assessing the risk of cardiovascular disease. The FBC can easily identify anaemia, a known risk factor for ischaemic heart disease and a comment observation in patients with acute coronary syndrome (ACS) and heart failure. A decreased haemoglobin concentration is an independent risk factor for cardiovascular morbidity and mortality. Anaemia is also associated with hypertension, arrhythmia and risk of stroke (Mozos, 2015). An elevation in the white blood cell (WBC) count confers predictive risk for coronary heart disease, and many studies have reported increased mortality in patients with ACS presenting with elevated WBC count (Madjid and Fatemi, 2013).

COAGULATION MARKERS

Patients in the ICU often demonstrate haemostatic abnormalities, ranging from thrombocytopenia or prolonged global clotting tests to complex defects, such as disseminated intravascular coagulation (DIC). Patients may be admitted with coagulation abnormalities or develop such pathologies whilst in intensive care (Levi and Sivapalaratnam, 2015). Hypercoagulable states are a risk for the development of thrombus-related pathologies and an increased risk of mortality in the ICU. The major causes of coagulopathies in the ICU include (but are not restricted to) sepsis and septic shock, DIC, cardiopulmonary bypass, major/multiple trauma and blood loss, or drug-induced. Assessment of coagulation can be determined with APTT, PT, thrombin time as well as clotting factor activities (Levi and Opal, 2006). D-dimer is a small protein fibrin degradation product found in the circulation following fibrinolysis. It is primarily used to diagnose the presence of thrombosis such as deep vein thrombosis (DVT), DIC and pulmonary embolism, and is associated with increased mortality. Increased D-dimer is associated with atrial thromboembolism, AF, ACS and stroke (Sathe and Patwa, 2014).

CARDIAC MARKERS

Cardiac biomarker measurements have been central to the diagnosis of CVD since the mid-1950s. Early biomarkers such as myoglobin and creatine kinase lacked cardiac specificity and are often elevated in non-cardiac pathologies, normally associated with skeletal muscle diseases. Although no longer advocated as biomarkers of cardiac damage, they remain useful in the assessment of general systemic muscle injury.

The late 1990s saw the emergence of potential markers with higher cardiospecificity. These are derived from proteins of the contractile apparatus in cardiomyocytes. The cardiac isoforms of troponin T (cTnT) and troponin I (cTnI) can be easily measured by robust immunoassay or point-of-care methodologies. The success of these biomarkers for cardiac injury has resulted in a number of definitions and clinical guidelines for the diagnosis and prognosis of acute coronary syndromes including AMI (Thygesen *et al.*, 2018). As detection technology and assay performance characteristics have improved, the detection of low-level cardiac troponin is now reliable, and values above the assay-specific clinical cut-off (99th percentile) confer risk for all causes of cardiac-related mortality. The evolution of the high sensitivity methods has expanded the clinical utility of these tests. Many pathological conditions (Table 13.1) have a concomitant cardiovascular involvement and associated elevation of cTnT or cTnI. At face value, these could cause clinical confusion in the critical care setting. However, with an appropriate understanding of the release kinetics by serial measurement and interpretation along with other biochemical/haematological parameters and clinical presentation, an understanding of the pathobiology of cardiovascular dysfunction in the critically ill patient becomes easier. The most recent definition of MI recognises this with inclusion of the term acute myocardial injury as well as recognising secondary causes of myocardial damage (Thygesen *et al.*, 2018).

The definition of AMI requires a distinctive rise and/or fall of cardiac troponin above the 99th percentile with clinical evidence of ischaemia. This is useful for the assessment of new AMI in critically ill patients. Prolonged elevation of cardiac troponin is suggestive of ongoing myocyte ischaemia/necrosis due to a non-atherothrombotic pathology. Fluctuations can still exist due to the severity of the underlying condition and response to therapy or a worsening clinical state. Elevation of cardiac troponin in critically ill patients in ICU, independent of the presence or absence of overt coronary artery disease pathology as the causative aetiology, is associated with an increased length of ICU stay and an almost three-fold higher risk of death (Collinson and Gaze, 2005).

Further to the markers of ischaemia and necrosis, the natriuretic peptides that regulate osmotic and cardiovascular homeostasis, such as atrial natriuretic peptide (ANP), b-type natriuretic peptide (BNP) and its N-terminal leader sequence NT-pro-BNP, are indicators of global cardiac

Table 13.1   Conditions Manifested in ICU Patients Associated with Elevated Cardiac Troponin

Acute kidney injury

Arrhythmia

Aortic dissection

Coronary vasospasm

Cardiomyopathy

Cardiac contusion

Chronic kidney disease

COVID-19

Hypertensive crisis

Myocarditis

Multi-organ failure

Neurological pathology

Pericarditis

Pulmonary embolism

Pulmonary hypertension

Sepsis and septic shock

Systemic inflammatory response syndrome

Vasculitides

stress and play a useful role in the diagnosis, prognosis and management of patients with acute or chronic heart failure. Although there was much early interest in ANP, BNP and NTproBNP have become the markers of choice in the clinical setting with both immunoassay techniques in a centralised laboratory or using POCT.

Whilst useful in assessing critically ill patients, interpretation of values of the natriuretic peptides must consider age, sex (Tooth et al., 2018) and the importance of multiple comorbid conditions, such as renal failure and sepsis, in such patients, as concentrations may be elevated in the absence of heart failure (McLean and Huang, 2012). In addition, direct use of BNP as a therapeutic agent has resulted in the suggestion that NT-proBNP may be the marker of choice.

FUTURE DIRECTIONS

The value of measurement of markers to assess critically ill patients is well established and mainstream for critical care clinicians. No single biomarker can effectively determine cardiovascular dysfunction in the ICU, and there is importance in assessing the totality of laboratory data and interpreting it in the appropriate clinical setting.

Central or peripheral catheters make sampling easy in the ICU; however, there is a need to consider appropriate intervals for testing, with evidence suggesting there is an overuse of laboratory tests with recommendations from the literature to reduce testing frequency (Devis et al., 2024).

Technologies for continuous monitoring (Bockholt et al., 2022) have proved beneficial in the ICU but are associated with increased overall testing costs. In addition, new and disruptive analytical technologies such as cardiac-specific microRNA analysis may offer superior clinical value along with advanced detection methods such as magnetic sensors, mass spectrometry POCT and advances in microfluidics. AI and machine learning could offer non-human assessment of continuous monitoring of biochemical data and offer real-time diagnostic and prognostic outcomes, similar to the manual method of periodically calculating risk scores. This may give rise to earlier warnings of deviation of global changes to the physiological state of the critically ill patient.

KEY POINTS

- Clinical assessment is vital to determine appropriate testing to assess the cardiovascular system in the ICU.

- Laboratory tests need to be interpreted in the appropriate clinical context.

- Interpretation should consider confounding factors such as age, sex and multi-organ involvement in critically ill patients.

- Appropriate testing at appropriate intervals will aid in the management of the critically ill patient.

REFERENCES

Adams KFJ, Fonarow GC, Emerman CL, LeJemtel TH, Costanzo MR, Abraham WT, Berkowitz RL, Galvao M, Horton DP; ADHERE Scientific Advisory Committee and Investigators. Characteristics and outcomes of patients hospitalized for heart failure in the United States: rationale, design, and preliminary observations from the first 100,000 cases in the Acute Decompensated Heart Failure National Registry (ADHERE). *Am Heart J.* 2005;149(2):209–216.

Bockholt R, Paschke S, Heubner L, Ibarlucea B, Laupp A, Janicijevic Z, Klinghammer S, Balakin S, Maitz MF, Werner C, Cuniberti G, Baraban L, Spieth PM. Real-time monitoring of blood parameters in the intensive care unit: state-of-the-art and perspectives. *J Clin Med.* 2022;11(9):2408.

Collinson P, Gaze D. Cardiac troponins in intensive care. *Critical Care (London, England).* 2005;9(4):345–346.

Devis L, Catry E, Honore PM, Mansour A, Lippi G, Mullier F, Closset M. Interventions to improve appropriateness of laboratory testing in the intensive care unit: a narrative review. *Annal Intensive Care.* 2024;14(1):9-y.

Levi M, Opal SM. Coagulation abnormalities in critically ill patients. *Critical Care (London, England).* 2006;10(4):222.

Levi M, Sivapalaratnam S. Hemostatic abnormalities in critically ill patients. *Int Emer Med.* 2015;10(3):287–296.

Loftus TJ, Filiberto AC, Ozrazgat-Baslanti T, Gopal S, Bihorac A. Cardiovascular and renal disease in chronic critical illness', *J Clin Med.* 2021;10(8):1601.

Loubser J, Bronislawski LP, Fonarov I, Casadesus D. Sine-wave electrocardiogram rhythm in a patient on haemodialysis presenting with severe weakness and hyperkalaemia. *BMJ Case Rep CP,* 2023;16(3):e255007.

Madjid M, Fatemi O. Components of the complete blood count as risk predictors for coronary heart disease: in-depth review and update. *Texas Heart Instit J.* 2013;40(1):17–29.

McLean AS, Huang SJ. Cardiac biomarkers in the intensive care unit. *Annal Intensive Care.* 2012;2:8.

Mozos I. Mechanisms linking red blood cell disorders and cardiovascular diseases. *BioMed Resh Int.* 2015; 2015:682054.

Sathe PM, Patwa UD. D Dimer in acute care. *Int J Crit Illness Inj Sci.* 2014;4(3):229–232.

Pearson TA, Mensah GA, Wayne Alexander R, Anderson JL, CannonIII RO, Criqui M, Fadl YY, Fortmann SP, Hong Y, Myers GL, Rifai N, SmithJr SC, Taubert K, Tracy RB, Vinicor F. Markers of inflammation and cardiovascular disease. *Circulation.* 2003;107(3):499–511.

Thygesen K, Alpert JS, Jaffe AS, Chaitman BR, Bax JJ, Morrow DA, White HD. ESC Scientific Document Group Fourth universal definition of myocardial infarction. *Eur Heart J.* 2018;40(3):237–269.

Tooth L, *et al.* Biochemistry' *Core Topics in Preoperative Anaesthetic Assessment and Management* Cambridge: Cambridge University Press, 2018, pp. 220–226.

Vallabhajosyula S, Patlolla SH, Dunlay SM, Prasad A, Bell MR, Jaffe AS, Gersh BJ, Rihal CS, Holmes DRJ, Barsness GW. Regional variation in the management and outcomes of acute myocardial infarction with cardiogenic shock in the United States. *Circulat Heart Failure.* 2020;13(2):e0066611.

Walker DM, West NEJ, Ray SG; British Cardiovascular Society Working Group on Acute Cardiac Care. From coronary care unit to acute cardiac care unit: the evolving role of specialist cardiac care. *Heart (British Cardiac Society).* 2012;98(5):350–352.

14 Neurological Disorders

Arun Koul and Abha Sharma

INTRODUCTION

As with any other medical speciality, history and examination are key to making a diagnosis in a patient presenting to the neurology emergency. Since it is often impossible to gather direct history from the patient in the ICU setting and the neurological examination isn't completely reliable in such cases, the importance of laboratory diagnosis can't be overemphasised. The chapter begins with a brief overview of the major lab tests done in the intensive care units. It is followed by a brief description of the common conditions encountered by a neurointensivist and their lab diagnosis. The chapter ends with a summary and some clinical pearls.

NEUROIMAGING IN THE INTENSIVE CARE [1, 2]

A non-contrast brain CT scan is often obtained in the emergency department or the ICU because of the widespread availability and ease of getting done. It is indispensable when acute stroke, subarachnoid haemorrhage, hydrocephalus, or mass lesions are strongly suspected. Although MRI is a better diagnostic tool, a plain CT scan may also show global brain oedema in severe cases of anoxic-ischaemic brain injury and in patients with severe hyperammonaemia. A brain MRI is also much more useful in cases like viral and autoimmune encephalitis and in posterior circulation strokes (where CT has limited utility). However, it is important to remember that even repeated negative MRIs do not exclude irreversible brain disease severe enough to keep the patient comatose, as happens in some cases after cardiac arrest and in some cases of autoimmune encephalitis. In such cases, the only tell-tale sign may be the progressive brain atrophy noticed on serial imaging. In some instances, it is necessary to obtain an angiogram (SAH, RCVS, dissections) or venogram (cerebral venous thrombosis) of the intracranial circulation.

CSF TESTING IN THE ICU [1, 3]

When lumbar puncture is indicated, it should be generally performed without delay. This statement is particularly true for suspected infectious aetiologies like meningitis and encephalitis. Not only does it guide treatment in case of infections, but it can provide invaluable information like intracranial pressure, which is vital for patient management. Even in non-infectious aetiologies like acute subarachnoid haemorrhage, the time-honoured three-tap test is used when imaging is negative and suspicion is high. It remains pertinent to remember that brain imaging (CT or MRI) is generally indicated before proceeding with lumbar puncture in suspected meningitis patients who are comatose, immunosuppressed, have a focal deficit or have signs of raised intracranial pressure.

EEG IN INTENSIVE CARE [1, 2, 4]

Patients who remain comatose after having clinically overt seizures can have a broad differential diagnosis including but not restricted to a persistent prolonged postictal state, an undiagnosed head injury, drug toxicity or non-convulsive status epilepticus. An EEG should be done to exclude non-convulsive status epilepticus as the cause of the persistent unresponsiveness which, if untreated, can result in permanent neurological damage and sometimes death. While that indication is clear, there is debate in the literature regarding the indication of electroencephalography (EEG) in comatose patients without high suspicion of seizures, as the EEG changes don't always mean a clinical or even a subclinical seizure. More importantly, it is unproven if treatment with anti-seizure medications can improve the outcomes of patients showing epileptiform abnormalities.

COMMON CLINICAL SCENARIOS IN THE NEUROINTENSIVE CARE [1, 2, 5]

Altered Sensorium

Evaluating a patient with altered sensorium is done by neurologists on a daily basis. The extent of the differential diagnoses in such a patient and the gravity of missing a treatable disease can become overwhelming. In each and every case of coma, a basic blood biochemistry should be obtained. Searching for drug intoxication should always be considered, but the extent of the workup is always determined by the clinical context. Special investigations like arterial blood

Table 14.1 Suspected Aetiology of Altered Sensorium/Coma and Intial Lab Tests

Suspected Aetiology of Altered Sensorium/Coma	Initial Lab Test
Massive hemispheric infarction/ICH	CT brain
Status epilepticus	EEG
Intraparenchymal mass lesions	CECT
Subdural/epidural hematoma	CT brain
Acute hydrocephalus	CT brain
Meningitis/encephalitis	CSF/CECT brain
Autoimmune encephalitis	MRI brain/CSF/autoimmune and paraneoplastic profile/EEG
Venous sinus thrombosis	CT/MRI/CT or MR venography
Posterior reversible encephalopathy	MRI/MRA
Drug intoxications	Toxic screen
Carbon monoxide poisoning	ABG
Hypoglycaemia/hyperglycaemia	Blood biochemistry
Uraemia	Blood biochemistry
Hyperammonaemia	Arterial ammonia levels
Pituitary apoplexy	CT/MRI/hormonal profile
Myxoedema coma/Hashimoto's encephalopathy	Thyroid status/ANA
Wernicke's encephalopathy	RBC transketolase, serum thiamine levels

EEG: electroencephalography; **MRA**: magnetic resonance angiography; **CSF**: cerebrospinal fluid
CT: computed tomography scan; **MRI**: magnetic resonance imaging; **ANA**: antinuclear antibody

Table 14.2 CSF Patterns in Meningitis

Aetiology	Cell Count/mm³/predominant Cell Type	Sugar	Protein mg/dlt
Normal	<5/lymphocytes	>40% serum	1–35
Bacterial	>500/Polymorphonuclear	<40% serum	>100
Viral	10–500/lymphocytes	>40% serum	<120
Tubercular	10–100/lymphocytes	<40% serum	>50

gases, serum ammonia and calculation of osmolar gap are also pertinent in many cases. The main concern when a patient presents with coma is to try and find a reversible cause (Table 14.1).

CNS Infections [1, 6–8]

Infections must, be considered in the differential diagnosis for any possible neurologic emergency presentation including but not restricted to meningitis, encephalitis, focal or multifocal brain lesions, myelopathy, myopathy and even neuropathy. Meningitis is a true neurological emergency wherein the appropriate treatment should be initiated within an hour of the patient reaching the hospital. CSF studies are invaluable in determining the aetiology, as shown in Tables 14.2, 14.3 and 14.4.

Seizures [10]

Status epilepticus (SE) (greater than 5 minutes of continuous seizure activity or greater than two episodes without return to baseline) demands rapid diagnosis and management. SE is associated not only with prolonged hospitalisation but can lead to permanent neurologic injury. Despite its ominous consequences, patients are commonly undertreated on initial presentation. Convulsive status is easy to diagnose as the manifestations are motor. But sometimes the patient may slip into non-convulsive status epilepticus without any major motor manifestations. Such cases demand prolonged EEG monitoring and sometimes an empirical anti-seizure drug trial. A very significant cause of prolonged status epilepticus is non-infectious autoimmune and paraneoplastic encephalitis. Many tests done on serum and CSF are available that help with the diagnosis of non-infectious encephalitis.

Table 14.3 Baseline Investigations in Suspected Meningitis

Infection Type	Microscopy/Culture/Direct Antigen Test [6–8]	Serology
Bacterial meningitis CSF and serum studies	2 ml CSF by LP; external ventricular drain or shunt fluid; blood (5–10 ml); urine	Acute phase and convalescent phase 5ml blood/serum
Usual tests	Gram stain; ZN (for AFB); routine bacterial culture and sensitivity; automated MGIT culture/LJ culture for Mycobacteria; antigen by latex agglutination; ICT	IgM/IgG antibody detection by ELISA; ICT
Interpretation	Gram-positive diplococci suggestive of *Streptococcus pneumoniae.* Gram-negative diplococci suggestive of *Neisseria meningitides.* Gram-negative bacilli suggestive of *E coli/Enterobacteriaceae.* Gram-positive bacilli suggestive of *Listeria.* Gram-negative coccobacilli suggestive of *Haemophilus influenzae.* Culture gives confirmatory diagnosis of pyogenic meningitis due to common bacterial agents Latex agglutination in CSF for capsular antigen confirm diagnosis of: *S pneumoniae/N meningitides/E coli/H influenza* C-polysaccharide. Antigen detection in urine by ICT confirms diagnosis of *S. pneumoniae*	better for difficult-to-culture bacteria. Useful for seroprevalence and not diagnosis – in c/o Meningococci Tp antibody by ICT-specific test for syphilis, confirms diagnosis of syphilis (all stages).
Viral meningitis/encephalitis Samples	CSF fluid aspirate/stool/blood/nasopharyngeal swabs/tissue biopsy/skin scrapings Test for presence of viral particles/inclusion bodies in clinical sample.	Second week of infection, i.e., acute phase first sample; convalescent phase second sample
Test and Interpretation	Direct demonstration of virus in clinical sample by electron microscopy confirms diagnosis of *rabies/pox virus/adenovirus/Ebola* Direct immunofluorescence microscopy detects virus particles in samples and confirms diagnosis of *herpes/adenoviruses/rabies* Demonstration of inclusion bodies by light microscopy in clinical samples confirms diagnosis: Negri bodies – *Rabies* Intranuclear inclusion bodies –*HSV/CMV/Poliovirus/Adenovirus/Measles*	blood/serum IgM/IgG by ELISA; antibody detection by ICT/HA; IgG avidity ELISA antigen by ELISA/ICT/HA/IF. Presence of IgM antibody or four-fold rise in titre of IgG (in two samples taken one week apart) suggestive of recent infection. Presence of only IgG without rise in titre indicates past or chronic infection: in *measles/Japanese encephalitis/Zika virus.* IgG avidity decreased in primary infection, increased in secondary infection: in *measles/Dengue/CMV.* Presence of viral antigen confirms early infection: NS1 antigen in dengue P24 antigen for HIV CMV antigen rabies antigen in skin biopsies

(Continued)

Table 14.3 (Continued)

Infection Type	Microscopy/Culture/Direct Antigen Test [6–8]	Serology
Parasitic and Fungal infections of CNS Sample Test and Interpretation	CSF (2–5 ml)/blood (5 ml)/skin scraping/tissue biopsy/stool For parasitic infections: Routine stool microscopy for ova/cyst/larva/trophozoites CSF/tissue for *tapeworm* hooklets/free-living *amoebae* trophozoites Blood peripheral smear (Giemsa stain) for *malarial parasite, tachyzoites of Toxoplasma gondii.* Biopsy tissue for tissue cyst (*Toxoplasma*) Test for malaria antigen by ICT For fungal infections: Gram stain for fungal elements India ink examination of CSF for *Cryptococcus neoformans* KOH mount for fungal elements Histopathology (H&E stain) of biopsy for fungal elements esp. dimorphic fungi/moulds Fungal antigen test by fluorescent antibody staining. Latex agglutination for cryptococcal antigen in CSF. Sample for fungal culture and sensitivity.	Blood/serum/plasma (5 ml): paired sera, one each in acute and convalescent phase For parasitic infection- IgM/IgG ELISA for *toxoplasma/hydatid disease/Taenia inf.* For fungal infections- Ig G/IgM/IgA antibody by ELISA especially for systemic mycoses. Galactomannan/1,3-beta-D-glucan antigen by ELISA for invasive mycoses
	Presence of parasite in clinical sample confirms diagnosis. Presence of fungal element gives presumptive diagnosis of fungal infection, however positive histopathology is confirmatory. Significance of fungal isolate in culture depends on source. Positive culture for dimorphic fungi like *Histoplasma* and *Cocci diodes* is confirmatory. For opportunistic/commensal fungi like yeast or *Aspergillus spp.* – repeat samples should be sent to confirm diagnosis along with clinical correlation and serological tests.	Presence of IgM or Rise in IgG antibody titre between acute and convalescent sera confirms diagnosis: *Toxoplasma infection* *Dimorphic fungi* IgG avidity ELISA to differentiate recent from past infection in *Toxoplasmosis.* Positive malarial antigen by ICT confirms malaria For fungal infections: positive serology confirms diagnosis for systemic mycoses due to dimorphic fungi-invasive candidiasis. Positive fungal antigen test confirms diagnosis: *Cryptococcal meningitis* *Invasive Aspergillosis* *Invasive Candidiasis*

ZN: Zeil Neilson stain; MGIT: Mycobacterium Growth Indicator Tube; ICT: Immunochromatographic test; IF: Immunofluorescence; HA: Hemagglutination

Headache

Headache is a common concern in emergency departments and accounts for over 2% of emergency visits. The main concern in a headache patient is to rule out a secondary headache. Table 14.6 gives a list of causes that should never be missed in an emergency setting.

Neuromuscular Emergencies [1, 12]

Patients with acute progressive neuromuscular weakness are often encountered by neurointensivists. Recognition of the severity of acute respiratory failure and timely intervention matching the degree of impairment is the initial step in managing these patients. Although the spectrum of neuromuscular emergencies is quite broad, we will restrict the discussion to the commonest

Table 14.4   Advance Laboratory Tests for Targeted Microbial Testing [7, 8]

Infection Type	Name of Test	Clinical Specimen	Application
Bacterial meningitis	16s rRNA PCR	CSF	Identify specific pathogens by detection of 16s ribosomal RNA
	Nucleic acid amplification tests (single plex/multiplex)	Blood/CSF/ nasopharyngeal swab/shunt fluid	RT-PCR and LAMP Assays for particular pathogens: Streptococcus pneumonia Neisseria meningitidis Haemophilus influenza Listeria monocytogenes Streptococcus agalactiae
	MALDI-TOF MS	Blood/CSF	
Tubercular meningitis	GeneXpert (Cartridge-based PCR)	CSF	Mass spectrometry
		CSF	identification based on weight
	GeneXpert ultra (Cartridge-based PCR)	CSF	
	TRUENAT (Chip-based micro real-time PCR)		Identification of *Mycobacterium tuberculosis* and Isoniazid/ rifampicin resistance
Viral meningitis/ encephalitis	16s rRNA amplification and Nucleic acid amplification tests (singleplex/multiplex)	Blood/CSF/ Nasopharyngeal swab/shunt fluid	Identify specific pathogens by detection of 16s ribosomal RNA and real-time PCR assays
Syndromic approach	BioFire film array ME panel Metagenomic next-generation sequencing (mNGS)	CSF CSF; Brain tissue	Real-time micro PCR detects multiple pathogens. Neural panel includes BACTERIA: *Escherichia coli* K1 *Haemophilus influenzae* *Listeria monocytogenes* *Neisseria meningitidis* *Streptococcus agalactiae Streptococcus pneumonia* VIRUSES: Cytomegalovirus (CMV) Enterovirus (EV) Herpes simplex virus 1 (HSV-1) Herpes simplex virus 2 (HSV-2) Human herpesvirus 6 (HHV-6) Human parechovirus (HPeV) Varicella zoster virus (VZV) YEAST: *Cryptococcus (C. neoformans/C. gattii)* Nucleic acid detection of any pathogen: viral and fungal meningitis especially.

Table 14.5   Laboratory Tests for Autoimmune and Paraneoplastic Encephalitis in Serum/CSF [9]

Name of Test	Application
Detection of autoantibodies	Screening: Tissue/cell-based assays for synaptic antibodies: anti-NMDA/AMPA/GABAb/ GABAa/mGLUR5/ Dopamine 2 receptor Specific: Immunoblot assay for intracellular paraneoplastic antibodies: anti-Hu/Ri/Yo/ Ma/CRMP5/amphiphysin
CSF analysis	Mild pleocytosis; protein 50–100 mg/dl; raised IgG
MRI/EEG/whole body PET scan	To exclude other causes/occult cancer

Table 14.6 Headache in Intensive Care [11]

Aetiology	Chief Complaints	Examination Findings	Initial Lab Tests	Additional Lab Tests
Subarachnoid haemorrhage	Thunderclap headache, severe neck pain, loss of consciousness	Signs of meningeal irritation	CT brain/MRI Brain	DSA/CSF
Reversible cerebral vasoconstriction syndrome	Thunderclap headache	Variable, at times focal deficits due to associated stroke	CT/MRI brain	CT or MR Angiography
Cervical artery dissection	Neck pain prominent, dizziness	Horner's syndrome, focal deficits due to associated stroke	MRI brain and neck	CT or MR Angiography
Cerebral venous sinus thrombosis	Headache, seizures	Focal deficits as per the site, optic disc oedema	CECT brain/CEMRI	CT or MR Venography
Hypertensive encephalopathy/posterior reversible encephalopathy syndrome	Headache, seizures, visual symptoms	Examination findings depending on the area affected, mostly posterior circulation involvement	CT/MRI brain	Ambulatory BP monitoring
Meningitis/encephalitis	Fever, neck pain, photophobia, altered sensorium	Signs of meningeal irritation	CT brain/CSF	Blood and CSF cultures
Brain abscess	Headache, fever	Focal deficits as per the site	CECT/CEMRI	Culture sensitivity of the aspirate
Brain tumour	Headache with features suggestive of raised intracranial pressure	Focal deficits as per the site/Disc oedema	CECT/CEMRI	MRS
Extra axial hematoma SDH/EDH	Head injury can present spontaneously. Also high index of suspicion in the elderly	Focal deficits as per the site/progressive decline in mental status	CT brain	MRI
Intraparenchymal haemorrhage	Headache, focal deficits	Focal deficits as per the site	CT brain	MRI/CT or MR Angiography in selected cases
Colloid cyst of the third ventricle	Positional headache and at times positional loss of consciousness	Non-specific examination findings	CT brain	MRI/CEMRI
Idiopathic intracranial hypertension	Headache (more in recumbent position) diplopia tinnitus transient visual obscurations	Sixth nerve palsy/optic disc oedema/field defects	CEMRI brain	MR Venography
Spontaneous intracranial hypotension	Headache (mostly in sitting position)	No specific clinical finding	CEMRI brain	MR Cisternography
Acute angle closure glaucoma	Eye pain, decreased vision	Painful red eye/raised intraocular tension	Tonometry	
Giant cell arteritis	Temple pain, vision loss	Optic disc oedema/temporal artery thickened and tender	Temporal artery Doppler/MRI brain and temporal artery	PET brain
Carbon monoxide toxicity	Headache temporally related to source of exposure	Findings mostly as per severity of exposure, from dizziness to coma Cherry red spot on fundus examination	Arterial blood gas analysis	

Table 14.7   Lab Diagnosis of Neuromuscular Diseases in the Intensive Care

GBS
CSF
Elevated protein without pleocytosis (i.e., albumin cytologic dissociation), though CSF may be normal early.
  Pleocytosis > 50 cells/microliter suggests an alternative diagnosis Electrophysiology:
AIDP: Prolonged motor conduction velocity and distal latencies, conduction block, temporal dispersion,
  prolonged F waves, normal sural nerve testing
AMAN/AMSAN: Decreased CMAP amplitude (and SNAP amplitudes in AMSAN) without demyelinating
  features, absent F waves, reversible conduction block
May be normal early in the disease course

MG
Serum antibody testing:
85% of patients have antibodies to AChR
MuSK, LRP-4 and agrin testing can be positive in AChR seronegative patients
Electrophysiology:
CMAP decrement > 10% on repetitive nerve stimulation
Increased jitter and blocking on single-fibre EMG (95% sensitive)

CINM
Electrophysiology
CIP: Reduced amplitude CMAP and SNAP without demyelinating features, neuropathic changes on EMG
CIM: Reduced amplitude CMAPs with prolonged durations, myopathic changes on EMG Peroneal nerve test:
  Two standard deviation drop in CMAP amplitude 100% sensitive but not specific for diagnosis

  GBS: Guillain-Barré syndrome; MG: myasthenia gravis; CINM: critical illness neuromyopathy; CSF:
    cerebrospinal fluid; CMAP: compound muscle action potential; SNAP: sensory nerve action potential; AIDP:
    acute inflammatory demyelinating polyneuropathy; AMAN: acute motor axonal neuropathy; AMSAN: acute
    motor and sensory axonal polyneuropathy; AChR: acetylcholine receptor; MuSK muscle-specific tyrosine
    kinase; LRP-4: low-density lipoprotein receptor-related protein 4; EMG: electromyography

Table 14.8   Neurological Emergencies (Movement Disorders and Demyelinating Disorders)

Neurological Emergency	Initial Lab Tests
Acute parkinsonism	Non-specific*
Neuroleptic malignant syndrome	CBC/CPK
Serotonin syndrome	CBC
Status dystonicus	Non-specific*
Myoclonic status	MRI brain/EEG
ADEM	MRI brain/CSF
Acute attack of MS	MRI brain/CSF/VEP/OCT
NMOSD	MRI brain and spine Antibodies against Aquaporin 4
MOGAD	MRI brain and spine Antibodies against myelin oligodendrocyte protein

*Tests done mostly to rule out precipitating causes

causes seen in our hospital setting: Guillain-Barré syndrome (GBS), myasthenia gravis (MG) and critical illness neuromyopathy (CINM).

Apart from the already mentioned emergencies a neurologist usually encounters emergencies due to demyelinating disorders but rarely movement disorders. An initial lab approach to these conditions is given in Table 14.8.

CLINICAL PEARLS

1. All lab investigations are guided by clinical history and examination.

2. In patients with coma, always look for a reversible cause.

3. In a patient with suspected ischaemic stroke, a CT is mostly done to rule out contraindications of thrombolysis. In eligible patients, start thrombolytic therapy as soon as possible.

4. In cases of suspected meningitis, draw the CSF as early as possible. The patient should receive the first dose of antibiotic within an hour of reaching the hospital.

5. Never miss a secondary headache in the ER. A detailed fundus examination and BP measurement will help rule out the most important secondary causes.

6. GBS and myasthenia may require ventilation at any stage; keep a close watch.

7. Lab tests change at a great pace in the ICU; follow up regularly.

8. Time and the brain are critically linked: a delay of one minute can mean the loss of millions of neurons!!

SUMMARY

Laboratory tests should be directed to prove or disprove the hypothesis that a certain disease is responsible for the condition in the patient. They should not be used as a "fishing expedition." When used judiciously, lab tests will help the clinician arrive at a diagnosis. However one should be aware of the fact that every biological measurement in a population varies over a normal range, which usually is defined as plus or minus 2 or 3 standard deviations (SDs) from the mean value; 2 SDs encompass 96%, and 3 SDs encompass 99% of the measurements from a normal population. Even with 3 SDs, one normal person in 100 has a value outside the normal range. Therefore, an abnormal result may not indicate the presence of a disease. Thus, all tests need to be interpreted in the appropriate clinical context. Interpreting the tests without a clinical history and examination would be like putting the cart before the horse!

REFERENCES

1. Plum F, Posner JB. *The Diagnosis of Stupor and Coma*, FA Davis Company, Philadelphia, PA, 1982, p. 177.

2. Finelli PF, Uphoff DF. Magnetic resonance imaging abnormalities with septic encephalopathy. *J Neurol Neurosurg Psychiatry*. 2004;75:1189.

3. Brouwer MC, Thwaites GE, Tunkel AR, van de Beek D. Dilemmas in the diagnosis of acute community-acquired bacterial meningitis. *Lancet*. 2012;380:1684.

4. Brenner RP. The electroencephalogram in altered states of consciousness. *Neurol Clin*. 1985;3:615.

5. Ely EW, Stephens RK, Jackson JC, *et al*. Current opinions regarding the importance, diagnosis, and management of delirium in the intensive care unit: a survey of 912 healthcare professionals. *Crit Care Med*. 2004;32:106.

6. Dorsett M, Liang SY. Diagnosis and treatment of central nervous system infections in the emergency department. *Emerg Med Clin North Am*. 2016;34(4):917–942.

7. Hussin SADS,Chua AL, Al-Talib H, Sekaran SD, and Wang SM. An overview of laboratory diagnosis of CNS viral infections. *J Pure Appl Micobiol*. 2022;16(4):2225–2245.

8. Ramachandran PS, Wilson MR. Metagenomics for neurological infections — expanding our imagination. *Nat Rev Neurol*. 2020;16:547–556.

9. Lee SK, Lee ST. The laboratory diagnosis of autoimmune encephalitis. *J Epilepsy Res*. 2016;6(2):45–50.

10. Glauser T, Shinnar S, Gloss D, *et al*. Evidence-based guideline: treatment of convulsive status epilepticus in children and adults: report of the guideline committee of the american epilepsy society. *Epilepsy Curr*. 2016;16:48.

11. Edlow JA. Managing patients with nontraumatic, severe, rapid-onset headache. *Ann Emerg Med*. 2018;71:400.

12. Juel VC, Bleck TP. Neuomuscular disorders in critical care. In: *Textbook of Critical Care*, Grenvik A, Ayres SM, Holbrook PR, Shoemaker WC (Eds), WB Saunders, Philadelphia, PA, 2000, p. 1886.

15 Enhancing Diagnostic Precision

Interpreting Laboratory Findings for Gastrointestinal Diseases in Intensive Care

Anuupama Suchiita, Binita Goswami and Nikhil Gupta

INTRODUCTION

In the high-stakes environment of intensive care units (ICUs), monitoring the gastrointestinal (GI) system is crucial. The GI system, vital for digestion, nutrient absorption, and immune defence, faces disruptions in critically ill patients. Complications like bleeding, infections, and organ dysfunction can significantly impact outcomes.

The reasons for monitoring the GI system in ICUs include early detection of complications, nutritional support optimisation, infection prevention, and managing organ dysfunction. Laboratory tests are pivotal in assessing GI function and diagnosing disorders in ICU patients. Blood tests (complete blood count (CBC), LFTs, electrolyte panels) offer insights into GI health, detecting issues like anaemia, liver dysfunction, and inflammation. Stool tests (faecal occult blood test (FOBT), stool cultures) identify bleeding and infectious pathogens. Imaging modalities (abdominal ultrasound, CT scans, MRI) visualise the GI tract, aiding in diagnosis. Endoscopic procedures (EGD, colonoscopy) allow direct visualisation and biopsy sampling.

Monitoring the GI system in ICUs optimises patient care, and laboratory tests guide clinical decisions, facilitating early intervention. Leveraging advanced diagnostic tools improves outcomes for critically ill patients in the ICU.

GI SYSTEM OVERVIEW AND FUNCTION

The GI tract, comprising organs like the oesophagus, stomach, small intestine, and large intestine, works collectively for digestion, nutrient absorption, and waste elimination. Each organ has specific functions vital to this process. Gastrointestinal processes are regulated by hormonal and neural mechanisms, with hormones like gastrin and cholecystokinin regulating acid secretion and bile production. Neural signals coordinate activities such as peristalsis and sphincter control. Maintaining gut integrity is crucial, as disruptions can lead to complications like bacterial translocation and sepsis. The GI tract plays a critical role in immune surveillance and defence. Strategies like enteral nutrition and probiotic supplementation are essential in preventing complications in critically ill patients. Understanding these regulatory mechanisms helps healthcare providers appreciate the GI system's importance and develop targeted interventions in intensive care settings.

LABORATORY TESTS FOR GASTROINTESTINAL FUNCTIONS

These tests and procedures collectively provide comprehensive insights into haematological parameters, liver health, electrolyte balance, gastrointestinal bleeding, infections, and structural abnormalities, aiding in the identification and management of gastrointestinal issues (Table 15.1). [1]

COMMON GASTROINTESTINAL DISORDERS IN INTENSIVE CARE [2]

Gastrointestinal Bleeding

GI bleeding refers to bleeding that occurs anywhere along the digestive tract, from the oesophagus to the rectum. It can manifest as overt bleeding with visible blood in the stool or vomit (hematemesis or melena) or as occult bleeding.

GI bleeding has diverse origins, including peptic ulcers, oesophageal varices, Mallory-Weiss tears, colorectal issues, and angiodysplasia. Peptic ulcers often result from H. pylori infection or NSAID use, causing upper GI bleeding. Oesophageal varices, linked to liver cirrhosis, lead to severe upper GI bleeding. Mallory-Weiss tears, from intense vomiting, cause upper GI bleeding. Colorectal polyps, inflammatory bowel disease (IBD), and cancer contribute to lower GI bleeding. In older adults, diverticulosis can lead to lower GI bleeding, and abnormal blood vessels like angiodysplasia may rupture. Symptoms vary based on location, severity, and cause, including hematemesis, melena, haematochezia, abdominal pain, dizziness, weakness, hypotension, and tachycardia.

DOI: 10.1201/9781003449713-15

Table 15.1 Overview of Laboratory Tests for Gastrointestinal Function

Category	Tests	Purpose and Significance
Routine Blood Tests	Complete blood count (CBC)	• Provides information about blood components, including red blood cells (RBCs), white blood cells (WBCs), and platelets. • Detects anaemia related to gastrointestinal bleeding or malabsorption. • Indicates infection through abnormalities in WBC count and differential.
	Liver function tests (LFTs)	• Assesses liver health by measuring enzymes (such as ALT, AST), bilirubin, and proteins (like albumin). • Detects liver damage, inflammation, or impaired synthetic function impacting the GI system. • Helps diagnose conditions such as liver cirrhosis, hepatitis, or liver failure.
	Electrolyte panel	• Measures levels of electrolytes (sodium, potassium, chloride, bicarbonate) in the blood. • Identifies electrolyte imbalances affecting GI function, such as nausea, vomiting, or alterations in motility and absorption. • Helps in managing conditions like diarrhoea, dehydration, or metabolic disorders.
Stool Tests	Faecal occult blood test (FOBT)	• Screens for the presence of hidden blood in the stool, which may indicate gastrointestinal bleeding. • Detects conditions such as ulcers, inflammatory bowel disease (IBD), colorectal cancer, or haemorrhoids. • Can be used for routine screening or as part of diagnostic evaluation for GI symptoms.
	Stool culture	• Identifies bacterial, viral, or parasitic pathogens causing gastrointestinal infections. • Enables targeted treatment with appropriate antimicrobial therapy. • Helps in diagnosing conditions such as bacterial gastroenteritis, parasitic infections, or viral enteritis.
Category	Tests	Purpose and Significance
Imaging Studies	Abdominal ultrasound	• Utilises high-frequency sound waves to create real-time images of abdominal organs. • Aids in detecting abnormalities like gallstones, liver masses, pancreatic cysts, or abdominal fluid accumulation (ascites). • Provides initial assessment for patients presenting with abdominal pain, jaundice, or suspected liver or gallbladder pathology.
	Computed tomography (CT) scan	• Employs X-rays and computer processing to generate detailed cross-sectional images of the abdomen. Detects conditions such as tumours, inflammation, trauma, or vascular abnormalities. • Offers superior spatial resolution compared to ultrasound, aiding in the characterisation of lesions and guiding treatment decisions.
Endoscopic Procedures	Esophagogastroduodenoscopy (EGD) (upper endoscopy)	• Involves the insertion of a flexible endoscope through the mouth to visualise the upper GI tract (oesophagus, stomach, duodenum). • Facilitates diagnosis of conditions like ulcers, inflammation, tumours, strictures, and varices. • Allows for tissue sampling (biopsy) and therapeutic interventions (e.g., dilation, haemostasis).

(Continued)

Table 15.1 (Continued)

Category	Tests	Purpose and Significance
	Colonoscopy	• Uses a flexible colonoscope inserted through the rectum to examine the entire colon and terminal ileum. • Enables detection of abnormalities such as polyps, tumours, inflammation, or vascular lesions. • Allows for biopsy and removal of polyps (polypectomy) during the procedure. • Gold standard for colorectal cancer screening and surveillance.
	Capsule endoscopy	• Ingestible capsule equipped with a camera to visualise the entire small intestine. • Useful for diagnosing conditions like obscure gastrointestinal bleeding, Crohn's disease, or small bowel tumours.
Category	Tests	Purpose and Significance
		• Provides high-resolution images without the need for sedation or intubation. • May require further investigation or intervention based on findings.

(*Aderinto-Adike & Quigley, 2014; Camilleri et al., 1998; 'Contemporary Practice in Clinical Chemistry', 2020; Suchodolski & Steiner, 2003; Watson et al., 2019*).

Laboratory examinations play a vital role in the diagnosis and ongoing monitoring of GI bleeding by evaluating haematological parameters and identifying indicators of blood loss or underlying pathology. Noteworthy findings encompass:

1. **Anaemia:** Characterised by diminished haemoglobin (Hb) and haematocrit (Hct) levels, indicative of blood loss.

2. **Liver or kidney dysfunction:** Detected through abnormalities in LFTs and renal function tests (BUN, creatinine).

3. **Coagulopathies or thrombocytopenia:** Identified by abnormalities in coagulation parameters like prothrombin time (PT), activated partial thromboplastin time (aPTT), and platelet count.

4. **Concealed blood in stool:** Indicated by positive results in FOBT, suggestive of lower GI bleeding.

5. **Iron deficiency anaemia:** Assessed through serum iron, ferritin, and total iron-binding capacity (TIBC) levels, reflecting chronic GI bleeding.

In addition to initial diagnosis, laboratory tests play a crucial role in monitoring patients with GI bleeding to assess the efficacy of interventions, guide transfusion therapy, and identify complications such as hypovolemic shock or multiorgan dysfunction. Serial measurements of haemoglobin, haematocrit, and other haematological parameters help track changes in blood loss and hemodynamic stability over time, guiding clinical decision-making and optimising patient care.

Inflammatory Bowel Disease (IBD)

IBD is a group of chronic inflammatory disorders of the gastrointestinal tract characterised by recurrent episodes of inflammation and tissue damage. Its main subtypes, Crohn's disease and ulcerative colitis, exhibit distinct clinical features, inflammation patterns, and management approaches.

Crohn's disease affects any GI tract segment, often the terminal ileum and colon, featuring transmural inflammation leading to complications like strictures, fistulas, and abscesses.

Symptoms include abdominal pain, diarrhoea, weight loss, fever, and extraintestinal manifestations like arthritis and skin lesions.

Ulcerative colitis, confined to the colon and rectum, primarily involves the mucosal layer, showcasing symptoms like bloody diarrhoea, abdominal pain, urgency, and rectal bleeding. Inflammation starts in the rectum, extending proximally in a continuous fashion, leading to diffuse mucosal ulceration and inflammation.

Key laboratory markers that play a crucial role in the diagnosis and monitoring of disease activity in patients with Crohn's disease and ulcerative colitis include:

1. **C-Reactive protein (CRP) and erythrocyte sedimentation rate (ESR):** CRP and ESR are acute-phase reactants that increase in response to inflammation. Elevated levels of CRP and ESR are indicative of active inflammation in IBD and can help assess disease severity and response to treatment. However, CRP and ESR levels may also be influenced by factors such as infection, surgery, or medications, and should be interpreted in conjunction with clinical findings.

2. **Faecal calprotectin:** Faecal calprotectin is a marker of intestinal inflammation and neutrophil activation. Elevated levels of faecal calprotectin are highly specific for active inflammation in IBD and correlate well with endoscopic disease activity. Faecal calprotectin testing is particularly useful for monitoring disease activity, predicting relapse, and assessing response to therapy in patients with Crohn's disease and ulcerative colitis.

3. **Blood tests:** Routine blood tests, including CBC and serum albumin levels, may provide supportive evidence of inflammation, anaemia, or malnutrition in patients with IBD. Anaemia, leucocytosis, and thrombocytosis may be seen in active disease, while hypoalbuminemia may indicate malnutrition or protein-losing enteropathy.

4. **Stool studies:** Stool tests, including FOBT and stool cultures, may be performed to rule out infectious causes of gastrointestinal symptoms and assess for occult bleeding in patients with IBD. Additionally, stool studies for pathogens such as C. difficile may be indicated in patients with suspected infectious colitis or disease exacerbation.

5. **Serological markers:** Serological markers, such as anti-Saccharomyces cerevisiae antibodies (ASCA) and anti-neutrophil cytoplasmic antibodies (ANCA), may be elevated in subsets of patients with Crohn's disease and ulcerative colitis, respectively. These markers may aid in distinguishing between the two subtypes of IBD and predicting disease behaviour or response to therapy in some cases.

These tests provide valuable information about the inflammatory burden, disease severity, and response to treatment, guiding clinical decision-making and optimising patient care in the management of IBD.

Acute Pancreatitis

Acute pancreatitis is sudden inflammation of the pancreas, ranging from mild to life-threatening. It involves premature activation of pancreatic enzymes, causing tissue damage and systemic inflammation. Causes include gallstones, alcohol, medications, and trauma.

Complications may include pancreatic necrosis, pseudocysts, and organ failure. Symptoms include severe abdominal pain, nausea, vomiting, epigastric tenderness, fever, and potential jaundice. Severe cases can lead to hypotension, shock, and multiorgan failure due to systemic inflammation or sepsis.

Laboratory tests for diagnosis and prognostication of acute pancreatitis include serum amylase and lipase levels.

1. **Serum amylase:** Serum amylase is an enzyme produced by the pancreas that aids in the digestion of carbohydrates. In acute pancreatitis, damaged pancreatic cells release elevated levels of amylase into the bloodstream. Serum amylase levels typically rise within 6–24 hours of symptom onset, peak within 48 hours, and gradually decline over 3–5 days. Elevated serum amylase levels are a sensitive but nonspecific marker for acute pancreatitis and may also be elevated in other conditions such as salivary gland disorders, bowel obstruction, or renal failure.

2. **Serum lipase:** Serum lipase is another pancreatic enzyme involved in the breakdown of fats. Like amylase, lipase levels increase in acute pancreatitis due to pancreatic injury. Lipase is more specific for pancreatitis than amylase and remains elevated for a longer duration, making it a preferred marker for diagnosis and monitoring. Serum lipase levels typically rise concurrently with amylase levels but may remain elevated for a longer period, providing a more reliable indicator of pancreatic injury and disease severity.

Various other laboratory tests are employed to evaluate pancreatic function, inflammation, and organ status in acute pancreatitis. These include CBC to detect leucocytosis, anaemia, or thrombocytopenia, LFTs to assess for biliary issues or liver injury, and serum electrolytes and renal function tests to monitor electrolyte balance and kidney function. Additionally, arterial blood gas (ABG) analysis may be conducted to identify metabolic abnormalities or respiratory issues, particularly in severe cases.

Liver Failure

Liver failure is a life-threatening condition characterised by the inability of the liver to perform its vital functions adequately, leading to systemic complications and multiorgan dysfunction. It can manifest as acute liver failure (ALF), which develops rapidly over days to weeks, or chronic liver failure (CLF), which occurs gradually over months to years.

Causes and Manifestations

1. **Acute liver failure (ALF):**

   - ALF may result from various aetiologies, including viral hepatitis (e.g., hepatitis A, B, or E), drug-induced liver injury (e.g., acetaminophen overdose), autoimmune hepatitis, acute fatty liver of pregnancy, ischaemic hepatitis (shock liver), or acute exacerbation of underlying chronic liver disease.

   - The clinical presentation of acute liver failure is characterised by rapid-onset jaundice, coagulopathy (manifested as prolonged prothrombin time or INR), hepatic encephalopathy (neurological impairment due to elevated ammonia levels), ascites, and signs of hepatic decompensation such as hepatic encephalopathy, gastrointestinal bleeding, or hepatorenal syndrome.

2. **Chronic liver failure (CLF):**

   - CLF typically develops as a consequence of progressive liver injury and fibrosis due to chronic liver diseases such as viral hepatitis (hepatitis B or C), alcoholic liver disease, non-alcoholic fatty liver disease (NAFLD) or non-alcoholic steatohepatitis (NASH), autoimmune hepatitis, primary biliary cholangitis (PBC), primary sclerosing cholangitis (PSC), or genetic liver disorders.

   - The manifestations of chronic liver failure vary depending on the underlying aetiology and stage of liver disease. Common features include jaundice, ascites, hepatic encephalopathy, coagulopathy, portal hypertension (manifested as variceal bleeding, splenomegaly, or portosystemic shunts), hepatorenal syndrome, and hepatopulmonary syndrome.

Interpretation of LFTs and Other Laboratory Parameters

LFTs are a panel of blood tests that assess various aspects of liver function, injury, and biliary function. Key LFTs and other laboratory parameters used in assessing liver function and diagnosing liver failure include:

1. **Alanine aminotransferase (ALT) and aspartate aminotransferase (AST):** ALT and AST are enzymes primarily found within hepatocytes. Elevated levels of ALT and AST indicate hepatocellular injury or inflammation. The AST/ALT ratio may help differentiate between different aetiologies of liver disease (e.g., AST/ALT ratio >1 in alcoholic liver disease).

2. **Bilirubin:** Bilirubin is a breakdown product of haemoglobin metabolism, and elevated serum bilirubin levels result in jaundice. Elevated bilirubin levels may indicate impaired bilirubin excretion (e.g., obstructive jaundice) or hepatocellular injury.

3. **Alkaline phosphatase (ALP) and gamma-glutamyl transferase (GGT):** ALP and GGT are enzymes involved in bile duct function. Elevated ALP and GGT levels suggest cholestasis or biliary obstruction.

4. **Albumin and prothrombin time (PT/INR):** Decreased serum albumin levels and prolonged PT/INR indicate impaired synthetic function of the liver, often seen in advanced liver disease with synthetic dysfunction and coagulopathy.

5. **Serum ammonia:** Elevated serum ammonia levels may occur in liver failure and hepatic encephalopathy due to impaired ammonia metabolism and detoxification by the liver.

6. **Serum electrolytes and renal function tests:** Monitoring serum electrolytes (e.g., sodium, potassium) and renal function (e.g., creatinine) is important in assessing complications such as hepatorenal syndrome and electrolyte imbalances in liver failure.

Along with LFTs, imaging studies (e.g., ultrasound, CT/MRI) and liver biopsy may be performed to further evaluate liver structure, assess for hepatic fibrosis or cirrhosis, and guide management decisions in liver failure.

Early recognition, prompt intervention, and multidisciplinary management are crucial in optimising outcomes and preventing complications in liver failure.

FUTURE PERSPECTIVES AND RESEARCH DIRECTIONS [3]
Emerging Technologies in Laboratory Diagnostics for the Gastrointestinal System

■ Microbiome analysis: Advancements in metagenomic sequencing and bioinformatics have enabled comprehensive analysis of the gut microbiome, leading to a better understanding of its role in health and disease. Future research may focus on developing microbiome-based diagnostic tests for gastrointestinal disorders and assessing the impact of microbiome modulation on patient outcomes.

■ Point-of-care testing (POCT): Advances in POCT technologies allow for rapid and decentralised testing of gastrointestinal biomarkers, facilitating early diagnosis and timely intervention in critical care and outpatient settings. Miniaturised devices and smartphone-based platforms enable real-time analysis of stool, blood, and breath samples, enhancing the accessibility and efficiency of diagnostic testing.

■ Liquid biopsy: Liquid biopsy techniques, such as circulating tumour DNA (ctDNA) analysis and extracellular vesicle profiling, hold potential for non-invasive detection of gastrointestinal malignancies and monitoring treatment response. Liquid biopsy-based assays may complement traditional tissue biopsies and provide valuable prognostic information in cancer patients.

These technologies in GI lab diagnostics will transform disease diagnosis, risk assessment, and treatment choices. Utilising emerging tech and personalised medicine, clinicians can enhance patient care and outcomes. Collaborative research and interdisciplinary partnerships are key for translating discoveries into clinical solutions in GI medicine.

MULTIORGAN DYSFUNCTION SYNDROME AND GASTROINTESTINAL INVOLVEMENT [4]

Multiorgan dysfunction syndrome (MODS) is a severe condition marked by dysfunction in two or more organs, common in critically ill patients. Gastrointestinal issues are frequent in MODS, impacting lab diagnosis and patient care. It stems from systemic inflammation triggered by severe illness, injury, infection, or shock, leading to organ failure. Gastrointestinal involvement includes ischaemia, barrier dysfunction, and bacterial translocation, worsening inflammation and organ dysfunction. This delves into the connection between MODS, gastrointestinal involvement, and laboratory diagnostics:

1. Laboratory diagnosis in MODS with gastrointestinal involvement:

   • Inflammatory markers: Laboratory tests, including C-reactive protein (CRP), procalcitonin (PCT), and interleukin-6 (IL-6), reflect the degree of systemic inflammation and may be elevated in MODS with gastrointestinal involvement. Serial measurements of inflammatory markers help assess disease severity, monitor treatment response, and guide therapeutic interventions.

   • Organ-specific biomarkers: Biomarkers of gastrointestinal injury, such as intestinal fatty acid-binding protein (I-FABP), citrulline, or D-lactate, may indicate gut barrier dysfunction and predict the development of MODS. Elevated levels of these biomarkers correlate with mucosal damage, bacterial translocation, and subsequent organ dysfunction.

   • Coagulation profile: Abnormalities in coagulation studies, including prolonged PT, aPTT, and disseminated intravascular coagulation (DIC) parameters, may indicate coagulopathy associated with MODS and gastrointestinal involvement. Monitoring coagulation parameters helps identify patients at increased risk of bleeding or thrombosis and guides anticoagulation therapy.

- Organ-specific function tests: Laboratory tests assessing organ function, such as LFTs, renal function tests, and markers of cardiac injury (e.g., troponin), provide valuable information about the extent of organ dysfunction in MODS. Abnormalities in these tests reflect impaired organ perfusion, cellular injury, and metabolic derangements, guiding treatment decisions and prognostication.

- Microbiological studies: Blood cultures, stool cultures, and polymerase chain reaction (PCR) assays for pathogens, help identify infectious aetiologies contributing to MODS and gastrointestinal involvement. Early detection and targeted antimicrobial therapy are essential for managing sepsis and preventing further organ dysfunction in critically ill patients.

2. Management considerations

- Hemodynamic optimisation: Early intervention with fluid resuscitation and vasopressors stabilises tissue perfusion, crucial for preventing organ dysfunction in MODS.

- Supportive care: Utilising mechanical ventilation, renal replacement therapy, and nutritional support aids in managing MODS and associated gastrointestinal issues. Continuous monitoring of organ function guides the adjustment of supportive measures.

- Source control: Swift identification and treatment of underlying causes like sepsis or trauma are vital for preventing organ dysfunction escalation. Source control methods, such as antimicrobial therapy and surgical intervention, target the primary pathology, reducing systemic inflammation.

In summary, MODS with gastrointestinal involvement presents significant challenges in laboratory diagnosis and patient management in intensive care settings.

NOVEL BIOMARKERS AND DIAGNOSTIC TECHNIQUES IN LABORATORY DIAGNOSIS IN INTENSIVE CARE

In recent years, advancements in laboratory diagnostics have introduced novel biomarkers and diagnostic techniques that hold promise for improving the management of critically ill patients in intensive care settings. These innovations provide valuable insights into disease pathophysiology, enable early detection of complications, and facilitate personalised treatment strategies. Some emerging biomarkers and diagnostic techniques are described below:

1. **Biomarkers of organ injury and dysfunction:** [5]

- **Intestinal fatty acid-binding protein (I-FABP):** I-FABP is a biomarker of intestinal epithelial cell damage and mucosal barrier dysfunction. Elevated serum levels of I-FABP indicate gastrointestinal injury, bacterial translocation, and increased risk of systemic inflammation and organ dysfunction in critically ill patients. Monitoring I-FABP levels helps identify patients at risk of multiorgan dysfunction and guide therapeutic interventions.

- **Trefoil factor 3 (TFF3):** TFF3 is a protein secreted by intestinal goblet cells, crucial for maintaining and repairing the intestinal lining. It protects against damage, aids in mucosal repair, and has anti-inflammatory properties. TFF3 levels serve as biomarkers for assessing mucosal integrity and diagnosing gastrointestinal disorders like IBD and colorectal cancer, offering insights into disease progression and treatment response.

2. **Point-of-care testing (POCT):** [6]

- **Lactate measurement:** Point-of-care lactate testing enables rapid assessment of tissue perfusion and oxygenation status in critically ill patients. Elevated blood lactate levels reflect tissue hypoperfusion, anaerobic metabolism, and increased mortality risk. POCT devices for lactate measurement facilitate timely resuscitation efforts, guide fluid therapy, and improve patient outcomes in septic shock and other critical conditions.

- **Procalcitonin (PCT) testing:** Point-of-care PCT testing aids in the early diagnosis of bacterial infections and sepsis in critically ill patients. PCT levels rise rapidly in response to bacterial toxins and correlate with the severity of infection and systemic inflammation. POCT devices for PCT measurement facilitate rapid decision-making regarding antimicrobial therapy initiation, de-escalation, or discontinuation, leading to more judicious antibiotic use and improved patient outcomes.

3. **Molecular diagnostics and genomic testing:** [7]

- **SeptiCyte™ LAB assay:** The SeptiCyte™ LAB assay is a molecular diagnostic test that quantifies the expression of host response genes in whole blood samples to differentiate sepsis from non-infectious systemic inflammation. SeptiCyte™ technology uses biomarker signatures to evaluate how a patient's immune system responds to infections. By analysing gene expression patterns associated with the immune response, the SeptiCyte™ LAB assay provides accurate and rapid sepsis diagnosis, guiding appropriate treatment and improving patient outcomes.

- **Next-generation sequencing (NGS):** NGS technology allows for comprehensive analysis of microbial DNA/RNA in clinical samples, enabling rapid identification of pathogens and antimicrobial resistance genes in critically ill patients with suspected infections. NGS-based metagenomic sequencing provides valuable information about the microbiome composition, pathogen diversity, and genetic determinants of antimicrobial resistance, guiding targeted antimicrobial therapy and infection control measures.

4. **Biomarker panels and multiplex assays:**

- **Cytokine panels:** Multiplex immunoassays for cytokine profiling enable simultaneous measurement of multiple inflammatory mediators in patient samples, providing a comprehensive assessment of immune dysregulation and systemic inflammation in critically ill patients. Profiling cytokine patterns helps stratify patients based on disease severity, predict clinical outcomes, and identify potential therapeutic targets for immunomodulatory therapies.

- **Sepsis biomarker panels:** Biomarker panels incorporating multiple markers of inflammation, coagulation, and organ dysfunction offer enhanced diagnostic accuracy and prognostic value for sepsis and septic shock. Combining biomarkers such as procalcitonin, CRP, lactate, and interleukins improves the sensitivity and specificity of sepsis diagnosis, facilitating early intervention and personalised treatment approaches.

These novel biomarkers and diagnostic techniques have the potential to revolutionise laboratory diagnosis in intensive care settings, enabling early detection of organ dysfunction, guiding targeted therapy, and improving patient outcomes. Incorporating these innovative approaches into clinical practice requires interdisciplinary collaboration, robust validation studies, and ongoing research efforts to optimise their utility and impact on patient care in the critical care setting.

GASTROINTESTINAL MOTILITY DISORDERS IN INTENSIVE CARE [8]

Gastrointestinal motility disorders encompass a spectrum of conditions characterised by abnormal movement patterns of the gastrointestinal tract, leading to symptoms such as dysphagia, reflux, abdominal pain, bloating, and altered bowel habits. In the ICU, critically ill patients may experience gastrointestinal motility disturbances due to various factors, including underlying medical conditions, surgical procedures, medications, and systemic illness.

Laboratory diagnosis plays a crucial role in identifying and managing these disorders. Here's an overview of gastrointestinal motility disorders and their laboratory diagnosis in the ICU:

1. Types of gastrointestinal motility disorders:

- **Achalasia:** Achalasia is a primary motility disorder characterised by impaired relaxation of the lower oesophageal sphincter (LES) and absent peristalsis in the oesophageal body, leading to dysphagia, regurgitation, and chest pain.

- **Gastroparesis:** Gastroparesis refers to delayed gastric emptying without mechanical obstruction, often secondary to autonomic dysfunction or neuropathy. Patients may present with early satiety, nausea, vomiting, and bloating.

- **Intestinal pseudo-obstruction:** Intestinal pseudo-obstruction is a syndrome characterised by symptoms of bowel obstruction without mechanical obstruction. It can affect the stomach, small intestine, or colon and presents with abdominal distension, pain, and vomiting.

- **Chronic idiopathic constipation:** Chronic idiopathic constipation encompasses various disorders characterised by infrequent bowel movements, difficulty passing stools, and incomplete evacuation.

- **Functional diarrhoea:** Functional diarrhoea refers to chronic diarrhoea without identifiable structural or metabolic abnormalities, often associated with altered colonic motility or secretion.

2. Laboratory diagnosis:

- **Serum biomarkers:** Although there are no specific serum biomarkers for gastrointestinal motility disorders, laboratory tests may help identify underlying causes or complications. For example, elevated white blood cell count and C-reactive protein levels may indicate inflammatory processes such as acute diverticulitis or inflammatory bowel disease.

- **Electrolyte imbalance:** Gastrointestinal motility disturbances can lead to electrolyte imbalances such as hypokalaemia or hypomagnesaemia, which may be detected in routine blood tests. Monitoring electrolyte levels is essential for managing complications such as arrhythmias or muscle weakness.

- **Faecal biomarkers:** Faecal biomarkers such as calprotectin may be elevated in inflammatory bowel disease or infectious gastroenteritis, which can contribute to gastrointestinal motility disturbances. Stool studies may also be performed to rule out infectious causes of diarrhoea.

- **Imaging studies:** Imaging modalities such as abdominal X-rays, barium studies, and abdominal ultrasound may be utilised to evaluate structural abnormalities or complications associated with gastrointestinal motility disorders, such as bowel dilation or obstruction.

- **Manometry studies:** Oesophageal manometry, gastric emptying studies, and colonic transit studies are invasive procedures used to assess gastrointestinal motility and transit times. These studies provide valuable diagnostic information regarding the function of the oesophagus, stomach, and intestines.

3. Management strategies:

- **Pharmacological therapy:** Medications such as prokinetic agents (e.g., metoclopramide, erythromycin), antispasmodics, and laxatives may be prescribed to improve gastrointestinal motility and alleviate symptoms.

- **Dietary modifications:** Dietary changes such as small, frequent meals, low-fat meals, and avoidance of gas-producing foods may help manage symptoms of gastrointestinal motility disorders.

- **Enteral feeding:** In severe cases of gastroparesis or intestinal pseudo-obstruction, enteral feeding via nasogastric or nasojejunal tubes may be necessary to provide nutrition and medications.

- **Surgical intervention:** Surgical options such as oesophageal dilation, pyloroplasty, or intestinal decompression surgery may be considered in refractory cases or complications such as bowel obstruction.

- **Multidisciplinary approach:** Managing gastrointestinal motility disorders in the ICU often requires a multidisciplinary approach involving gastroenterologists, surgeons, nutritionists, pharmacists, and critical care specialists to optimise patient care and outcomes.

GASTROINTESTINAL COMPLICATIONS OF CRITICAL ILLNESS [9]

In intensive care settings, critically ill patients are susceptible to a range of GI complications that can significantly impact their prognosis and management. Laboratory diagnosis plays a crucial role in identifying and managing these complications promptly and effectively. Below is a summary of prevalent GI issues related to critical illness and their laboratory diagnosis within the ICU:

1. Stress ulcers:

- Stress ulcers, also known as stress-related mucosal damage (SRMD), can occur in critically ill patients due to factors such as mechanical ventilation, shock, sepsis, and coagulopathy. They present with upper GI bleeding, often manifesting as hematemesis or melena.

Laboratory tests such as CBC and FOBT may reveal anaemia and occult blood in the stool, suggestive of GI bleeding. Additionally, LFTs and coagulation profiles help assess the severity of liver dysfunction and coagulopathy contributing to bleeding risk.

2. Ileus:

- Ileus, characterised by impaired bowel motility, abdominal distension, and lack of bowel sounds, commonly occurs in critically ill patients following surgery, trauma, or severe illness. While laboratory tests do not directly diagnose ileus, monitoring serum electrolytes (e.g., potassium) and renal function is essential to identify electrolyte imbalances and renal dysfunction, which may exacerbate ileus. Imaging studies such as abdominal X-rays or CT scans help confirm the diagnosis by demonstrating bowel dilation and air-fluid levels.

3. Ischaemic bowel disease:

- Ischaemic bowel disease, including mesenteric ischaemia and ischaemic colitis, can occur secondary to hypoperfusion, embolic events, or thrombosis in critically ill patients. It presents with abdominal pain, bloody diarrhoea, and signs of systemic sepsis. Laboratory tests such as lactate levels and ABG analysis aid in the assessment of tissue hypoperfusion and metabolic acidosis, suggestive of ischaemic insult. Imaging studies, including abdominal CT angiography and mesenteric duplex ultrasound, help confirm the diagnosis by demonstrating bowel wall thickening, pneumatosis, or vascular abnormalities.

4. Gastrointestinal infections:

- Critically ill patients are susceptible to gastrointestinal infections, including Clostridium difficile-associated colitis, viral gastroenteritis, and bacterial translocation. These infections present with diarrhoea, abdominal pain, and systemic signs of infection. Stool studies, including stool cultures and Clostridium difficile toxin assays, are essential for identifying the causative pathogens. Additionally, FOBT may help differentiate infectious from non-infectious causes of GI bleeding.

5. Acute pancreatitis:

- Acute pancreatitis can occur in critically ill patients due to factors such as gallstones, alcohol abuse, or medication-induced injury. It presents with severe epigastric pain, nausea, vomiting, and elevated serum pancreatic enzymes (amylase, lipase). Serum amylase and lipase levels are elevated in acute pancreatitis, aiding in the diagnosis and prognostication of the condition. Additionally, imaging studies such as abdominal ultrasound or CT scans may reveal pancreatic inflammation or fluid collections.

Gastrointestinal complications are common in critically ill patients in the ICU and require prompt recognition and management to prevent adverse outcomes. Laboratory diagnosis, in conjunction with clinical assessment and imaging studies, plays a vital role in identifying these complications and guiding appropriate interventions in intensive care settings.

CONCLUSION

In conclusion, this chapter has provided a comprehensive overview of interpreting laboratory findings for gastrointestinal diseases in intensive care settings. We explored various laboratory tests specific to the gastrointestinal system, essential for diagnosing and monitoring common disorders encountered in ICU patients. Furthermore, we discussed future perspectives and emerging technologies in laboratory diagnostics, highlighting the potential for advancements in precision medicine. Understanding multiorgan dysfunction syndrome and its gastrointestinal involvement is crucial for effective patient management. Finally, we examined novel biomarkers, diagnostic techniques, motility disorders, and complications of critical illness, underscoring the importance of ongoing research and interdisciplinary collaboration in optimising diagnostic precision and patient outcomes in intensive care settings.

REFERENCES

1. Suchodolski JS, Steiner JM. Laboratory assessment of gastrointestinal function. *Clin Tech Small Anim Pract.* 2003;18(4):203–210.

2. Aderinto-Adike AO, Quigley EMM. Gastrointestinal motility problems in critical care: a clinical perspective. *J Dig Dis.* 2014;15(7):335–344.

3. Ju M, Gao Z, Li K, Wang Z. Partial advances in the diagnosis and treatment of gastrointestinal cancer. *Chronic Diseases Translat Med.* 2023;9(1):1–4.

4. Klingensmith NJ, Coopersmith CM. The gut as the motor of multiple organ dysfunction in critical illness. *Critical Care Clin.* 2016;32(2):203–212.

5. Balanza N, López-Varela E, Baro B, Bassat Q. Biomarkers of intestinal injury and dysfunction: adding new possibilities to current methods for risk stratification of children with malaria disease. *mBio.* 2022;13(6):e0222222.

6. Lin CT, Lu JJ, Chen YC, Kok VC, Horng JT. Diagnostic value of serum procalcitonin, lactate, and high-sensitivity C-reactive protein for predicting bacteremia in adult patients in the emergency department. *PeerJ.* 2017;5:e4094.

7. Montero MM, Hardy-Werbin M, Gonzalez-Gallardo S, Torres E, Rueda R, Hannet I, *et al.* Evaluation of the host immune response assay SeptiCyte RAPID for potential triage of COVID-19 patients. *Sci Rep.* 2023;13(1):944.

8. Grajecki D, Tacke F. Gastrointestinal motility disorders in critically ill patients. *Deutsche Medizinische Wochenschrift.* 2022;147(11):696–704.

9. El Moheb M, Naar L, Christensen MA, Kapoen C, Maurer LR, Farhat M, *et al.* Gastrointestinal Complications in Critically Ill Patients with and without COVID-19. *JAMA.* 2020;324(18):1899–1901.

16 Bone and Joint Diseases

Anirban Bhattacharjee and Ankit Patowary

INTRODUCTION

Patients with bone and joint diseases are often admitted to the intensive care units (ICU) either for the disease or for secondary complications. Some diseases like connective tissue disorders can have multisystem involvement with features of chronic immunosuppressive therapy, while some autoimmune disorders can cause periodic flare-ups, secondary infections, and organ dysfunction (Table 16.1). Therefore an intensivist should have a comprehensive understanding of the pathophysiology of diseases and knowledge of their management. In this regard, the correct interpretation of laboratory tests is an essential skill that benefits patients in many ways.

COMMON LABORATORY TESTS AND THEIR INTERPRETATION

1. Blood tests

   a. Complete Blood Count and Blood Smear Examination: Anemia is a common finding in all CTDs. Autoimmune hemolytic anemia is common in systemic lupus erythematosus (SLE). Microangiopathic hemolytic anemia with schistocytosis is seen in Thrombotic thrombocytopenic purpura (TTP) (associated with SLE or mixed connective tissue disease (MCTD)), catastrophic antiphospholipid syndrome (CAPS), and scleroderma renal crisis. Thrombocytopenia can be seen in ITP associated with SLE and in catastrophic antiphospholipid syndrome (CAPS). Leukopenia can be seen in SLE and rheumatoid arthritis (RA). Pancytopenia in a critically ill patient with multiorgan dysfunction and very high ferritin levels should raise the suspicion of macrophage activation syndrome (MAS).

   b. Urinalysis: The presence of microscopic hematuria with RBC casts and proteinuria indicates glomerulonephritis (lupus nephritis, ANCA-associated vasculitis).

   c. Inflammatory markers: C-reactive protein (CRP) is elevated in most disease flare-ups and remains low in SLE unless there is a coexisting infection or serositis.

   d. Muscle enzymes (CPK, AST) are elevated in inflammatory myopathies.

   e. Coagulation: aPTT is prolonged in APS.

   f. Liver function test: Elevation of liver enzymes may be seen in SLE and vasculitis. It is frequently seen in macrophage activation syndrome.

2. Immunological tests

   a. Antinuclear antibodies (ANAs): These are directed at nuclear targets. They can be subdivided into four categories based on their targets: DNA, histones, non-histone proteins bound to RNA, and nucleolar antigens.

      Indirect immunofluorescence (IIF) microscopy in human cellular extract (HEp-2) is the gold standard approach for screening for ANA. Based on the targets of the autoantibodies, the different immunofluorescence patterns (categorized as nuclear, cytoplasmic, and mitotic) are seen and reported as per the International Consensus on ANA Patterns (ICAP) (available at www.anapatterns.org). An IIF report includes the pattern of immunofluorescence (nuclear/cytoplasmic/mitotic) and the positivity titer. A cut-off titer of 1:80 is used as an entry criterion in the 2019 EULAR/ACR classification for further testing with sub-serology, although care must be taken about the fact the specificity of the test at 1:80 titer is poor (74.7%) [6], and therefore, ANA can be positive in about 25% of normal healthy populations. Therefore, pre-test clinical probability is of paramount importance to avoid a false-positive diagnosis.

      A positive ANA screening by IIF, along with strong clinical suspicion, is followed by anti-extractable nuclear antigens (ENA) assays by enzyme immunoassays to detect specific auto-antibodies (Table 16.2). IIF with Hep-2 cells may be false negative in some cases (Sjögren's syndrome, for example) that can be diagnosed with an ENA assay.

DOI: 10.1201/9781003449713-16

Table 16.1 Multiorgan Complications of Connective Tissue Disorders

Organ System	Complications	Associated Connective Tissue Disorders
Central nervous system	Delirium or psychosis	SLE
	Seizure	SLE
	Stroke	SLE, APS, SSc
Respiratory system	Interstitial lung disease	RA, SSc, SLE, PM/DM
	Pleural effusion	SLE, RA, SSc
	Diffuse alveolar hemorrhage	SLE, APS
Cardiovascular system	Tamponade	SLE, RA, SSc, MCTD
	Endocarditis	SLE, RA
	VTE/PE	APS, SLE, SSc
	Cardiogenic shock	SLE, APS, SSc
Renal system	Glomerulonephritis	SLE, RA
	Thrombosis	SLE, APS
	Scleroderma renal crisis	SSc

APS: Antiphospholipid syndrome; DM: Dermatomyositis; PM: Polymyositis; RA: Rheumatoid arthritis; SLE: Systemic lupus erythematosus; SS: Sjögren syndrome; SSc: Systemic sclerosis

Table 16.2 Common Autoantibodies Seen in Connective Tissue Disorders

Antibody	Associated Conditions
Antinuclear antibodies	Highly sensitive for SLE (98%); repeated negative tests rule out diagnosis. Poor specificity at lower titer cut-offs
Anti-dsDNA	High titers are specific for SLE; correlates with disease activity and lupus nephritis
Anti-Smith	Specific for SLE
Anti-histone	Most frequently positive in drug-induced lupus
Antiphospholipid antibodies	Present in one-third of SLE patients (only 5–10% develop antiphospholipid syndrome)
Anti-U1-RNP	Not specific for SLE; seen in mixed connective tissue disorder
Anti-Ro (SS-A) and Anti-La (SS-B)	Not specific for SLE; associated with Sjögren syndrome; correlates with decreased risk of lupus nephritis
Antiribosomal P	May correlate with CNS lupus
Anti-centromere	Limited cutaneous systemic sclerosis
Anti-topoisomerase (Scl-70), anti-RNA polymerase III	Diffuse cutaneous systemic sclerosis

b. Anti-double stranded DNA: Anti-ds DNA (with or without Anti-Sm) is highly specific for SLE, but the sensitivity is low (approximately 60%). The presence of anti-ds-DNA correlates with disease activity and lupus nephritis.

c. Complement: Low serum levels of C3 and C4, often with increased anti-ds DNA titers indicate active SLE, particularly lupus nephritis.

d. Rheumatoid factor (RF) and anti-CCP antibody: The laboratory diagnosis of RA is made by detecting rheumatoid factor (RF) and anti-CCP antibodies in serum. Serum IgM RF is positive in 75–80% of cases with RA; therefore, a negative test doesn't exclude RA. The test may be false positive in the presence of other connective tissue diseases (CTDs), such as primary Sjögren's disease and SLE, and with non-rheumatic diseases such as chronic hepatitis B and C infections. Serum anti-CCP antibody has similar sensitivity as RF but higher specificity (~95%) and, therefore, is helpful in differentiating RA from other inflammatory arthritis.

e. Antiphospholipid antibodies and lupus anticoagulant: The tests for specific antiphospholipid antibodies include:

  i. IgG and IgM Anticardiolipin antibodies (aCL) ELISA

 ii. IgG and IgM Anti-beta2 glycoprotein I (anti-beta2GPI) antibodies ELISA

iii. Lupus anticoagulant (LA), using a three-step functional coagulation assay:

   i. Screen: Prolonged dRVVT (dilute Russell viper venom test) or an optimized aPTT

   ii. Mix: Mixing plasma from normal individuals fails to correct the dRVVT or aPTT

   iii. Confirmatory test: Addition of excess phospholipid corrects the dRVVT or aPTT

If the patient has had an acute thrombotic event or is on anticoagulants, the coagulation-based tests will be unreliable. ELISA for aCL and anti-beta2GPI can be reliably used in such patients. Two tests for antiphospholipid antibodies should be positive 12 weeks apart to confirm the diagnosis.

 f. Myositis-specific antibodies:

   i. Ro/Ku/U1-RNP/PM-Scl: Polymyositis/dermatomyositis overlap syndromes

   ii. HMG-CoA reductase: Dermatomyositis, immune-mediated necrotizing myopathy related to statins

   iii. Anti-MDA5: Dermatomyositis with a high risk of progressive interstitial lung disease (ILD)

   iv. Anti-Jo-1, PL-7, PL-12, EJ, OJ: Anti-synthetase syndrome

   v. Anti-cytoplasmic 5' nucleotidase 1A: Inclusion body myositis

   vi. Anti-Mi 2, anti-TIF1, anti-NXP-2, anti-SAE: Dermatomyositis

SPECIFIC DISORDERS

Systemic Lupus Erythematosus

SLE is a multisystem autoimmune disorder involving autoantibodies that cause tissue injury by immune complex deposition or direct binding of antibodies to cells and tissues (Figure 16.1). Patients are classified as SLE as per the 2019 European League Against Rheumatism/American College of Rheumatology (EULAR/ACR) classification criteria if they fulfill the entry criterion of ANA positivity, at least one clinical criterion, and an overall score of 10 or more in clinical and immunological domains (see Table 16.3) [8].

Lupus Nephritis

Lupus Nephritis is a serious complication seen in 50-60% of patients with SLE. Diagnosis is made by the presence of hematuria and/or proteinuria in urinalysis, antinuclear antibody screen, and renal biopsy. Nephritis is often associated with raised anti-ds-DNA titers with decreased serum

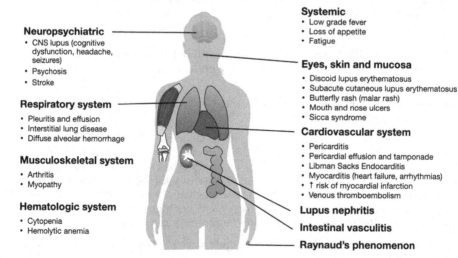

Figure 16.1   Clinical manifestations of systemic lupus erythematosus.

Table 16.3   2019 EULAR/ACR Criteria for Diagnosis of SLE

Entry Criterion	Clinical Domains and Criteria (score)	Immunological Domains and Criteria (score)
At least one ANA positive report at any point in life	Fever [2]	Anti-ds-DNA or Anti-Sm positivity [6]
	Hematologic Leukopenia [3] Thrombocytopenia [4] AIHA [4]	Complement levels Low C3 or low C4 [3] Low C3 and low C4 [4]
	Mucocutaneous Oral ulcers [2] Non-scarring alopecia [2] SCLE or DLE [4] Acute cutaneous lupus [6]	Antiphospholipid antibodies positivity [2]
	Neuropsychiatric Delirium [2] Psychosis [3] Seizure [5]	
	Serositis Pleural/pericardial effusion [5] Acute pericarditis [6]	Diagnosis of SLE requires: • Positive entry criterion • > 1 clinical criteria • Total score > 10 (Only the highest weighted criteria in each domain is counted; do not consider a criterion as positive if an alternate cause is more likely than SLE)
	Renal Proteinuria > 500mg in 24 hours [4] Class II or V lupus nephritis [8] Class III/IV lupus nephritis [10]	
	Joint symptom [6]	

(Adapted from Ref. [8]).

complement levels. Lupus nephritis is classified as per the International Society of Nephrology (ISN) and the Renal Pathology Society (RPS) classification (2003) into five classes [10,11]:

■ Class I: Minimal mesangial lupus nephritis

■ Class II: Mesangial proliferative lupus nephritis

■ Class III: Focal lupus nephritis (proliferative or sclerosing or both)

■ Class IV: Diffuse lupus nephritis (proliferative or sclerosing or both; segmental or global)

■ Class V: Membranous lupus nephritis

■ Class VI: Advanced sclerosis lupus nephritis (> 90% of glomerular units are sclerosed globally)

Antiphospholipid Syndrome (APS)

APS is an acquired thrombophilia caused by autoantibodies against phospholipids and phospholipid-binding plasma proteins. It can occur as primary APS or in association with other autoimmune diseases, mainly SLE.

Laboratory evidence includes mild thrombocytopenia, increased activated partial thromboplastin time, and biological false-positive serological tests for syphilis. Testing for antiphospholipid antibodies is done to confirm the diagnosis. Two tests 12 weeks apart should be positive to confirm the diagnosis.

Catastrophic antiphospholipid syndrome (CAPS) is an acute and severe form of APS characterized by widespread microvascular thrombosis induced by the activation of prothrombotic pathways by antiphospholipid antibodies.

Clinical suspicion of CAPS arises primarily in female patients of reproductive age presenting with organ failures such as acute kidney injury (AKI) or respiratory failure or thrombotic complications, evidence of microangiopathic hemolytic anemia, thrombocytopenia or pancytopenia, prolonged activated partial thromboplastin time (aPTT) in vitro, and a false-positive Venereal Disease Research Laboratory (VDRL) test [14]. Additional findings may include disseminated intravascular coagulation and elevated serum ferritin levels.

Rheumatoid Arthritis

Rheumatoid arthritis (RA) is a chronic autoimmune inflammation of synovial joints with many extra-articular organ manifestations. The diagnosis of RA is done in the presence of clinical signs and symptoms of inflammatory small joint polyarthritis with features of synovitis involving hands and feet. The 2010 American College of Rheumatology/European League Against Rheumatism (ACR/EULAR) classification criteria (Table 16.4) may be used as a guide to diagnosis; a score of 6 or more out of 10 indicates the diagnosis of RA [22]. A general approach to evaluation of arthritis is outlined in Figure 16.2.

Table 16.4 2010 Rheumatoid Arthritis Classification Criteria: An American College of Rheumatology/European League against Rheumatism Collaborative Initiative

Entry Criteria:

Atleast 1 joint involvement with definite clinical synovitis not better explained by alternate disease

		Score
Joint involvement	• 1 large joint	0
	• 2–10 large joints	1
	• 1–3 small joints	2
	• 4–10 small joints	3
	• >10 joints (at least 1 small joint)	5
Serology	Negative RF, negative anti-CCP Ab	0
	Low + RF or anti-CCP Ab	2
	High + RF or anti-CCP Ab	3
Acute-phase reactants	Normal CRP and ESR	0
	Abnormal CRP or ESR	1
Symptom duration	< 6 weeks	0
	> 6 weeks	1

(Adapted from Ref [22]).

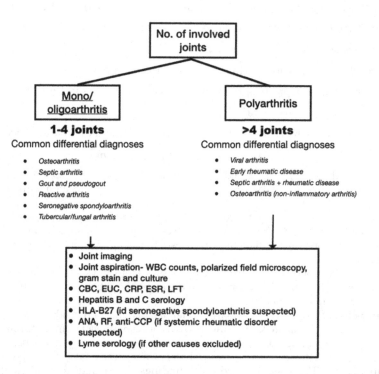

Figure 16.2 Differential diagnoses and diagnostic workup of arthritis.

The laboratory diagnosis is made by detecting rheumatoid factor (RF) and anti-CCP antibodies in serum as previously discussed. Normocytic normochromic anemia is frequent, and non-specific inflammatory markers such as erythrocyte sedimentation rate (ESR), and CRP are also elevated [23].

The incidence of ILD in RA is 4–68%, depending on the screening test applied [20]. Usual interstitial pneumonia (UIP) and non-specific interstitial pneumonia (NSIP) are prevalent radiologic patterns. Pericarditis and cardiomyopathy (due to granulomatous myocarditis and coronary artery disease) are the cardiac manifestations of the disease. Rheumatoid vasculitis can complicate 2–5% of cases and present as cutaneous signs (petechiae, purpura), vasculitis ulcers, and/or sensorimotor polyneuropathies [21]. Intensivists are also needed to have the knowledge of potential serious toxicities of disease-modifying anti-rheumatoid drugs (DMARDs), as outlined in Table 16.5.

Systemic Sclerosis

Systemic sclerosis (SSc) is a chronic connective tissue disorder characterized by fibrosis of the skin and internal organs. Two types are recognized: limited (~80% of patients) and diffuse (~20%). Organ involvement is seen in both types. In general, the prognosis of limited disease is better than diffuse disease.

The antinuclear antibody test is almost always positive. The anti-SCL 70 or anti-topoisomerase I antibody is found more frequently in diffuse systemic sclerosis but can be positive in up to 20% of patients with limited disease. Anti-SCL-70 indicates a poor prognosis, with a higher risk of developing ILD. Anticentromere antibody is highly specific for limited systemic sclerosis but may be present in overlap syndromes. Anti-RNA polymerase III antibodies are detected in 10–20% of cases and are associated with rapidly progressive skin changes and renal crises [23,27].

Scleroderma renal crisis (SRC) occurs in approximately 10–15% of patients with systemic sclerosis. It usually presents as accelerated hypertension with rapidly progressive oliguric renal failure, although ~10% of patients may be normotensive. The pathophysiology involves obliterative renal vasculopathy leading to reduced renal blood flow. Reduction in RBF causes activation of RAS, resulting in further vasoconstriction, setting up a vicious cycle that results in hypertension and renal failure.

The diagnosis of SRC is based on the clinical presentation of progressive oliguric renal failure and accelerated hypertension. Urinalysis shows mild proteinuria, microscopic hematuria, and granular casts. Moderate thrombocytopenia with features of microangiopathic hemolytic anemia is often seen, and TTP becomes a close differential diagnosis; renal biopsy and ADAMTS13 assay may be required to differentiate between the two conditions. SRC should be differentiated from ANCA-positive rapidly progressive glomerulonephritis, as the management of the two conditions is different.

Immune-Mediated Inflammatory Myopathies

This group of disorders is characterized by progressive muscle weakness with elevated serum muscle enzymes, myopathic changes on electromyography, and characteristic muscle biopsy findings. Major types of inflammatory myopathies include dermatomyositis (DM), polymyositis (PM), inclusion body myositis (IBM), immune-mediated necrotizing myopathy (IMNM), and anti-synthetase syndrome (ASS) (Table 16.6).

Serum creatine phosphokinase is always raised in uncontrolled PM. CPK is often normal in patients with IBM and may be normal in up to 20% of patients with DM. ANA is often positive, especially in patients with other coexisting connective tissue diseases (CTDs). RF may be positive in a minority of cases. Several myositis-specific antibodies are found in patients with inflammatory myopathies and are often associated with specific clinical features of the disease. Anemia is uncommon, and ESR and CRP are mostly normal. EMG shows a myopathic pattern of muscle weakness. Muscle biopsy is often required to aid the diagnosis.

SPECIAL SCENARIOS IN RHEUMATOLOGY
Macrophage Activation Syndrome

Macrophage activation syndrome (MAS) is one of the dreaded complications of autoimmune diseases with a high mortality rate. MAS resembles sepsis with multiorgan failure and is often not diagnosed early, thereby contributing to high mortality. The pathophysiology involves excessive T-cell and macrophage activation and proliferation, leading to a life-threatening systemic inflammatory cascade. MAS belongs to a group of disorders called hemophagocytic lymphohistiocytosis.

Table 16.5   Serious Toxicities and Monitoring of Disease-Modifying Anti-Rheumatic Drug Therapy

Drugs	Serious Toxicities	Initial Screening and Laboratory Monitoring Required
Hydroxychloroquine	• Irreversible retinal damage • Cardiotoxicity (QT prolongation) • Agranulocytosis • Neuropathy and myopathy	• Visual field testing at initiationMonitoring of visual field testing every year
Methotraxate	• Hepatotoxicity • Myelosuppression • Interstitial pneumonitis • Teratogenicity	• CBC, LFT, viral hepatitis, pregnancy screen at initiation • CBC, LFT, creatinine monitoring every 2–3 months
Sulfasalazine	• Granulocytopenia • Hemolytic anemia (with G6PD deficiency) • Allergic reaction including Steven Johnson syndrome/Toxic Epidermal Necrolysis	• CBC, LFT, and G6PD screen at initiation • CBC: First monitoring at 4–6 weeks of initiation, then every 3 months
Leflunomide	• Hepatotoxicity • Myelosuppression • Teratogenicity	• CBC, LFT, viral hepatitis screen before initiation • CBC, LFT, creatinine monitoring every 2–3 months
TNF-α inhibitors (Infliximab, Etanercept, Adalimumab etc.)	• Increased risk of bacterial/fungal infections • TB reactivation • Infusion site reaction	• Skin test (purified protein derivative) before initiation • Screening for latent TB before initiation • LFTs periodically
Abatacept	• Increased risk of bacterial/viral infections	• PPD skin test before initiation
Rituximab	• Infections • Infusion reaction • Cytopenia • Hepatitis B reactivation	• CBC and viral hepatitis screen before initiation • Regular CBC monitoring
Tocilizumab	• Risk of infection • Infusion reaction • Cytopenias • LFT elevation	Regular CBC and LFT monitoring

Table 16.6 Immune-Mediated Inflammatory Myopathies

Disorder	Epidemiology	Clinical Features	Investigations
PM	Typically presents in early adulthood and is more common in women than in men.	Symmetrical and proximal more than distal muscle weakness, with/without associated heart, lung and joint involvement. Patients have increased risk of developing cancer than normal population, with a lower risk than DM.	• Highly elevated CPK (approximately 50x normal value or more) • Muscle biopsy shows endomysial monomuclear inflammatory infiltrate.
DM	DM can start in childhood (juvenile DM) or adulthood, and is more common in women than men.	Symmetrical muscle weakness (proximal more than distal) associated with characteristic heliotropic rash, Shawl sign, Gottron's papules and Gottron's sign. Patients may develop myocarditis, vasculitis and interstitial lung diseases, or overlap with other CTDs. Patients are at increased risk of developing malignancies.	• Highly elevated CPK in classic DM (may be normal in amyopathic DM) • Various MSAs (anti-MDA5, anti-TIF1, anti-Mi-2, anti-NXP2) • Muscle biopsy shows monomuclear inflammatory infiltration, predominantly in perimyseal connective tissue and around blood vessels. Perifascicular atrophy, if found, is characteristic.
IBM	IBM always presents in adulthood, typically in elderly male beyond 50 years age.	Slowly progressive weakness with early involvement of wrist and fingers. The weakness is often asymmetrical. There is no increased risk of malignancy.	• Normal or mildly increased CPK • Anti-CN-1a antibody • Endomysial inflammatory infiltration similar to PM on biopsy, along with the presence of intracellular "rimmed vacuoles"
IMNM	Can develop in childhood and adulthood, with the median age of onset about 40–50 years. Females are affected approximately thrice as commonly as males.	Acute or insidious onset of symmetrical muscle weakness (proximal > distal). HMCGR Antibody-positive cases can be triggered by statins.	• Elevated CPK; anti-HMGCR or anti-SRP antibodies. • Muscle necrosis with minimal inflammatory infiltrate on biopsy
ASS	Can develop in childhood and adulthood, and affects female more than males.	ASS presents as proximal myositis and extramuscular manifestations: interstitial lung disease, fever, inflammatory arthritis, "mechanic's hand" and Raynaud's phenomenon. An erythematous rash may sometimes be seen.	• Elevated CPK with anti-synthetase antibodies • Perimysial and perivascular inflammatory infiltrate

DM: Dermatomyositis; IBM: inclusion body myositis; IMNM: immune-mediated necrotizing myopathy; ASS: anti-synthetase syndrome; MSA: Myositis-specific antibodies; PM: Polymyositis

Most reported in juvenile idiopathic arthritis and adult-onset Still's disease, MAS can also complicate SLE, MCTD, and juvenile dermatomyositis.

A decline in two or three blood cell lines (RBC/WBC/platelets) due to increased destruction from phagocytosis and consumption in systemic inflammation is a frequent and early indicator of the disease. Profound hyperferritinemia, often exceeding 10,000 ng/ml, is a distinctive feature of MAS, and a normal ferritin level below 500 ng/ml makes the diagnosis unlikely. Ferritin level also correlates with the disease activity and response to the treatment. Additional supportive findings include hypertriglyceridemia, elevated liver enzymes, mildly increased bilirubin levels, and hypofibrinogenemia. Although CRP levels are typically elevated, the ESR paradoxically decreases. Hemophagocytosis in bone marrow biopsy is often a delayed finding and, therefore, not essential for the clinical diagnosis. The clinical and laboratory features of HLH and MAS are outlined in Figure 16.3. Specific serum markers of HLH activity, the soluble CD25 and CD23, are elevated. HLH-2004 criteria, primarily used for the diagnosis of primary HLH, may be used for the diagnosis. A

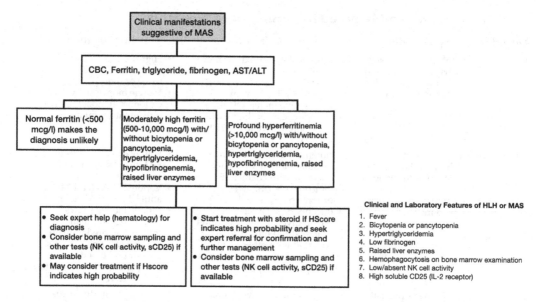

Figure 16.3 Diagnosis of macrophage activation syndrome (Adapted from Ref. [31]).

scoring system called HScore has been developed to estimate the probability of HLH, available online (https://saintantoine.aphp.fr/score/) [30]. Immediate treatment with methylprednisolone of 1 g per day with or without intravenous immunoglobulin. Further treatment with anakinra and etoposide is given in consultation with hematology colleagues. Unlike patients with primary HLH, a hematopoietic stem cell transplant is rarely required [31].

Pulmonary-Renal Syndrome

Pulmonary-renal syndrome (PRS) manifests as rapidly progressive glomerulonephritis and diffuse alveolar hemorrhage, developing from vasculitis affecting pulmonary and renal microvasculature. Predominantly, approximately 70% of cases are linked with ANCA-associated vasculitis, with a further 20% attributed to anti-glomerular basement membrane (anti-GBM) disease. Less than 10% of instances may arise from conditions such as double-positive disease (both ANCA and anti-GBM positive), antiphospholipid syndrome (APS), SLE-associated vasculitis, and IgA vasculitis (Henoch-Schönlein purpura) [32,33]. Half of the affected patients require mechanical ventilation due to acute respiratory failure.

Diagnostic confirmation is done by bronchoscopic alveolar lavage (BAL), revealing progressive blood staining and hemosiderin-laden macrophages in sequential samples, coupled with hematuria and proteinuria evident in urinalysis, and autoimmune antibodies. BAL also helps in ruling out pulmonary infections. A hemogram typically demonstrates normocytic normochromic anemia with an acute decline in hemoglobin levels during diffuse alveolar hemorrhage (DAH). Chest radiography is universally performed, indicating bilateral infiltrative opacification patterns, occasionally having a slight predilection for mid-zone involvement with apical sparing. High-resolution computed tomography (CT) surpasses chest radiography in discerning mild cases with localized ground-glass opacifications, particularly when accompanied by additional findings such as pleural effusion [5,14].

CONCLUSION

Most of the investigations to diagnose emergencies in rheumatologic disorders are specific and time-sensitive, and they are conducted to confirm the diagnosis, monitor the response to treatment, and prognosticate the family members of outcomes.

REFERENCES

1. Goldenberg DL. Septic arthritis and other infections of rheumatologic significance. *Rheum Dis Clin North Am.* 1991;17(1):149–156.

2. Margaretten ME, Kohlwes J, Moore D, Bent S. Does this adult patient have septic arthritis? *JAMA.* 2007;297(13):1478–1488.

3. Papanicolas LE, Hakendorf P, Gordon DL. Concomitant septic arthritis in crystal monoarthritis. *J Rheumatol.* 2012;39(1):157–160.

4. Mathews CJ, Weston VC, Jones A, Field M, Coakley G. Bacterial septic arthritis in adults. Lancet. 2010 Mar 6;375(9717):846-55. doi: 10.1016/S0140-6736(09)61595-6. PMID: 20206778

5. Dumas G, Arabi YM, Bartz R, Ranzani O, Scheibe F, Darmon M, Helms J. Diagnosis and management of autoimmune diseases in the ICU. Intensive Care Med. 2024 Jan;50(1):17–35. doi: 10.1007/s00134-023-07266-7. Epub 2023 Dec 19. PMID: 38112769.

6. Leuchten N, Hoyer A, Brinks R, Schoels M, Schneider M, Smolen J, *et al.* Performance of antinuclear antibodies for classifying systemic lupus erythematosus: a systematic literature review and meta-regression of diagnostic data. *Arthritis Care Res (Hoboken).* 2018;70(3):428–438.

7. Cojocaru M, Cojocaru IM, Silosi I, Vrabie CD. Manifestations of systemic lupus erythematosus. *Maedica (Bucur).* 2011;6(4):330–336.

8. Aringer M, Costenbader K, Daikh D, Brinks R, Mosca M, Ramsey-Goldman R, *et al.* European league against rheumatism/American College of Rheumatology classification criteria for systemic lupus erythematosus. *Arthritis Rheumatol.* 2019;71(9):1400–1412.

9. Fanouriakis A, Kostopoulou M, Alunno A, Aringer M, Bajema I, Boletis JN, *et al.* 2019 update of the EULAR recommendations for the management of systemic lupus erythematosus. *Ann Rheum Dis.* 2019;78(6):736–745.

10. Weening JJ, D'Agati VD, Schwartz MM, Seshan S V, Alpers CE, Appel GB, *et al.* The classification of glomerulonephritis in systemic lupus erythematosus revisited. *Kidney Int.* 2004;65(2):521–530.

11. Weening JJ, D'Agati VD, Schwartz MM, Seshan S V, Alpers CE, Appel GB, *et al.* The classification of glomerulonephritis in systemic lupus erythematosus revisited. *J Am Soc Nephrol.* 2004;15(2):241–250.

12. Rovin BH, Ayoub IM, Chan TM, Liu ZH, Mejía-Vilet JM, Floege J. KDIGO 2024 clinical practice guideline for the management of lupus nephritis. *Kidney Int.* 2024;105(1):S1–S69.

13. Tektonidou MG, Andreoli L, Limper M, Amoura Z, Cervera R, Costedoat-Chalumeau N, *et al.* EULAR recommendations for the management of antiphospholipid syndrome in adults. *Ann Rheum Dis.* 2019;78(10):1296–1304.

14. Gutiérrez-González LA. Rheumatologic emergencies. *Clin Rheumatol* [Internet]. 2015 [cited 2024 Feb 13];34(12):2011–2019.

15. Erkan D. Expert perspective: management of microvascular and catastrophic antiphospholipid syndrome. *Arthrit Rheumatol.* 2021;73(10):1780–1790.

16. Wolfe AM, Kellgren JH, Masi AT. The epidemiology of rheumatoid arthritis: a review. II. Incidence and diagnostic criteria. *Bull Rheum Dis.* 1968;19(3):524–529.

17. Cross M, Smith E, Hoy D, Carmona L, Wolfe F, Vos T, *et al*. The global burden of rheumatoid arthritis: estimates from the global burden of disease 2010 study. *Ann Rheum Dis.* 2014;73(7):1316–1322.

18. Amaya-Amaya J, Rojas-Villarraga A, Mantilla RD, Anaya JM. Rheumatoid arthritis. 2013 [cited 2024 Mar 1]. Available from: https://www.ncbi.nlm.nih.gov/books/NBK459454/

19. Turesson C, Jacobsson LTH. Epidemiology of extra-articular manifestations in rheumatoid arthritis. *Scand J Rheumatol* [Internet]. 2004 [cited 2024 Mar 1];33(2):65–73.

20. Kim EJ, Collard HR, King TE. Rheumatoid arthritis-associated interstitial lung disease: the relevance of histopathologic and radiographic pattern. *Chest* [Internet]. 2009 [cited 2024 Mar 1];136(5):1397.

21. Cojocaru M, Cohocaru IM ihaela, Chico B. New insight into the rheumatoid vasculitis. *Rom J Intern Med* [Internet]. 2015 [cited 2024 Mar 1];53(2):128–132.

22. Aletaha D, Neogi T, Silman AJ et al. 2010 Rheumatoid arthritis classification criteria: an American College of Rheumatology/European League Against Rheumatism collaborative initiative. *Arthritis Rheum* 2010;62: 256981.

23. Rheumatoid Arthritis | Harrison's Principles of Internal Medicine, 21e | AccessMedicine | McGraw Hill Medical [Internet]. [cited 2024 Mar 1]. Available from: https://accessmedicine .mhmedical.com/content.aspx?bookid=3095&sectionid=265438014

24. Fraenkel L, Bathon JM, England BR, St.Clair EW, Arayssi T, Carandang K, *et al*. American College of Rheumatology guideline for the treatment of rheumatoid arthritis. *Arthritis Rheumatol* [Internet]. 2021 [cited 2024 Mar 1];73(7):1108–1123.

25. Bussone G, Mouthon L. Interstitial lung disease in systemic sclerosis. *Autoimmun Rev* [Internet]. 2011 [cited 2024 Mar 1];10(5):248–255.

26. Chaisson NF, Hassoun PM. Systemic sclerosis-associated pulmonary arterial hypertension. *Chest* [Internet]. 2013 [cited 2024 Mar 1];144(4):1346.

27. Rheumatoid Arthritis | Current Medical Diagnosis & Treatment 2024 | AccessMedicine | McGraw Hill Medical [Internet]. [cited 2024 Mar 1]. Available from: https://accessmedicine .mhmedical.com/content.aspx?bookid=3343&sectionid=279931084

28. Kowal-Bielecka O, Fransen J, Avouac J, Becker M, Kulak A, Allanore Y, *et al*. Update of EULAR recommendations for the treatment of systemic sclerosis. *Ann Rheum Dis* [Internet]. 2017 [cited 2024 Mar 1];76(8):1327–1339.

29. Oldroyd AGS, Lilleker JB, Amin T, Aragon O, Bechman K, Cuthbert V, *et al*. British Society for Rheumatology guideline on management of paediatric, adolescent and adult patients with idiopathic inflammatory myopathy. *Rheumatology* [Internet]. 2022 [cited 2024 Mar 1];61(5):1760–1768.

30. Fardet L, Galicier L, Lambotte O, Marzac C, Aumont C, Chahwan D, *et al*. Development and validation of the HScore, a score for the diagnosis of reactive hemophagocytic syndrome. *Arthritis Rheumatol.* 2014;66(9):2613–2620.

31. Carter SJ, Tattersall RS, Ramanan AV. Macrophage activation syndrome in adults: recent advances in pathophysiology, diagnosis and treatment. *Rheumatology (Oxford).* 2019 Jan 1;58(1):5–17. doi: 10.1093/rheumatology/key006. PMID: 29481673.

32. West SC, Arulkumaran N, Ind PW, Pusey CD. Pulmonary-renal syndrome: a life threatening but treatable condition. *Postgrad Med J.* 2013 May;89(1051):274-83. doi: 10.1136/postgradmedj-2012-131416. Epub 2013 Jan 24. PMID: 23349383.

33. Boyle N, O'Callaghan M, Ataya A, Gupta N, Keane MP, Murphy DJ, McCarthy C. Pulmonary renal syndrome: a clinical review. *Breathe (Sheff).* 2022 Dec;18(4):220208. doi: 10.1183/20734735.0208-2022. Epub 2023 Jan 10. PMID: 36865943; PMCID: PMC9973488.

17 Interpreting Laboratory Diagnosis in Intensive Care *Urinary System*

Urmila Anandh, Divya Bajpai and Barnali Das

INTRODUCTION

The kidneys are extremely vulnerable to various kinds of damage, including in the intensive care unit. Worsening underlying disease, various medical and surgical interventions, multiple medications and their nephrotoxic potential both by themselves and also because of complex drug interactions create a milieu where kidneys become damaged. One of the major manifestations of kidney issues is the development of acute kidney injury.

Acute kidney injury (AKI) is defined as the sudden decline in the glomerular filtration rate, which manifests as a rise in serum creatinine and a drop in urine output in the patient [1, 2]. AKI is a heterogenous clinical syndrome with multiple underlying etiology, severity, and outcomes and is considered a part of a group of diseases known as acute kidney disorders (AKD). In some patients, it is transient, whereas in others, it is persistent and can lead to the development of chronic kidney disease. AKI is noted in 15% of all hospital admissions and in intensive care; almost half of admitted patients have/develop AKI [3]. The development of AKI in intensive care not only worsens electrolyte and acid-base abnormalities but is also responsible for increasing mortality [4, 5]. AKI also has significant prognostic implications. Current literature suggests that a significant percentage of patients eventually go on to develop chronic kidney disease (CKD) [6, 7]. The development of CKD in these patients increases their risk of other comorbidities, and there is an increased risk and incidence of coronary events in these patients [8]. In fact, AKI, AKD, and CKD are often considered as a continuum of a process (Figure 17.1).

DIAGNOSIS

Over the years, multiple diagnostic criteria for the diagnosis of AKI have been developed. The initial diagnostic criteria were that of RIFLE [9] and AKIN [10]. In 2012, Kidney Disease Improving Global Outcomes (KDIGO) developed the guidelines for the diagnosis of AKI, and a standardized grading of the severity of AKI was developed [11]. The KDIGO definition attempts to correct the confusion and challenges faced by clinicians and researchers taking care of patients with AKI. However, the definition of AKI is dependent on the baseline serum creatinine, which often is not available in the critical care unit. In the presence of renal functional reserve and long half-life, there are concerns about using serum creatinine as an indicator of estimated glomerular filtration rate (eGFR) [12]. Measurement of timed creatinine clearance, kinetic eGFR based on two serial measurements, utilization of iohexol clearance, and cystatin C-based eGFR measurements are suggested [13]. Many studies have cited issues in urine output measurements in the ICU and the utilization of these criteria in the diagnosis of AKI [14]. There are also concerns about the validity of the baseline creatinine level based on which the diagnosis of AKI is made [15–17].

These caveats are addressed in Table 17.1.

BASIC ROUTINE LABORATORY AND POINT-OF-CARE TESTS
Serum Creatinine Assay

Over the past fifty years, serum creatinine has been one of the fundamental parameters used in laboratory investigation, for assessing kidney function. In routine chemistry laboratories, the two primary creatinine assays commonly utilized are: (i) Jaffe alkaline picrate method, and (ii) enzymatic methodologies [18]. Conventional Jaffe methods are known for their reduced accuracy, often exhibiting false increase. Hence, rate kinetic and rate-blank kinetic alkaline picrate methods have been developed, to address challenges associated with method specificity and interference, arising from substances such as proteins, glucose and acetoacetate. Enzymatic methods demonstrate reduced interference and improved analytical sensitivity and specificity in comparison to Jaffe assays. Point-of-care testing (POCT) assays for direct measurement of creatinine in whole blood are widespread. Challenges inherent in creatinine methods encompass assay imprecision, calibration variability and susceptibility to interferences.

The use of serum creatinine as a measurement of kidney function brings about many issues. Initially, creatinine was not considered the ideal candidate for the measurement of glomerular filtration rate (GFR). As creatinine is generated from muscle, there are physiological variations in its level based on gender, ethnicity, and age. This is addressed by using the analyte in various standard equations to derive an estimated GFR as the measure of kidney function. One reason was

DOI: 10.1201/9781003449713-17

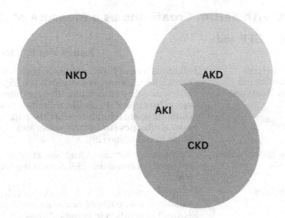

Figure 17.1   Acute kidney disorders and their link to chronic kidney disease.

Table 17.1   Challenges in the Diagnosis of AKI

Issue	Caveats
Available baseline serum creatinine (SCr)	An outpatient SCr is a better marker than inpatient values. There are many confounding variables in the measurement of SCr in the intensive care unit (catabolic state, fluid overload, nutritional status, drugs interfering in measurement). If multiple SCr levels are available, the lowest value should be considered for the diagnosis of AKI.
Unavailable outpatient Baseline SCr	In such a situation, the creatinine value corresponding to a GFR of 75 ml/min using the MDRD formula should be used. This leads to sensitivity and specificity issues in diagnosis, as eGFR is age-dependent. Also, the assumption that the patients had no renal dysfunction is fallacious.
Urine output criteria	Often the urine output measurement is inadequate in most ICUs and varies based on fluid resuscitation, use of diuretics, etc.
Body weight assessment	Often difficult in sick patients in the ICU. A dynamic number and using ideal or measured bodyweight has its own advantages and disadvantages. For research interventions, using ideal body weight may be more appropriate.

that the measurement of creatinine was done with Jaffe's reaction, and there were many endogenous substances (acetate, pyruvate) that were responsible for a positive reaction [18]. This led to an overestimation of 21%, which is compensated by the fact that there is approximately 28% tubular secretion in normal individuals [19]. This "accommodation" between the laboratory estimation and renal physiology is acceptable as long as renal function is normal. In uremic individuals, there is a significant extra-renal elimination (gut), which leads to a slower rise in creatinine commensurate with the decline in the GFR [20]. In addition, there are other laboratory methodology issues and pathophysiologic states where creatinine estimation does not give an accurate estimation of GFR (Table 17.2). Clinicians in the intensive care unit should be aware of these situations impacting creatinine estimation. A spurious estimation can lead to inappropriate drug dosing in ICUs. To overcome these limitations, newer laboratory techniques are being utilized in the estimation of this analyte [21–23]. Many authors also suggest the use of serum cystatin C in the diagnosis of kidney dysfunction.

Cystatin C in the Diagnosis of AKI in the ICU

Cystatin C (Scys), a cysteine protease inhibitor that has a half-life of 90 minutes, can be of help in the early diagnosis of AKI in ICUs. It can be easily measured, but it is also modified by age, gender, muscle mass, smoking status, inflammation, and malignancy [37]. In ICUs, this marker is of major advantage, as its level rises earlier than serum creatinine, and hence it is useful in early diagnosis of acute kidney injury [38, 39]. It also has a better performance in clinical situations

Table 17.2   Issues with Serum Creatinine as a Measure of Kidney Function

Serum Creatinine-Based eGFR and Kidney Function	Issues and Fallacies
Interference in the tenuous balance between laboratory estimation and tubular secretion of serum creatinine	Fallacious loss of function in situations with Waldenstrom's macroglobulinemia, ketoacidosis [24, 25]. Fallacious gain in function with hyperbilirubinemia [26]. Loss in function if drugs like trimethoprim-sulfamethoxazole, and cimetidine, are administered to the patient [27, 28]. Many antibiotics (aminoglycosides and cephalosporins) can cause a rise in creatinine [29].
Analytic interference of the Jaffe reaction	Dopamine, dobutamine, and N-acetylcysteine cause spurious reduction of creatinine [30] accounting for their "reno-protective" effect.
Interference in the production of creatinine	Overproduction in clinical situations of rhabdomyolysis [31] and situations where fenofibrate is administered [32]. Reduced generation in hepatic disease [33].
Physiologic limitations of creatinine	Impact of the muscle mass (in malnutrition, obesity) [34]. Dietary intake of cooked red meat increases serum creatinine levels [35, 36].

like extremes of age [40], patients with chronic liver disease, and malnourished individuals. In a meta-analysis of prospective cohort studies, Scys performed as a better marker of AKI in the ICU and was not significantly influenced by gender and age [41]. Recent studies have shown that Scys is a better marker of eGFR in patients who have been in ICUs for a long time. This marker becomes important, as muscle loss is common in patients with prolonged critical illness [42]. Serum cystatin C may be the analyte preferred in clinical situations of sepsis and contrast-induced AKI [43], and a combination of both cystatin c and creatinine may give a better idea of kidney function [44].

Basic Laboratory Investigations Differentiating the Types of AKI

AKI is a collection of various clinical syndromes that often manifest in a similar way – the rise in creatinine! This overdependence on a single biochemical variable often hinders the appropriate evaluation and therapy of AKI. It is important to note that the KDIGO definition of the diagnosis of AKI does not elucidate or educate the clinicians about the possible type and cause of AKI. It is also important to understand that multiple systemic insults leading to AKI don't follow similar pathophysiology, and hence we don't have a "one size fits all" therapeutic approach [45–47].

Traditionally AKI is differentiated into pre-renal, renal, and post-renal AKI (Figure 17.2). There are multiple causes for the various forms of AKI, and often one cause is responsible for more than one form of AKI. To a certain extent, there are laboratory investigations that help us differentiate between the forms of AKI and help guide the treatment of AKI.

Biochemical Investigations Differentiating Types of AKI

Urinary biochemistry was utilized more than 50 years ago to discriminate between pre-renal AKI and established acute tubular necrosis [48]. The commonly used indices are

1. Fractional excretion of sodium (FeNa)

2. Fractional excretion of urea (FeUrea)

The use of FeNa ([U/P] Na/[U/P] creatinine x100) for distinguishing between pre-renal AKI and established acute tubular necrosis is based on the premise that tubular function is preserved in a pre-renal state leading to avid sodium absorption. Thus, a FeNa of < 1% is suggestive of pre-renal AKI. However, this investigation has its limitations (Table 17.3) and loses its discriminatory power in non-oliguric AKI and AKI patients who have received diuretics. In obstructive renal failure, the FeNa is also < 1% [49, 50].

Similarly, FeUrea ([U/P] Urea/ [U/P] creatinine x100) is used to differentiate pre-renal AKI from ATN, and because the site of absorption of urea is proximal, it is minimally influenced by thiazide and loop diuretics. FeUrea of < 35% is suggestive of pre-renal AKI, and a value > 50% is considered to be reflective of ATN [51]. This index also has been shown to have limitations [52, 53].

There are many caveats to the optimal utilization of urinary indices in the diagnosis of pre-renal AKI, and these investigations are often not used in hospital-acquired AKI [54].

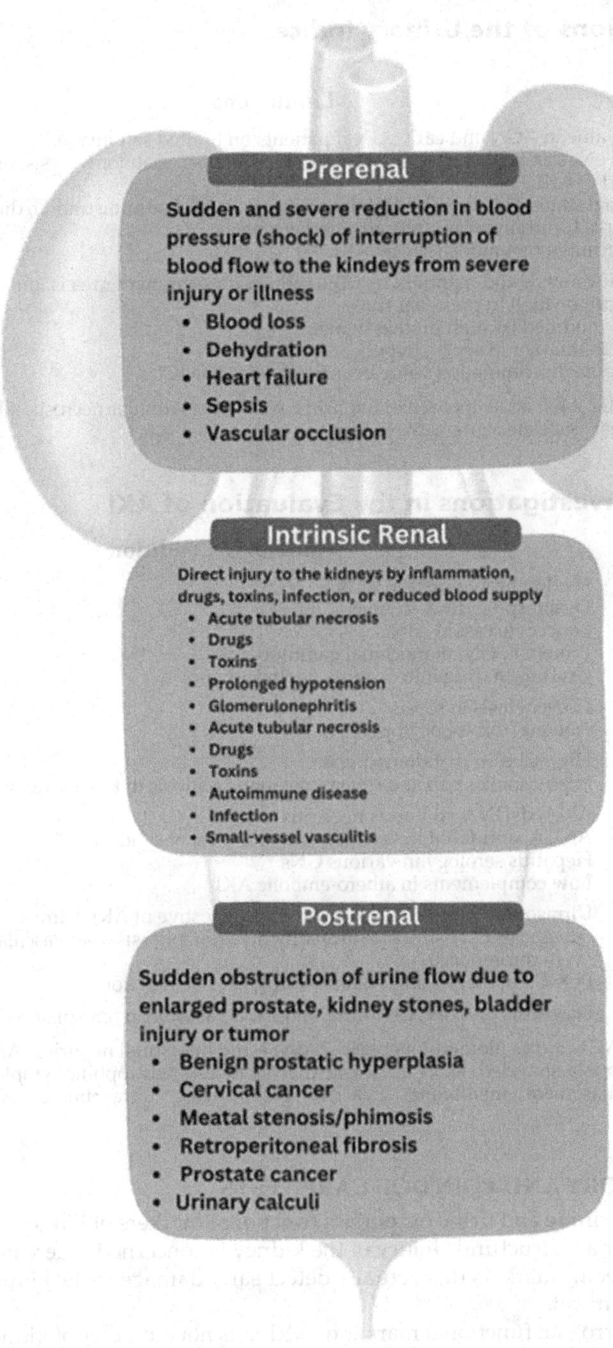

Prerenal

Sudden and severe reduction in blood pressure (shock) of interruption of blood flow to the kindeys from severe injury or illness
- Blood loss
- Dehydration
- Heart failure
- Sepsis
- Vascular occlusion

Intrinsic Renal

Direct injury to the kidneys by inflammation, drugs, toxins, infection, or reduced blood supply
- Acute tubular necrosis
- Drugs
- Toxins
- Prolonged hypotension
- Glomerulonephritis
- Acute tubular necrosis
- Drugs
- Toxins
- Autoimmune disease
- Infection
- Small-vessel vasculitis

Postrenal

Sudden obstruction of urine flow due to enlarged prostate, kidney stones, bladder injury or tumor
- Benign prostatic hyperplasia
- Cervical cancer
- Meatal stenosis/phimosis
- Retroperitoneal fibrosis
- Prostate cancer
- Urinary calculi

Figure 17.2 Various forms of AKI.

Laboratory Investigations in the Evaluation of the Cause of AKI

Besides basic biochemistry, various other investigations are performed to find the cause of AKI [55, 56].

These investigations are briefly outlined in Table 17.4. Urine microscopy is a useful tool but rarely used in ICUs. One of the reasons for the underutilization is that patients are often catheterized, and the urine microscopy results often are fallacious. However, in clinical situations, wherever possible, urine microscopy should be done. The reader is advised to refer to various reviews on this subject, as a microscopic examination is beyond the scope of this chapter [57].

Table 17.3 Limitations of the Urinary Indices

Urinary Indices	Limitations
FeNa	Limited value in AGN and early AIN if patients on limited salt intake.
	In ATN, FeNa can be low in sepsis, chronic liver disease, rhabdomyolysis, hemoglobinuric AKI, and C-AKI.
	In pre-renal states, FeNa can be high in intravenous fluid administration, diuretic use, glucosuria, bicarbonaturia, and salt wasting states.
	Less discriminating value in sepsis-AKI.
FeUrea	In osmotic diuresis and mannitol use, the tubular absorption of urea is impaired, hence FeUrea can be high in pre-renal states.
	FeUrea is modified by high protein intake.
	Not a useful marker in septic, hyper-catabolic states.
	Questionable discriminating value in critically ill in the ICUs.

AGN: acute glomerulonephritis; AIN: acute interstitial nephritis; ATN: acute tubular necrosis; AKI: acute kidney injury, C-AKI: contrast associate acute kidney injury

Table 17.4 Other Investigations in the Evaluation of AKI

Diagnostic Tests	Pathologic Condition
Urine microscopy	Muddy brown casts in ATN
	Dysmorphic RBCs in AGN
	Leucocyte cast in AIN
	Protein in GN, monoclonal gammopathy
	Crystals in drug intoxication, nephrolithiasis
Complete blood count	Leucocytosis in sepsis
	Anemia, thrombocytopenia is TMA
Other biochemical investigations	High CPK in rhabdomyolysis
	High osmolar gap and severe metabolic acidosis in toxin-induced AKI
Serologic investigations	ANA, dsDNA, in Lupus nephritis
	ANCA, anti-GBM in various pulmonary-renal syndromes
	Hepatitis serology in various GNs
	Low complements in athero-embolic AKI
Ultrasound with POCUS	Ultrasound: normal size kidneys are suggestive of AKI. Ultrasound helps in the diagnosis of obstructive uropathy (hydronephrosis) and vascular insults (renal vein thrombosis)
	POCUS in diagnosing volume status, cardiac function
Renal biopsy	Diagnosis of AGN, vasculitis, and AIN. Valuable in unexplained AKI

ATN: acute tubular necrosis; AGN: acute glomerulonephritis; AIN: acute interstitial nephritis; ANA: antinuclear antibody; dsDNA: double-stranded deoxy nucleic acid; ANCA: anti-neutrophilic cytoplasmic antibody; GBM: glomerular basement membrane; POCUS: point-of-care ultrasound; TMA: thrombotic microangiopathy

ADVANCED LABORATORY AND POINT-OF-CARE TESTS

Ironically, both serum creatinine and urine output are functional markers of kidney damage and hence are misnomers as far as "structural" injury of the kidney is concerned. There is hence an urgent requirement for specific markers that actually detect early damage to the kidneys before the functional changes manifest.

Serum creatinine is a surrogate functional marker of AKI. It is not a marker of kidney damage. In addition, the rise of serum creatinine is often late, and the diagnosis of AKI is often delayed. There is an urgent unmet need to have biomarkers that can diagnose AKI at an early stage.

Biomarkers in AKI

The need for biomarkers in acute kidney injury (AKI) arises from the fact that there is a significant time lag between the tubular injury and the rise in serum creatinine. Thus, various investigational biomarkers are being evaluated to detect tubular injury early in a patient with "sub-clinical AKI." Early detection will be especially valuable when causative factors for AKI can be alleviated, like exposure to iodinated contrast media or other nephrotoxins [58]. Also, biomarkers can reflect upon the pathogenesis of kidney injury and may aid the distinction between acute tubular injury and other conditions like acute interstitial nephritis, which will have therapeutic implications [59].

Moreover, biomarker profiles can unmask unique injury patterns (e.g., septic vs. ischemic), which can often have overlapping clinical findings [60]. To date, there is no effective treatment for AKI. Biomarkers can prove helpful in research settings for the early recruitment of patients and randomization to treatment arms [61]. This will facilitate the evaluation of novel therapeutic targets before the phase of established tubular necrosis. If effective treatment options for AKI become available in the future, early detection of AKI with the help of biomarkers will optimize the management of patients with AKI. Rarely, creatinine elevation might represent a defect in its excretion and not true AKI as in the case of vancomycin + piperacillin-tazobactam use. Here, normal values of biomarkers confirm pseudo-toxicity [62] (Figure 17.3). Various biomarkers available for the evaluation of AKI are described in Table 17.5.

Combination of Biomarkers

Evidence suggests that combining various biomarkers improves their sensitivity for early detection of AKI [81]. Thus, many manufacturers have now created panels and urinary scores for diagnosis and prognostication of AKI [82]. These can also be combined with traditional markers like serum creatinine. For example, Basu et al. evaluated a combination of urinary NGAL and cystatin C combined with creatinine and urea for predicting AKI in patients undergoing cardiac surgery [83]. Similarly, a panel of urinary NGAL and urinary KIM-1 predicted dialysis initiation or in-hospital death in patients at the emergency department [84]. In patients with liver cirrhosis and ATN, significantly higher values of NGAL, IL-18, KIM-1, L-FABP, and albumin were found [85].

Current Limitations in Clinical Use and Future Directions

There are significant technical challenges in standardizing and validating the biomarkers. It is vital that these tests have a minimal turn-around time when being used for early detection of AKI. They also need to be cost-effective to promote widespread use in resource-limited settings where the outcomes of AKI are severely compromised. It must be remembered that all the biomarkers available to date provide modest benefits over traditional clinical tools in AKI diagnosis and management [86]. There is a scarcity of controlled trials that demonstrate a measurable clinical benefit

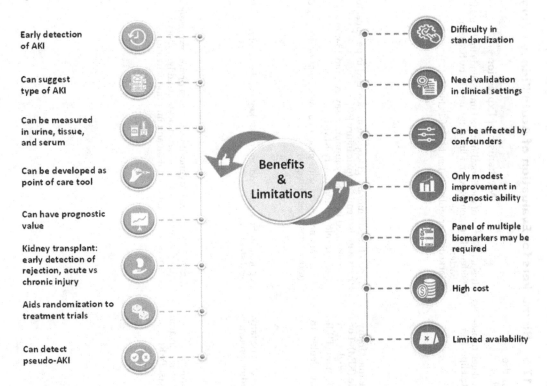

Figure 17.3 Biomarkers in AKI.

Table 17.5   Biomarkers for Evaluation of Acute Kidney Injury

Name of the Biomarker	Mechanism of Expression	Comments	Limitations
Neutrophil gelatinase-associated lipocalin (NGAL)	It is a member of the lipocalin superfamily, binds to the iron-siderophore complex, and limits the uptake by bacteria: bactericidal effect. Markedly upregulated after kidney ischemia [63]	Promising biomarker for early detection of acute tubular necrosis. Has been extensively evaluated in post-cardiac surgery and critically ill patients [64, 65]. Reported sensitivity and specificity for AKI diagnosis in cardiac surgery patients are 76% and 77% [66]. Can help to distinguish pre-renal AKI from ATN [67].	The threshold value for urinary NGAL is not very well-defined [68].
Urinary kidney injury molecule (KIM)–1 or T cell immunoglobulin mucin domain (TIM)-1	Type 1 transmembrane glycoprotein increased in proximal tubule cells with ischemic or toxic injury [69]. It is measured in urine by immunoassay. A rapid 15-min assay has been developed for urinary KIM-1.	In cardiac surgery patients, pre-operative KIM-1 and α-GST predicted AKI [70]. KIM-1 can aid distinction between ATN and other forms of AKI and CKD [69].	It is vulnerable to atherosclerotic vascular disease, diabetes, and hypertension.
Urinary interleukin-18 (IL-18)	An inflammatory cytokine produced by antigen-presenting cells (monocytes/macrophages)	Raised in pre-renal AKI, urinary tract infections, and CKD. Most of the data is from patients in intensive care units [71].	Suitable cut-off values are not well-defined. Conflicting evidence regarding its utility to predict AKI.
Urinary liver-type fatty acid-binding protein (L-FABP)	A potent antioxidant and one of the key regulators of free fatty acid stability.	Urinary excretion is increased in the stress of proximal tubular epithelial cells. Levels correlate with the severity of the ischemic tubular injury and can predict the need for dialysis and in-hospital mortality [72].	Liver function can affect values. Larger studies are needed for further validation.
Soluble urokinase plasminogen activator receptor (suPAR)	A glycosyl-phosphatidylinositol-anchored protein expressed on endothelial cells, podocytes, monocytes, and lymphocytes. A biomarker for inflammation and immune activation.	It triggers mitochondrial superoxide generation in kidney cells, causing a heightened energy demand, ultimately leading to kidney injury. It aids in the prediction of progressive decline in kidney function both in health and in CKD [73]. In critically ill patients, serum suPAR correlates with markers of organ dysfunction and guides prognosis [74].	It is also associated with infection, cardiovascular disease, liver disease, diabetes, and cancer.

Urinary low-molecular-weight proteins	They are α-1-microglobulin, β-2-microglobulin, urinary cystatin C, retinol-binding protein (RBP), and adenosine deaminase-binding protein (ABP).	In healthy individuals, they are completely reabsorbed with no secretion. Acute tubular injury leads to their urinary secretion [75].	Can also be present in mild reversible injury, which is clinically non-significant and has low specificity [76].
Urinary tubular enzymes	They are proximal renal tubular epithelial antigen (HRTE-1), αα–glutathione S-transferase (α-GST), pi-glutathione S-transferase (pi-GST), γ-glutamyl transpeptidase (γ-GT), alanine aminopeptidase (AAP), lactate dehydrogenase (LDH), N-acetyl glycosaminidase (NAG), and alkaline phosphatase (ALP).	They are released from proximal tubular cells within hours of injury.	Standardized detection methods and cut-offs are lacking.
Clusterin	Anti-apoptotic glycoprotein associated with cell adhesion and aggregation	Urinary clustering can serve as a marker for both glomerular and tubular injury [77].	More human data is needed.
Diagnostic and Prognostic markers			
Urinary insulin-like growth factor-binding protein 7 (IGFBP7) and tissue inhibitor of metalloproteinases-2 (TIMP2): Food and Drug Administration-approved test (NephroCheck).	IGFBP2 and TIMP2 are both inducers of G1 cell cycle arrest. Have tumor suppression properties.	In the Sapphire study, these outperformed other biomarkers in the identification and risk stratification of AKI in patients with sepsis (AUC = 0.82) or post-surgery (AUC = 0.85) [78].	The presence of proteinuria interferes with the assay. Also, raised urinary bilirubin > 7.2 g/dl invalidates the assay.
Urinary renin and angiotensinogen	Angiotensinogen is the substrate of the renin-angiotensin system (RAS). They regulate hemodynamics, natriuresis, aquaresis, cellular proliferation, fibrosis, and inflammation	In the cardiac surgery cohort, the urinary angiotensinogen to urinary creatinine ratio (uAnCR) and urine renin to creatinine ratio correlate with AKI severity and predict hospital stay [79].	Larger studies and validation of tests are needed.
Plasma NGAL		Plasma NGAL levels correlate with the severity of AKI. It aids the distinction between transient ischemia, AKI, and CKD [80].	Validation of cut-off is needed

of adding biomarkers in care management bundles. However, biomarkers have a definite role in some settings, like preventing drug-related AKI and identifying patients at high risk for adverse outcomes. Future studies must focus on moving the biomarkers from the bench to the bedside and exploring such therapeutic endpoints.

AKI ALERTS

Alerts from laboratory services aiding in the early detection of AKI can support clinicians in making therapeutic decisions, potentially facilitating early patient recovery. This approach is increasingly being implemented in various regions worldwide. AKI alerting systems are mandatory in several NHS hospitals in the UK. The algorithm is programmed into the laboratory system, and alerts are distributed through various communication modalities such as text messages to mobile devices and emails [87,88[. In some centers, the alert is also integrated into the electronic health record system. While many studies have not demonstrated significant overall benefits in outcomes, AKI alerts have heightened physicians' awareness of possible AKI risks in their patients. It has also led to specific behavioral changes among doctors, such as modifications in nephrotoxic medication use and adjustments in fluid management practices [89–91].

Interpretations by Authorities Defining AKI

Over the past few decades, a spectrum of over 35 distinct definitions of AKI have been utilized [92]. The vast number of definitions for AKI has led to significant variability in reported incidence rates, thereby posing challenges. This, at times, renders comparisons across available published research on AKI difficult or impractical [93–95]. Consequently, it has become imperative to develop a consensus-based and precise definition of AKI that can be universally adopted. Table 17.6 provides information on the diagnostic and staging criteria for AKI.

Table 17.6 Summary of Diagnostic and Staging Criteria for AKI

Classification	AKI Definition	Stage	SCr Criteria for Staging
RIFLE [96]	Rise in serum creatinine ≥ 50% in 7 days or urine volume < 0.5 mL/kg/h for 6–12 h	Risk	Increase in serum creatinine ≥ 1.5 times baseline or decrease in GFR ≥ 25%; or urine volume < 0.5 mL/kg/h for 6–12 h
		Injury	Increase in serum creatinine ≥ 2 times baseline or decrease in GFR ≥ 50%; or urine volume < 0.5 mL/kg/h for 12 h
		Failure	Increase in serum creatinine ≥ 3 times baseline or decrease in GFR ≥ 75%; or urine volume < 0.3 mL/kg/h for 24 h; or anuria for 12 h
		Loss	Complete loss of kidney function > 4 weeks
		End-stage kidney disease	Complete loss of kidney function > 3 months
AKIN [97]	Rise in SCr ≥ 0.3 mg/dl (26.5 μmol/L) or ≥ 50% increase in serum creatinine (1.5 times from baseline) in 48 hours or reduction in urine volume < 0.5 mL/kg/h for > 6 h	1	Increase in serum creatinine ≥ 0.3 mg/dL (26.5 mmol/L); or increase in blood creatinine to 1.5–2 times from baseline; or urine volume < 0.5 mL/kg/h for 6–12 h
		2	Increase in blood creatinine to 2–3 times from baseline; or urine volume < 0.5 mL/kg/h for 12 h
		3	Increase in blood creatinine to 3 times from baseline; or blood creatinine 4.0 mg/dL (354 mmol/L); or initiation of kidney replacement therapy; or urine volume < 0.3 mL/kg/h for 24 h; or anuria for 12 h

(Continued)

Table 17.6 (Continued)

Classification	AKI Definition	Stage	SCr Criteria for Staging
KDIGO 2012 [98]	Increase in serum creatinine by ≥ 0.3 mg/dL (26.5 mmol/L) within 48 h; or increase in blood creatinine to 1.5 times baseline, known or presumed to have occurred in the past 7 days; or urine volume < 0.5 mL/kg/h for 6 h	1	Increase in serum creatinine ≥ 0.3 mg/dL (26.5 mmol/L); or increase in blood creatinine to 1.5–1.9 times from baseline; or urine volume < 0.5 mL/kg/h for 6–12 h
		2	Increase in serum creatinine to 2.0–2.9 times from baseline; or urine volume < 0.5 mL/kg/h for 12 h
		3	Increase in serum creatinine to 3 times from baseline; or blood creatinine ≥ 4.0 mg/dL (354 mmol/L); or initiation of kidney replacement therapy; or decrease in eGFR to < 35 mL/min/1.73m2 in patients < 18 years; or urine volume < 0.3 mL/kg/h for 24 h; or anuria for 12 h
20/20 AACC AKI criteria [99]	The new AACC guidance recommends using a +0.20 mg/dL (~ 20 µmol/L) change in creatinine when the baseline is less than 1.00 mg/dL (~ 90 µmol/L), or a +20% change when baseline serum creatinine is greater than 1.0 mg/dL	Risk	Rise in serum creatinine 0.20 mg/dL, if < 1.00 mg/dL baseline or rise of 20% if baseline serum creatinine > 1.00 mg/dL

In April 2019, KDIGO convened a conference in Rome, Italy, titled "Acute Kidney Injury." Participants reviewed and analyzed information published since 2012, concerning the diagnosis, risk assessment, and management of AKI patients, sharing their perspectives on areas of consensus and divergence [100]. The objectives were to provide the research and clinical communities with a comprehensive overview of the current state of AKI diagnosis and management and to prepare for future revisions of the 2012 guidelines.

Need for AACC (Currently Academy of Diagnostic and Laboratory Medicine (ADLM)) Guidelines for AKI

In order to enhance patient outcomes and healthcare quality by promoting best practices, the AACC developed a guidance document [99]. This document was formulated with input from multidisciplinary experts, including laboratory scientists and nephrologists, and is grounded in the prevailing evidence. Its purpose is to guide laboratory practitioners and clinicians in the investigation of AKI. It is important to note that addressing scenarios where AKI may develop involves not only biomarker assessments but also the implementation of proactive measures to prevent its occurrence or reduce its severity. One of the principal recommendations in the guidance was to address a deficiency in the existing criteria for AKI identification, using creatinine testing, which was established by the KDIGO guidelines in 2012, as the primary diagnostic tool for this condition. Recent research has associated the application of KDIGO diagnostic criteria with an increased incidence of false-positive diagnoses of AKI. To rectify this issue, the AACC guidance recommends the adoption of novel diagnostic thresholds, termed the 20/20 AACC AKI criterion with creatinine tests, in order to evaluate the possible presence of AKI in patients.

The 20/20 AACC AKI guidance document, released by AACC, seeks to provide enhanced guidance to clinicians and diagnosticians in their assessments of AKI, with the objective of advancing best practices to enhance patient outcomes.

Sources of analytical variability in creatinine measurement encompass assay imprecision, calibration discrepancies (both inter-method and intra-method, day-to-day variability), and analytical interferences. Given that the definition and staging of AKI predominantly rely on fluctuations in blood creatinine levels, controlling assay imprecision and minimizing interferences are critical issues to be prioritized. Furthermore, ensuring minimal between-method bias is crucial when monitoring AKI using results obtained from multiple laboratories. The documented intra-individual biological variability of blood creatinine in healthy adults is reported to be 4.5%.

One significant recommendation of the guidance is the adoption of new diagnostic thresholds for AKI, known as the 20/20 AACC AKI criteria. The KDIGO guidelines, which define a +0.3 mg/dL change in baseline creatinine as indicative of AKI, have been associated with elevated rates of false-positive diagnoses, in as much as up to 30.5% of individuals with chronic kidney disease [101]. In contrast, the updated AACC guidance proposes employing a criterion of +0.20 mg/dL (~ 20 µmol/L) for creatinine changes when the baseline is below 1.00 mg/dL (~ 90 µmol/L), or a +20% change when baseline blood creatinine exceeds 1.00 mg/dL. These adjustments could potentially enhance sensitivity in detecting AKI. Evidence from a study involving 14,912 adult patients supports the adoption of these updated criteria, showing that same-day changes of 0.20 mg/dL or 20% are correlated with all-cause mortality [102].

The updated criteria aim to enhance the precision of AKI diagnosis. In populations such as geriatrics and pediatrics, where baseline creatinine levels are low, approximately 0.5 mg/dL, it may require more time to achieve a 0.3 mg/dL absolute increase. When baseline creatinine levels are high, approximately 4 mg/dL, a 0.3 mg/dL absolute change may be of limited significance, making the percentage change more meaningful. The 20/20 AACC AKI guidance document addresses the challenge of biological variability affecting diagnostic thresholds and the definition of "baseline" creatinine.

AKI Electronic Alerts

Over the past decade, the emergence of new electronic tools and biomarkers has facilitated the identification of patients at a higher risk of AKI and has enabled the early detection of AKI-associated changes. Nevertheless, human trials have questioned the efficacy of these electronic tools and biomarkers. Furthermore, universal access to technology has emerged as a significant barrier to its implementation.

Advanced analytical tools such as machine learning (ML) have empowered the development of robust support systems that facilitate efficient management in busy hospital settings. An E-alert system developed using a machine learning algorithm, aligned with AKI criteria defined by international standards, has the potential to promptly identify AKI patients and mitigate its effects effectively [103]. An algorithm was formulated based on the KDIGO 2012 criteria, with its logical framework, illustrated in Figure 17.4, to identify and flag patients exhibiting AKI in the dataset [95].

These outcomes can be evaluated in terms of mortality rates, length of hospital stay, and progression to CKD in individuals. The recently published "KDIGO 2024 Clinical Practice Guideline for the Evaluation and Management of Chronic Kidney Disease" suggests that clinicians should not define chronicity based on a single abnormal level for eGFR and urine albumin to creatinine ratio, as this could be due to a recent acute kidney injury event or acute kidney disease [104]. As already discussed, there is biological and analytical variability in serum creatinine assays. Thus, repeat testing to confirm the diagnosis is based on risk factors for CKD as well as concern for AKI/AKD.

In conclusion, it is essential to comprehend the underlying dynamics of biochemical factors and other disease-related variables to identify patients predisposed to developing AKI. This understanding will enable early intervention or control measures for such patients.

SOME CLINICAL PEARLS

1. Acute kidney injury (AKI) is defined as the sudden decline in the glomerular filtration rate which manifests as a rise in the serum creatinine and a drop in the urine output.

2. The basic laboratory investigation used over more than last 50 years in the assessment of kidney function has been serum creatinine.

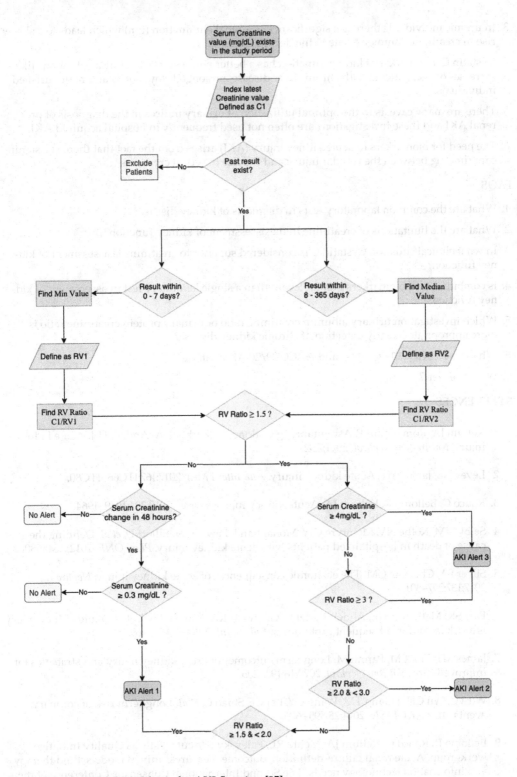

Figure 17.4 KDIGO 2012 logic for AKI flagging [95].

3. In uremic individuals there is a significant extra-renal elimination (gut) which leads to a slower rise in creatinine commensurate to the decline in the GFR.

4. Cystatin C as a marker of kidney function has a better performance in clinical situations like extremes of age, patients with chronic liver disease, prolonged stay in ICU and malnourished individuals.

5. There are many caveats to the optimal utilization of urinary indices in the diagnosis of pre-renal AKI and these investigations are often not used frequently in hospital acquired AKI.

6. The need for biomarkers in acute kidney injury (AKI) arises from the fact that there is a significant time lag between the tubular injury and the rise in serum creatinine.

FAQS

1. What are the common laboratory tests in diagnosis of kidney disease?

2. What are the limitations of creatinine in the assessment of kidney function?

3. In what clinical situation Cystatin C is considered superior to creatinine is assessment of kidney function?

4. Is combination of biomarkers more relevant than a single laboratory test in assessment of kidney functions?

5. Which investigation urinary albumin creatinine ratio or urinary protein creatinine ratio is more appropriate in early detection of chronic kidney disease?

6. What are KDIGO 2012 Criteria and AACC 20/20 AKI Criteria?

7. What is e alert?

REFERENCES

1. Kellum JA, Romagnani P, Ashuntantang G, Ronco C, Zarbock A, Anders H-J. Acute kidney injury. *Nature Rev Nephrol.* 2021;7:52.

2. Levey AS, James MT. Acute kidney injury. *Ann Intern Med.* 2017;167:ITC66–ITC80.

3. Ronco C, Bellomo R, Kellum JA. Acute kidney injury. *Lancet.* 2019;394:1949–1964.

4. Selby NM, Kolhe NV, McIntyre CW, Monaghan J, Lawson N, Elliott D, *et al.* Defining the cause of death in hospitalized patients with acute kidney injury. *PLoS ONE.* 2012;7:e48580.

5. Silver SA, Chertow GM. The economic consequences of acute kidney injury. *Nephron.* 2017;137:297–301.

6. Parr SK, Mathenly ME, Abdel -Kadel K, Greevy Jr RA, Bian A, Fly J, *et al.* Acute kidney injury is a risk factor for subsequent proteinuria. *Kidney Int.* 2018;93:460–469.

7. James MT, Bhatt M, Pannu M. Long term outcomes of acute kidney injury and strategies for improved care. *Nat Rev Nephrol.* 2020;16:193–205.

8. Wu VC, Wu CH, Huang TM, Wang CY, Lai CF, Shiao C, *et al.* Long-term risk of coronary events after AKI. *JASN.* 2014;25:595–605.

9. Bellomo R, Ronco C, Kellum JA, Mehta RL, Palevsky P; Acute Dialysis Quality Initiative workgroup. Acute renal failure-definition, outcome measures, animal models, fluid therapy and information technology needs. The Second International Consensus Conference of the Acute Dialysis Quality Initiative (ADQI) Group. *Crit Care.* 2004;8:R204–R212.

10. Mehta RL, Kellum JA, Shah SV, Mollitoris BA, Ronco C, Warnock DG, Levin A. Acute kidney injury network: report of an initiative to improve outcomes in acute kidney injury. *Crit Care*. 2007;11:R31.

11. Kellum JA. KDIGO clinical practice guideline for acute kidney injury, Section 2. AKI definition. *Kidney Int Suppl*. 2012;2:19–36.

12. Ronco C, Bellomo R, Kellum J. Understanding renal functional reserve. *Intensive Care Med*. 2017;43:917–920.

13. Chen S. Retooling the creatinine clearance equation to estimate GFR when the plasma creatinine is changing acutely. *J Am Soc Nephrol*. 2013;24:877–888.

14. Kellum JA, Silaneu FE, Murugan R, Lucko N, Shaw AD, Clemont G. Classifying AKI by urine output versus serum creatinine level. *J Am Soc Nephrol*. 2015;26:2231–2238.

15. Siew ED, Ikizler TA, Matheny ME, Shi Y, Schildcrout JS, Danciu I, *et al*. Estimating baseline kidney function in hospitaliszed patients with impaired kidney function. *Clin J Am Soc Nephrol*. 2012;7:712–719.

16. Siew ED, Matheny ME, Ikizler TA, Lewis JB, Miller RA, Waitman LR, *et al*. Commonly used surrogates for baseline renal function affect the classification and prognosis of acute kidney injury. *Kidney Int*. 2010;77:536–542.

17. Pickering JW, Endre ZH. Back-calculating baseline creatinine with MDRD misclassifies acute kidney injury in the intensive care unit. *Clin J Am Soc Nephrol*. 2010;5:1165–1173.

18. Dunea G, Freedman P. Serum creatinine. *JAMA*. 1968;204:163.

19. Diskin CJ. Creatinine and glomerular filtration rate: evolution of an accommodation. *Ann Clin Biochem*. 2007;44:16–19.

20. Carrie BJ, Golbetz HV, Michaels AS, Myers BD. Creatinine: an inadequate filtration marker in glomerular disease. *Am J Med*. 1980;69:177–182.

21. Panteghini M. Enzymatic assays for creatinine: time for action. *Scand J Clin Lab Invest Suppl*. 2008;241:84–88.

22. Cobbaert CM, Baadenhuijsen H, Weykamp CW. Prime time for enzymatic creatinine methods in pediatrics. *Clin Chem*. 2009;241:55:549–558.

23. Drion L, Cobbaert C, Groenier KH, Weykamp C, Bilo Henk JG, Wetzels JFM, *et al*. Clinical evaluation of analytical variations in serum creatinine measurements: why laboratories should abandon Jaffe techniques. *BMC Nephrol*. 2012;13:133.

24. Molitch ME, Rodman E, Hirsch CA, Dubinsky E. Spurious serum creatinine elevations in ketoacidosis. *Ann Intern Med*. 1980;93:280–281.

25. Hummel KM, von Ahsen N, Kuhn RB, Kaboth U, Grunewald RW, Oellerich M, *et al*. Pseudohypercreatininemia due to positive interference in enzymatic creatinine measurements caused by monoclonal IgM in patients with Waldenstrom's macroglobulinemia. *Nephron* 2000;86:188–189.

26. Halstead AC, Nanji AA. Artifactual lowering of serum creatinine levels in the presence of hyperbilirubinemia. *JAMA*. 1984;251:38–39.

27. Berglund F, Killander J, Pompeius R. Effect of trimethoprim-sulfamethoxazole on the renal excretion of creatinine in man. *J Urol*. 1975;114:802–808.

28. Burgess E, Blair A, Krichman K, Cutler RE. Inhibition of renal creatinine secretion by cimetidine in humans. *Ren Physiol*. 1982;5:27–30.

29. Syal K, Banerjee D, Srinivasan A. Creatinine estimation and interference. *Ind J Clin Biochem*. 2013;28:210–211.

30. Daly TM, Kempe KC, Scott MG. Bouncing creatinine levels. *N Engl J Med*. 1996;334:1749–1750.

31. Perrone RD, Madias NE, Levey AS. Serum creatinine as an index of renal function: new insights into old concepts. *Clin Chem*. 1992;38:1933–1953.

32. Hottelart C, El Asper N, Rose F, Achard JM, Fournier A. Fenofibrate increases creatininemia by increasing metabolic production of creatinine. *Nephron*. 2002;92:536–541.

33. Papadakis MA, Arieff AI. Unpredictability of clinical evaluation of renal function in cirrhosis. Prospective study. *Am J Med*. 1987;82:945–952.

34. Cook JG. Factors influencing the assay of creatinine. *Ann Clin Biochem*. 1975;12:219–232.

35. Preiss DJ, Godber IM, Lamb EJ, Dalton RN, Gunn IR. The influence of a cooked-meat meal on estimated glomerular filtration rate. *Ann Clin Biochem*. 2007;44:35–42.

36. Delanaye P, Cavalier E, Pottel H. Serum creatinine: not so simple. *Nephron*. 2017;136:302–308.

37. Bagshaw SM, Bellomo R. Cystatin C in acute kidney injury. *Curr Opin Crit Care*. 2010;16:533–539.

38. Dharnidharka V, Kwon C, Stevens G. Serum cystatin C is superior to serum creatinine as a marker of kidney function: a meta-analysis. *Am J Kidney Dis*. 2002;40:221–226.

39. Roos J, Doust J, Tett SE, Kirkpatrick. Diagnostic accuracy of cystatin C compared to serum creatinine for the estimation of renal dysfunction in adults and children—a meta-analysis. *Clin Biochem*. 2007;40:383–391.

40. Yang H, Lin C, Zhuang C, Chen J, Jia Y, Shi H, *et al*. Serum cystatin C as a predictor of acute kidney injury in neonates: a meta-analysis. *J Pediat*. 2022;98:230–240.

41. Yong Z, Pei X, Zhu B, Yuan H, Zhao W. Predictive value of serum cystatin C for acute kidney injury in adults: a meta-analysis of prospective cohort trials. *Sci Rep*. 2017;7:41012.

42. Haines RW, Fowler AJ, Liang K, Pearse RM, Larsson AO, Puthucheary Z, *et al*. Comparison of cystatin C and creatinine in the assessment of measured kidney function during critical illness. *CJASN* 2023;18:997–1005.

43. Pei Y, Zhou G, Wang P, Shi F, Ma X Zhu J.Serum cystatin C, kidney injury molecule-1, neutrophil gelatinase-associated lipocalin, klotho and fibroblast growth factor-23 in the early prediction of acute kidney injury in a Chinese emergency cohort study. *Eur J Med Res*. 2022;27:39.

44. Che M, Wang X, Xie B, Huang R, Liu S, Yan Y, *et al*. Use of both serum cystatin C and creatinine as diagnostic criteria for cardiac surgery-associated acute kidney injury and its correlation with long-term major adverse events. *Kidney Blood Press Res*. 2019;44:415–425.

45. Singbarti K, Kellum JA. AKI in the ICU: definition, epidemiology, risk stratification, and outcomes. *Kidney Int*. 2012;81:819–825.

46. Barasch J, Zager R, Bonventre JV. Acute kidney injury: a problem of definition. *Lancet*. 2017;389:779–781.

47. Kellum JA, Prowle JR. Paradigms of acute kidney injury in the intensive care setting. *Nat Rev Nephrol*. 2018;14: 217–230. https://doi.org/10.1038/snrneph.2017.184.

48. Espinel CH. The Fe Na test use in differential diagnosis of acute renal failure. *JAMA*. 1976;236:579–581.

49. Miller TR, Anderson RJ, Linas SL, Henrich WL, Berns AS, Gabow PA, *et al*. Urinary diagnostic indices in acute renal failure: a prospective study. *Ann Intern Med*. 1978; 89:47–50.

50. Pruc C, Kjellstrand C. Urinary indices and chemistries in the differential diagnosis of prerenal failure and acute tubular necrosis. *Semin Nephrol*. 1985;5:224–233.

51. Carvounis CP, Nisar S, Guro-Razuman S. Significance of the fractional excretion of urea in the differential diagnosis of acute renal failure. *Kidney Int*. 2002;62:2223–2229.

52. Pepin MN, Bouchard J, Legault L, Ethier J. Diagnostic performance of fractional excretion of urea and fractional excretion of sodium in the evaluations of patients with acute kidney injury with or without diuretic treatment. *Am J Kidney Dis*. 2007;50:566–573.

53. Lima C, Macedo E. Urinary biochemistry in the diagnosis of acute kidney injury. *Disease Markers*. 2018;2018:4907024. https://doi.org/10.1155/2018/4907024.

54. Diskin CJ, Stokes TJ, Dansby LM, Radcliff L, Carter TB. Toward the optimal clinical use of the fraction excretion of solutes in oliguric azotemia. *Ren Fail*. 2010;32:1245–1254.

55. Murithi AK, Nasr SH, Leung N. Utility of urine eosinophils in the diagnosis of acute interstitial nephritis. *CJASN*. 2013;8:1857–1862.

56. Thongprayoon C, Hansrivjit P, Kovvuru K, Kanduri SR, Torres-Ortiz A, Acharya P, *et al*. Diagnostics, risk factors, treatment and outcomes of acute kidney injury in a new paradigm. *J Clin Med*. 2020;9:1104.

57. Perazella MA, Coca SG. Traditional urinary biomarkers in the assessment of hospital-acquired AKI. *CJASN*. 2012;167–174.

58. Jamale TE, Hase NK. Acute kidney injury biomarkers: need to move from bench to bedside. *J Postgrad Med*. 2014;60:160.

59. Martinez Valenzuela L, Draibe J, Fulladosa X, Torras J. New biomarkers in acute tubulointerstitial nephritis: a novel approach to a classic condition. *Int J Mol Sci*. 2020;21:4690.

60. Molinari L, Del Rio-Pertuz G, Smith A, Landsittel DP, Singbarti K, Palevsky PM, *et al*. Utility of biomarkers for sepsis-associated acute kidney injury staging. *JAMA Netw Open*. 2022;5(5):e2212709.

61. Endre ZH, Walker RJ, Pickering JW, Shaw GM, Frampton CM, Henderson SJ, *et al*. Early intervention with erythropoietin does not affect the outcome of acute kidney injury (the EARLYARF trial). *Kidney Int*. 2010;77:1020–1030.

62. Miano TA, Hennessy S, Yang W, DunnTG, Weisman AR, Oniyide O, *et al*. Association of vancomycin plus piperacillin-tazobactam with early changes in creatinine versus cystatin C in critically ill adults: a prospective cohort study. *Intensive Care Med*. 2022;48:1144–1155.

63. Herget-Rosenthal S. One step forward in the early detection of acute renal failure. *Lancet Lond Engl*. 2005;365:1205–1206.

64. Haase M, Devarajan P, Haase-Fielitz A, Bellomo R, Cruz DN, Wagener G, *et al.* The outcome of neutrophil gelatinase associated lipocalin-positive subclinical acute kidney injury: a multicenter pooled analysis of prospective studies. *J Am Coll Cardiol.* 2011;57:1752–1761.

65. Mishra J, Dent C, Tarabishi R, Mitsnefes MM, Ma Q, Kelly CBS, *et al.* Neutrophil gelatinase-associated lipocalin (NGAL) a biomarker for acute renal injury after cardiac surgery. *Lancet Lond Engl.* 2005;365:1231–1238.

66. Haase M, Haase-Fielitz A, Bellomo R, Mertens PR. Neutrophil gelatinase-associated lipocalin as a marker of acute renal disease. *Curr Opin Hematol.* 2011;18(1):11–18.

67. Paragas N, Qiu A, Zhang Q, Samstein B, Deng SX, Schmidt-Ott KM, Viltard M, *et al.* The NGAL reporter mouse detects the response of the kidney to injury in real time. *Nat Med.* 2011;17:216–222.

68. Zou C, Wang C, Lu L. Advances in the study of subclinical AKI biomarkers. *Front Physiol.* 2022;13. https://www.frontiersin.org/articles/10.3389/fphys.2022.960059.

69. Han WK, Bailly V, Abichandani R, Thadhani R, Bonventre JV. Kidney Injury Molecule-1 (KIM-1): a novel biomarker for human renal proximal tubule injury. *Kidney Int.* 2002;62:237–244.

70. Koyner JL, Vaidya VS, Bennett MR, Qing M, Worcester E, Akhter SA, *et al.* Urinary biomarkers in the clinical prognosis and early detection of acute kidney injury. *CJASN.* 2010;5:2154–2165.

71. Parikh CR, Abraham E, Ancukiewicz M, Edelstein CL. Urine IL-18 is an early diagnostic marker for acute kidney injury and predicts mortality in the intensive care unit. *JASN.* 2005;16:3046–3052.

72. Susantitaphong P, Siribamrungwong M, Doi K, Noiri E, Terrin N, Jaber BL. Performance of urinary liver-type fatty acid-binding protein in acute kidney injury: a meta-analysis. *Am J Kidney Dis.* 2013;61:430–439.

73. Hayek SS, Leaf DE, Samman Tahhan A, Raad M, Sharma S, Waikar SS, *et al.* Soluble urokinase receptor and acute kidney injury. *N Engl J Med.* 2020;382:416–426.

74. Backes Y, van der Sluijs KF, Mackie DP, Tacke F, Koch A, Jyrki JT, *et al.* Usefulness of suPAR as a biological marker in patients with systemic inflammation or infection: a systematic review. *Intensive Care Med.* 2012;38:1418–1428.

75. Herget-Rosenthal S, Poppen D, Hüsing J, Marggraf G, Pietruck F, Heinz-Gunther J, *et al.* Prognostic value of tubular proteinuria and enzymuria in nonoliguric acute tubular necrosis. *Clin Chem.* 2004;50:552–558.

76. Trof RJ, Di Maggio F, Leemreis J, Groeneveld ABJ. Biomarkers of acute renal injury and renal failure. *Shock Augusta Ga.* 2006;26:245–253.

77. Musiał K, Augustynowicz M, Miśkiewicz-Migoń I, Kałwak K, Ussowicz M, Zwolińska D. Clusterin as a new marker of kidney injury in children undergoing allogeneic hematopoietic stem cell transplantation—a pilot study. *J Clin Med.* 2020;9:2599.

78. Kashani K, Al-Khafaji A, Ardiles T, *et al.* Discovery and validation of cell cycle arrest biomarkers in human acute kidney injury. *Crit Care Lond Engl.* 2013;17:R25.

79. Alge JL, Karakala N, Neely BA, *et al*. Urinary angiotensinogen and risk of severe AKI. *CJASN*. 2013;8:184–193.

80. Soto K, Papoila AL, Coelho S, *et al*. Plasma NGAL for the diagnosis of AKI in patients admitted from the emergency department setting. *CJASN*. 2013;8:2053–2063.

81. Han WK, Wagener G, Zhu Y, Wang S, Lee HT. Urinary biomarkers in the early detection of acute kidney injury after cardiac surgery. *CJASN*. 2009;4:873–882.

82. Hall IE, Coca SG, Perazella MA, *et al*. Risk of poor outcomes with novel and traditional biomarkers at clinical AKI diagnosis. *CJASN*. 2011;6:2740–2749.

83. Basu RK, Wong HR, Krawczeski CD, *et al*. Combining functional and tubular damage biomarkers improves diagnostic precision for acute kidney injury after cardiac surgery. *J Am Coll Cardiol*. 2014;64:2753–2762.

84. Nickolas TL, Schmidt-Ott KM, Canetta P, *et al*. Diagnostic and prognostic stratification in the emergency department using urinary biomarkers of nephron damage: a multicenter prospective cohort study. *J Am Coll Cardiol*. 2012;59:246–255.

85. Belcher JM, Sanyal AJ, Peixoto AJ, *et al*. Kidney biomarkers and differential diagnosis of patients with cirrhosis and acute kidney injury. *Hepatol Baltim Md*. 2014;60:622–632.

86. Schaub JA, Parikh CR. Biomarkers of acute kidney injury and associations with short- and long-term outcomes. *F 1000 Res*. 2016;5:986.

87. Colpaert K, Hoste EA, Steurbaut K, Benoit D, van Hoecke S, Turck F, *et al*. Impact of real-time electronic alerting of acute kidney injury on therapeutic intervention and progression of RIFLE class. *Crit Care Med*. 2012;40:1164–1170.

88. Porter CJ, Juurlink I, Bisset LH, Bavakunji R, Mehta RL, Devonald AAJ. Real time electronic alert to improve detection of acute kidney injury in a large teaching hospital. *Nephrol Dial Transplant*. 2014;29:1888–1893.

89. McCoy AB, Waitman LR, Gadd SC, Danciu J, Smith JP, Lewis JB, *et al*. A computerised provider order entry intervention for medication safety during acute kidney injury: a quality improvement report. *Am J Kidney Dis*. 2010;56:832–841.

90. Al-Jaghbeer M, DEalmeida D, Bilderback A, Ambrosino R, Kellum JA. Clinical decision support for in-hospital AKI. *JASN*. 2018;29:654–660.

91. Atia J, Evison F, Gallier S, Hewins P, Ball S, Gavin J, *et al*. Dose acute kidney injury alerting improve patient outcomes? *BMC Nephrol*. 2023;24:14.

92. Kellum John A, *et al*. Developing a consensus classification system for acute renal failure. *Curr Opin Crit Care*. 2002;8:509–514.

93. Schaefer JH, *et al*. Outcome prediction of acute renal failure in medical intensive care. *Intensive Care Med*. 1991;17:19–24.

94. Silvester W, *et al*. Epidemiology, management, and outcome of severe acute renal failure of critical illness in Australia. *Crit Care Med*. 2001;29:1910–1915.

95. Bhat L, Das B, Clinical validation and comparative study between the KDIGO 2012 AKI criteria and the AACC guidance document 2020. *Indian J Clin Biochem*. Published online on 06 September 2024. https://doi: 10.1007/s12291-024-01263-3

96. Bellomo R, *et al.* Acute renal failure - definition, outcome measures, animal models, fluid therapy and information technology needs: the Second International Consensus Conference of the Acute Dialysis Quality Initiative (ADQI) Group. *Crit Care.* 2004;8:R204–R212.

97. Mehta RL, *et al.* Acute Kidney Injury Network: report of an initiative to improve outcomes in acute kidney injury. *Crit Care.* 2007;11:R31.

98. Khwaja, A. KDIGO clinical practice guidelines for acute kidney injury. *Nephron Clin Pract.* 2012;120:c179–c184.

99. El-Khoury JM, *et al.* AACC guidance document on laboratory investigation of acute kidney injury. *Journal Appl Lab Med.* 2021;6:1316–1337.

100. Ostermann M, *et al.* Controversies in acute kidney injury: conclusions from a Kidney Disease: Improving Global Outcomes (KDIGO) Conference. *Kidney Int.* 2020:98:294–309. https://doi:10.1016/j.kint.2020.04.020.

101. Lin J, *et al.* False-Positive rate of AKI using Consensus Creatinine-Based Criteria. *Clin J Am Soc Nephrol.* 2015;10: 1723–1731. https://doi:10.2215/CJN.02430315.

102. Yeh HC, *et al.* 24-hour serum creatinine variation associates with short- and long-term all-cause mortality: a real-world insight into early detection of acute Kidney injury. *Sci. Rep.* 2020;10:6552. https://doi:10.1038/s41598-020-63315-x.

103. Tomašev N, *et al.* A clinically applicable approach to continuous prediction of future acute kidney injury. *Nature.* 2019;572:116–119. https://doi:10.1038/s41586-019-1390-1.

104. Levin A, *et al.* Executive summary of the KDIGO 2024 Clinical Practice Guideline for the Evaluation and Management of Chronic Kidney Disease: known knowns and known unknowns. *Kidney Int.* 2024;105:684–701. https://doi:10.1016/j.kint.2023.10.016.

18 Haematological Disorders

Anirban Hom Choudhuri and Santvana Kohli Arora

INTRODUCTION

Although haematological disorders are common secondary manifestations in many diseases in the intensive care unit (ICU), primary haematological disorders (HDs) are not uncommon admissions and carry higher all-cause mortality risk than patients without haematological disorders [1]. Advancements in the diagnosis and management of haematological disorders leading to better outcomes have led to an increased admission of such patients in ICUs. While the less common non-malignant haematological disorders present usually with leucocytosis and coagulopathies, the more common malignant haematological disorders present more often with anaemia and bleeding disorders. However, patients of both malignant and non-malignant aetiology can run a rapid downhill course due to immune-mediated reactions [2]. Hence, early recognition of the disorder helps in its management to give better outcomes. The right laboratory tests and their right interpretation play a big role in this.

Table 18.1 exhibits the common haematological disorders (both malignant and non-malignant) encountered in the ICU.

COMMON LABORATORY TESTS AND THEIR INTERPRETATION

Some common laboratory tests for detecting haematological disorders are mentioned below. Table 18.2 enlists the common haematological disorders and the main laboratory changes seen in them.

1. Complete blood count (CBC)

CBC is the most common laboratory test, and its correct interpretation is essential for diagnosis and monitoring of the disease course. Circulating blood cells, including red blood cells (RBCs), white blood cells (WBCs), and platelets, are counted and sized electronically. The Coulter counter generates an electrical pulse when a blood cell passes through a small aperture surrounded by electrodes. Each electrical pulse represents an individual cell, and the pulse height indicates the cell volume. Therefore, the electronic counter registers the total cell count, as well as estimates the average cell volume and cell size. These measurements for RBC are referred to as the mean corpuscular volume (MCV) and the RBC distribution width. Modern electronic counters are capable of multimodal assessment of cell size and content, thus differentiating the various categories of WBCs including neutrophils, lymphocytes, monocytes, eosinophils, and basophils (i.e., 5-part differential).

Table 18.1 Common Haematological Disorders (Malignant and Non-Malignant) in ICU

Malignant	Non-Malignant
Acute myeloid leukaemia – affects the white blood cells known as myeloid cells	RBC disorders • Anaemia (nutritional anaemia, anaemia of chronic disease, anaemia of renal insufficiency, haemolytic anaemia, aplastic anaemia) • Polycythaemia vera
Acute lymphoid leukaemia – affects the white blood cells known as lymphocytes	Platelet disorders – Thrombocytopenia - Thrombocytosis
Chronic myeloid leukaemia – bone marrow makes too many white blood cells	White cell disorders – Leucocytosis - Leukopenia
Chronic lymphoid leukaemia – affects the white blood cells known as lymphocytes	Clotting disorders – acquired and inherited
Hodgkin's lymphoma – develops in the lymph nodes of the lymphatic system	Haemoglobinopathies – Sickle cell disease - Thalassemia
Non-Hodgkin's lymphoma – appears as a solid tumour in the glands, usually of the neck, chest, armpit or groin	Myeloproliferative disorders (MPDS)
Small lymphocytic lymphoma	Myelodysplastic syndrome (MDS)
Myeloma – malignancy of plasma cells	

DOI: 10.1201/9781003449713-18

Table 18.2   Laboratory Changes Observed in Common Haematological Disorders Seen in ICU

S. No.	Disorder	Common Laboratory Changes
1.	Iron deficiency anaemia	• Low haemoglobin and low RBC count • Microcytic hypochromic picture • Thrombocytosis • Low serum ferritin • High reticulocyte count with therapy
2.	B12/folate deficiency	• Macrocytosis with or without overt anaemia (MCV > 100 fL) • Hyper-segmented neutrophils (more than 5% of PMN with more than five lobes is required) • Megaloblasts in bone marrow • Increased methylmalonic acid and homocysteine concentration in blood
3.	Haemolytic anaemia	• Low haemoglobin and low RBC count • High LDH and reduced haptoglobin • High indirect bilirubin • High reticulocyte count • Sickle cells on peripheral smear in sickle cell disease • Target cells and teardrop cells on smear in thalassemia
4.	Anaemia of chronic disease	• Low haemoglobin and low RBC count • Microcytic picture • Unremarkable peripheral smear
5.	Aplastic anaemia	• Presence of ≥ 2 of the following: • Absolute neutrophil count < 0.5×10^9/L • Absolute reticulocyte count < 60×10^9/L) • Platelet count < 20×10^9/L • Bone marrow with < 25% cellularity (hypocellularity) • Very severe aplastic anaemia is defined as absolute neutrophil count < 200/microL (< 0.2×10^9/L)
6.	ITP	• Thrombocytopenia • Peripheral smear may show platelet fragments or large platelets • Increased production of megakaryocytes in the bone marrow • Diagnosis of exclusion
7.	TTP/HUS	• Thrombocytopenia • Peripheral smear shows schistocytes • Increased LDH level and decreased haptoglobin level • May be associated with increased creatinine levels
8.	Disseminated intravascular coagulation (DIC)	• Prolonged coagulation times • Thrombocytopenia • High levels of fibrin degradation products (FDPs) • Elevated D-dimer levels • Schistocytes on peripheral smear
9.	Myelodysplasia	• Blood picture may range from single cytopenia, bicytopenia, to pancytopenia in later stages • RBCs are usually macro-ovalocytes with punctate basophilia • Morphological abnormalities in granulocytes – bilobed or unsegmented nuclei (pseudo-Pelger-Huet abnormality) or hyper-segmentation on the nuclei (6–7 lobes) • Giant hypogranular platelets and megakaryocyte fragments • Bone marrow changes include hypercellularity with trilineage dysplastic changes
10.	Acute myeloid leukaemia	• Pancytopenia • Blast cells ≥ 20% of marrow nucleated cells or ≥ 20% of nonerythroid cells (may approach 90% of WBC count) • This is distinguished from ALL by presence of Auer rods (red staining, elongated needle-like inclusions) in the cytoplasm of AML myeloblasts
11.	Chronic myeloid leukaemia	• Granulocyte count elevated, usually ≤ 50×10^9/L in asymptomatic patients and 200×10^9/L to $1,000 \times 10^9$/L in symptomatic patients • Neutrophilia (a left-shifted white blood cell differential), basophilia, and eosinophilia are common • Thrombocytosis may be seen

(Continued)

Table 18.2 (Continued)

S. No.	Disorder	Common Laboratory Changes
12.	Acute lymphoid leukaemia	• Pancytopenia • Blast cells ≥ 20% of marrow nucleated cells or ≥ 20% of nonerythroid cells (may approach 90% of WBC count) • Blast cells in the bone marrow are typically between 25 and 95% in patients with ALL
13.	Chronic lymphoid leukaemia	• Absolute peripheral lymphocytosis of $> 5 \times 10^9$/L • Peripheral blood flow cytometry can confirm clonality in circulating B cells
14.	Multiple myeloma	• Neoplastic proliferation of a single clone of plasma cells derived from B cells in the bone marrow • Production of an abnormal immunoglobulin called monoclonal protein (M protein) and free light chain proteins designated as kappa or lambda • Serum protein electrophoresis – M protein is the tumour marker • Bone marrow aspiration – at least 10% of the bone marrow nucleated cells should be plasma cells

RBC: red blood cells; PMN: polymorphonuclear cells; MCV: mean corpuscular volume; LDH: lactate dehydrogenase; ITP: idiopathic thrombocytopenic purpura; TTP/HUS: thrombotic thrombocytopenic purpura/ haemolytic uraemic syndrome

a. Haemoglobin and RBCs

Any fall in the haemoglobin level and RBC count indicates anaemia. The type of anaemia can be microcytic (low mean cell volume), macrocytic (high mean cell volume), or normocytic (normal mean cell volume) [3].

If there is microcytic hypochromic anaemia, the flow chart in Figure 18.1 can be useful for workup. One major cause of microcytic hypochromic anaemia is iron deficiency, which is diagnosed by high serum ferritin, low serum iron plus high total iron-binding capacity, transferrin levels, red cell protoporphyrin levels, or staining of bone marrow aspirates for iron. The differential diagnosis of iron deficiency anaemia includes anaemia of chronic disease (also known as anaemia of inflammation). The clinical and laboratory features of inflammation or chronic infection may suggest this diagnosis, which is confirmed by the demonstration of normal or high serum ferritin and reduced serum iron, transferrin, and iron-binding capacity. Serum soluble transferrin receptors may distinguish iron deficiency anaemia from anaemia of chronic disease when ferritin levels are not level, though further research is needed to know the overall diagnostic accuracy of these tests.

Similarly, while evaluating normocytic anaemia (Figure 18.2), the first step is to exclude potentially treatable causes like bleeding, nutritional anaemia, anaemia due to renal insufficiency, and haemolysis. Initial laboratory tests on suspicion of haemolysis should include serum haptoglobin, lactate dehydrogenase (LDH), and indirect bilirubin and reticulocyte count.

Use of certain drugs (e.g., hydroxyurea, zidovudine) and alcohol consumption is associated with macrocytosis and should be excluded during evaluation for macrocytic anaemia (Figure 18.3). The next step is to rule out nutritional causes (B_{12} or folate deficiency).

b. Total and differential leucocyte count

Leucocytosis has many potential aetiologies, both malignant and non-malignant. It is important to use age- and pregnancy-specific ranges for the interpretation of WBC count. A repeat CBC with peripheral smear may reveal the type and maturity of WBCs, their uniformity, and the presence or absence of toxic granulations. Leucocytosis indicates infection, particularly bacterial, and should prompt physicians to identify other signs and symptoms, and also determine the site of infection. The peripheral WBC count can double within hours after certain stimuli because of the large bone marrow storage and intravascular marginated pools of neutrophils. Apart from infection, other stressors capable of causing acute leucocytosis include surgery, exercise, trauma, emotional stress, certain medications, asplenia, smoking, obesity, and chronic inflammatory conditions [4].

c. Platelet count

The quantification of platelets by automated cell analysers is sometimes imperfect, as in vitro micro and EDTA-induced aggregation may lead to low counts. This fallacy can be ruled out by

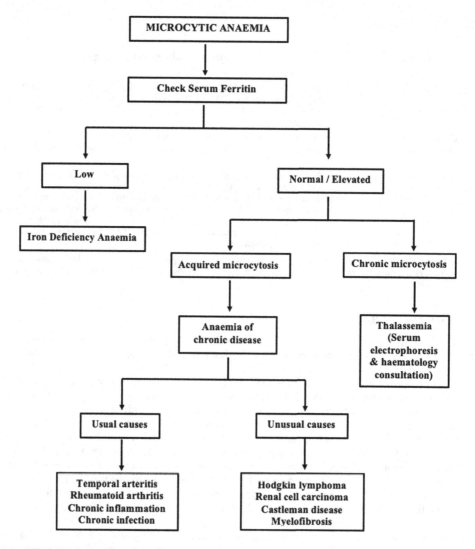

Figure 18.1 Diagnostic algorithm for microcytic anaemia.

recounting platelets in citrated blood. A platelet count $< 50 \times 10^9/L$ is associated with more risk of bleeding. A minimum target platelet count of $75 \times 10^9/L$ is appropriate in this situation.

Platelet function is traditionally tested by bleeding time. However, bleeding time may lack standardisation, be invasive, show subjective variations, and have low sensitivity and specificity in detecting mild disorders. Traditional assays, such as light transmittance aggregometry, are the gold standard for platelet function testing where platelet agonists are added to platelet-rich plasma and the increase of light transmittance is recorded as platelets start to aggregate.

Thrombocytopenia increases bleeding complications, and platelet transfusion is indicated prophylactically to reduce bleeding. Large multicentre studies on prophylactic platelet transfusions in thrombocytopenic non-ICU patients have found restrictive prophylactic platelet transfusion strategy to be safe, although the cut-off value is debatable (Figure 18.4) [5].

Thrombotic events may occur sometimes despite low platelet counts due to increased expression of procoagulant mediators by malignant cells, as in leukaemia [6]. Rapid cell death after chemotherapy can also increase the release of procoagulant factors into the bloodstream. Finally, central venous catheterisation is also a risk factor for thrombosis in patients with HMs.

2. Coagulation profile

Mostly, prothrombin time (PT) and activated partial thromboplastin time (aPTT) are the screening tests to detect abnormal haemostasis [7]. The INR, which is the PT ratio of a test sample compared

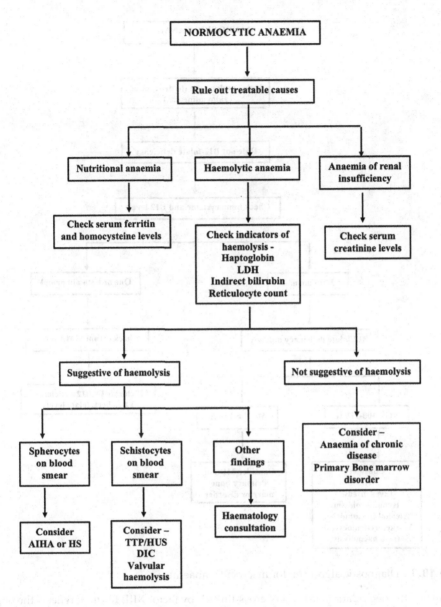

Figure 18.2 Diagnostic algorithm for normocytic anaemia.

with a normal PT, corrected for the sensitivity of the thromboplastin used in the test, is also reported. The PT measures the activity of the extrinsic pathway of coagulation and is dependent on the functional activity of factors II, V, VII, and X. It does not detect deficiencies in other coagulation factors. The PT is less sensitive to single-factor deficiency and remains normal until single-factor levels fall below 50%, but it is more sensitive to multiple-factor deficiencies. The aPTT measures the intrinsic and common pathways of the coagulation cascade and is sensitive to deficiencies of factors II, V, VIII, IX, XI, XII, high molecular weight kallikrein, and fibrinogen. It is most commonly used in ICU to monitor patients receiving unfractionated heparin. As with the PT, the aPTT is normal in mild factor deficiency, platelet dysfunction, mild von Willebrand disease, and factor XIII deficiency.

3. Fibrin degradation products and D-dimer

Fibrinogen (or fibrin) degradation products (FDPs) are released following plasmin-mediated degradation of fibrinogen or fibrin. The D-dimer is a specific fragment formed only upon degradation of cross-linked fibrin. The typical normal range is <10 µg/mL (serum) or <5 µg/mL (plasma) [8].

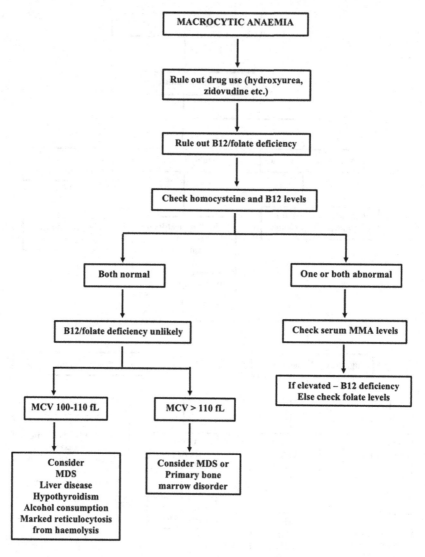

Figure 18.3 Diagnostic algorithm for macrocytic anaemia.

D-dimer is the degradation product of cross-linked (by factor XIII) fibrin. It reflects the ongoing activation of the haemostatic system. The reference concentration of D-dimer is < 250 ng/mL or < 0.4 μ/mL. Elevated D-dimer levels reflect ongoing activation of the haemostatic and thrombolytic system, identifying any of the following:

- Thromboembolic phenomena in the body
- Deep venous thrombosis (DVT)
- Monitoring anticoagulative therapy (a decreasing value indicating effective treatment)
- Disseminated intravascular coagulation (DIC)
- Snake venom poisoning

Additionally, D-dimer levels may be elevated in pregnancy, inflammation, malignancy, trauma, post-surgery, liver disease (decreased clearance), and heart disease [9]. It is also frequently high in hospitalised patients.

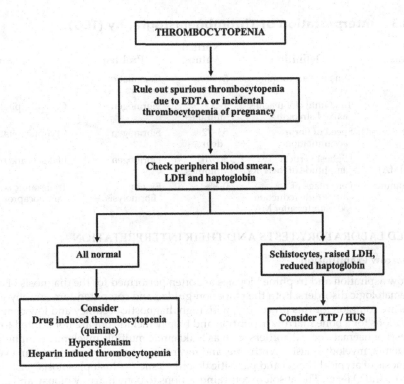

Figure 18.4   Diagnostic algorithm for thrombocytopenia.

4. Thromboelastography (TEG)

TEG visualises the viscoelastic changes that occur during coagulation in vitro and provides a graphic representation of clot formation and lysis [10]. Clinically, two devices are being used: the TEG® system (Haemoscope Corporation, Niles, Illinois, USA) and the ROTEM (Pentapharm GmbH, Munich, Germany). Although TEG® and ROTEM® traces look similar, the nomenclature and reference ranges are different, and the outcomes of both techniques are not interchangeable. TEG has the capability to assess bedside within 30 minutes the sum of platelet function, coagulation proteases and inhibitors, together with the fibrinolytic system, and is therefore considered helpful in various areas of haemostasis testing.

A normal TEG tracing is represented in Figure 18.5 and the common abnormalities seen are enlisted in Table 18.3.

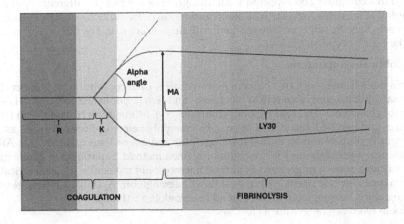

Figure 18.5   A normal thromboelastography trace.

Table 18.3   Interpretation of Thromboelastography (TEG)

Components	Definition	Normal Values	Problem	Treatment
R time	Time to start forming clot	5–10 minutes	Coagulation factors	FFP
K time	Time until clot reaches a fixed strength	1–3 minutes	Fibrinogen	Cryoprecipitate
Alpha angle	Speed of fibrin accumulation	53–72 degrees	Fibrinogen	Cryoprecipitate
Maximum amplitude (MA)	Highest vertical amplitude of the TEG	50–70 minutes	Fibrinogen	Platelets and/or DDAVP
Lysis at 30 minutes (LY30)	Percentage of amplitude reduction 30 minutes after MA	0–8%	Excess fibrinolysis	Tranexamic acid and/or aminocaproic acid

ADVANCED LABORATORY TESTS AND THEIR INTERPRETATION

1. Bone marrow examination

Bone marrow aspiration and trephine biopsies are often performed for the diagnosis of a multitude of haematologic disorders. Both the palpation-guided and computed-tomography-guided approaches are common for this procedure, with high diagnostic accuracy and low complication rates. Indications for a bone marrow aspiration and biopsy include but are not limited to a definitive diagnosis of haematologic disorders such as leukaemia, multiple myeloma, lymphoma, unexplained anaemia, myelodysplastic syndrome, and fever of unknown origin. They can even aid in the diagnosis of atypical fungal and parasitic disorders such as histoplasmosis, leishmaniasis, cryptococcus, and Q fever. The absolute contraindications to bone marrow biopsy and aspiration include severe bleeding diatheses such as severe haemophilia or severe DIC.

2. Flow cytometry

Flow cytometry is a laser-based technique used to detect and analyse the chemical and physical characteristics of cells or particles. It is most commonly used to evaluate bone marrow, peripheral blood, and other fluids in the body [11].

Flow cytometry may be used to characterise and count types of WBCs in the evaluation of infectious diseases, autoimmune disorders, or immunodeficiencies. It is also used to diagnose and classify haematological malignancies. This is especially true if initial testing showed an increased number of lymphocytes, abnormal cell counts, or the presence of immature blood cells. It can be used to predict how aggressive the cancer will be and to help determine if the cancer will respond to certain treatments or if the disease has relapsed after treatment.

A sample of blood, bone marrow, or tissue cells is placed in a suspension and injected into the flow cytometer machine. The cells are arranged in a single file line and then passed in front of a laser beam, scattered light, and fluorescent light. Next, the cells are counted and categorised. The data is stored in a computer and reported via a histogram or dot plot. If different types of cells are being tested at the same time, such as blood and tissue cells, multicolour flow cytometry is a useful approach. Specific cell types are marked with fluorescent dye. The flow cytometer machine then sorts the cells by type and colour.

3. Haemoglobin electrophoresis

Haemoglobin is a tetramer with two pairs of globin chains, each containing an identical heme group. Normal adult haemoglobin (HbA) has two α- and two β-globin chains ($\alpha_2 \beta_2$). Foetal haemoglobin (HbF) has two α- and two γ-globin chains ($\alpha_2 \gamma_2$). Minor adult haemoglobin (HbA$_2$) is made of two α- and two δ-globin chains ($\alpha_2 \delta_2$). Haemoglobin electrophoresis is used as a screening test to identify normal and abnormal haemoglobins and assess their quantity [12]. Alkaline and/or citrate agar electrophoresis is the commonly used method. Separation of haemoglobins is based on variable rates of migration of charged haemoglobin molecules in an electrical field. Haemoglobin types include haemoglobin A_1 (HbA$_1$), haemoglobin A_2 (HbA$_2$), haemoglobin F (HbF; foetal haemoglobin), haemoglobin C (HbC), and haemoglobin S (HbS).

Haemoglobin reference ranges are as follows:

Adult/elderly:

Percentage of total Hb

- HbA$_1$: 95–98%
- HbA$_2$: 2–3%
- HbF: 0.8–2%
- HbS: 0%
- HbC: 0%
- HbE: 0%

Children:

HbF

- Newborn: 50–80%
- < 6 months: < 8%
- >6 months: 1–2%

4. Platelet antibody and aggregation

A simple assay that assesses platelet function and antibody activity is **light transmission aggregometry**. This assay can be used to determine antibody activity in patients with disorders such as heparin-induced thrombocytopenia (HIT) and vaccine-induced thrombotic thrombocytopenia (VITT). First described by Born in the 1960s, light transmission aggregometry is considered a *gold standard* assay for platelet function, often assigned as the first step for analysing platelet dysfunction in haemorrhagic patients [13].

Briefly, for the detection of pathogenic antibodies, platelet-rich plasma (PRP) is treated with a specific agent (e.g., patient sera or purified patient antibodies) with constant stirring. Upon activation, platelets undergo a shape change and adhere to each other forming aggregates. This causes a reduction in opacity allowing more light to pass through PRP. Light transmission through the cuvette is proportional to the degree of platelet aggregation and is measured by the photocell over time. The advantage of this protocol is that it is a simple, reliable assay that can be applied to assess antibody activity in thrombotic conditions. Light transmission aggregometry does not require the use of radioactive reagents and is technically less demanding compared with ^{14}**C-serotonin release assay**. The ^{14}C-serotonin release assay (SRA) and the heparin-induced platelet activation (HIPA) test are also common assays used to test antibody activity.

Another method of analysing platelet activation is **whole-blood aggregometry**. This method measures the change in electrical impedance between two electrodes to indicate platelet aggregation. Although this process accounts for the effect of all blood cells on platelet function, it cannot determine with accuracy the direct or indirect contributions of other blood cells to the platelet activation observed. To avoid confounding factors in whole blood, light transmission aggregometry using PRP is an ideal, relatively simple, and reliable method to specifically determine platelet activity.

5. Antiphospholipid antibody (APLA) testing

Antiphospholipid syndrome (APS) is diagnosed in patients with recurrent thromboembolic events and/or pregnancy loss in the presence of persistent laboratory evidence for APLA. Diagnostic tests for the detection of APLA include laboratory assays that detect **anticardiolipin antibodies, lupus anticoagulant (LA),** and **anti-β$_2$-glycoprotein I antibodies**.

There are different classes (isotypes) of anticardiolipin antibodies, namely IgG, IgM, and IgA. IgG is the anticardiolipin antibody type most associated with complications. An enzyme-linked immunosorbent assay (ELISA) is used to test for anticardiolipin antibodies. High levels of the IgM isotype are associated with autoimmune haemolytic anaemia.

The activated partial thromboplastin time (aPTT) is often used to test for LA. If this test is normal, more sensitive coagulation tests are performed, including the modified Russell viper venom time (RVVT), platelet neutralisation procedure (PNP), and kaolin clotting time (KCT). Normally, two of these tests (the apt and the RVVT) are performed to detect whether LA is present.

6. Ristocetin-induced platelet aggregation (RIPA)

RIPA is used as an in vitro test to determine the presence and integrity of the platelet glycoprotein (GP) Ibα-V-IX complex and von Willebrand factor (VWF) interaction and is usually performed using platelet-rich plasma (PRP) [14].

Ristocetin is an antibiotic but was found to cause thrombocytopenia and so removed from the market. Ristocetin induces the binding of von Willebrand Factor (VWF) to the GpIb complex by an alteration of the electrostatic forces between GpIb and VWF in the micro-circulation. Low-dose (<0.5–0.7 mg/mL) ristocetin-induced platelet agglutination (RIPA) can be of value in identifying patients with Type 2B Von-Willbrand disease (VWD). In cases in which there is a low sensitivity to ristocetin in light transmission aggregometry, this can suggest Type 1, 3, 2A, or 2M VWD. Enhanced agglutination of ristocetin, i.e., high sensitivity, suggests either 2B VWD or PT-VWD.

To conclude, haematological disorders encompass a broad spectrum of disorders where selection of the right test at the right time is pivotal for establishing diagnosis and appropriate treatment.

REFERENCES

1. McCaughey C, Blackwood B, Glackin M, Brady M, McMullin MF. Characteristics and outcomes of haematology patients admitted to the intensive care unit. *Nurs Crit Care.* 2013;18(4):193–199.

2. Chen CL, Wang ST, Cheng WC, Wu BR, Liao WC, Hsu WH. Outcomes and prognostic factors in critical patients with hematologic malignancies. *J Clin Med.* 2023;12(3):958.

3. Tefferi A, Hanson CA, Inwards DJ. How to interpret and pursue an abnormal complete blood cell count in adults. *Mayo Clin Proc.* 2005;80(7):923–936.

4. Riley LK, Rupert J. Evaluation of patients with leukocytosis. *Am Fam Physician.* 2015;92(11):1004–1011.

5. Stanworth SJ, Estcourt LJ, Powter G, Kahan BC, Dyer C, Choo L, *et al.* TOPPS Investigators. A no-prophylaxis platelet-transfusion strategy for hematologic cancers. *N Engl J Med.* 2013;368(19):1771–1780

6. Russell L, Holst LB, Kjeldsen L, Stensballe J, Perner A. Risks of bleeding and thrombosis in intensive care unit patients with haematological malignancies. *Ann Intensive Care.* 2017;7(1):119.

7. Retter A, Barrett NA. The management of abnormal haemostasis in the ICU. *Anaesthesia.* 2015;70:121–e41.

8. Papageorgiou C, Jourdi G, Adjambri E, Walborn A, Patel P, Fareed J, *et al.* Disseminated intravascular coagulation: an update on pathogenesis, diagnosis, and therapeutic strategies. *Clin Appl Thromb Hemost.* 2018;24(9S):8S–28S.

9. Spring JL, Winkler A, Levy JH. The influence of various patient characteristics on D-dimer concentration in critically Ill patients and its role as a prognostic indicator in the intensive care unit setting. *Clin Lab Med.* 2014;34(3):675–686.

10. Woźniak D, Adamik B. Tromboelastografia, metoda szybkiej diagnostyki zaburzeń układu krzepniecia [Thromboelastography]. *Anestezjol Intens Ter.* 2011;43(4):244–247.

11. McKinnon KM. Flow cytometry: an overview. *Curr Protoc Immunol.* 2018;120:5.1.1–5.1.11.

12. Robinson AR, Robson M, Harrison AP, Zuelzer WW. A new technique for differentiation of hemoglobin. *J Laborat Clin Med.* 1957;50(5):745–752.

13. Leung HHL, Perdomo J, Ahmadi Z, Chong BH. Determination of antibody activity by platelet aggregation. *Bio Protoc.* 2023;13(17):e4804.

14. Frontroth JP, Favaloro EJ. Ristocetin-Induced Platelet Aggregation (RIPA) and RIPA mixing studies. *Methods Mol Biol.* 2017;1646:473–494.

19 Endocrine System

A. Zara Herskovits, Nina Raoof and Lakshmi V. Ramanathan

INTRODUCTION

Critically ill patients often have overlapping syndromes with varied differential diagnoses. Identifying the correct etiology is vital to ensure the best patient outcomes. Endocrinopathies may lead to syndromes that result in critical illness, such as diabetic ketoacidosis, or syndromes like adrenal insufficiency that can mimic other common reasons for ICU admission, such as sepsis. Those practicing in the ICU must develop a robust differential diagnosis and understand how to appropriately utilize the laboratory testing available for making an accurate diagnosis [1].

Laboratory support for the ICU patient can be performed at the point of care (POCT) or in a centralized laboratory. Blood gases, electrolytes, ionized calcium and lactate are often part of a panel of tests that can be performed on whole blood in the ICU setting or on samples sent to a central laboratory. Methodological issues related to endocrine tests performed in the clinical laboratory can result in extended turnaround times. Although several point-of-care platforms are used in Europe, they have not received approval from the FDA and are not used in the United States.

In this chapter, we will consider different endocrine emergencies presented in critical care medicine along with basic and advanced laboratory and point-of-care testing options. The limitations and challenges of endocrine test methodologies will also be discussed.

CLASSIFICATION OF DISEASE AND/OR SEVERITY

Diabetic Hyperglycemic Crisis

Diabetic hyperglycemic crisis is a relatively common endocrinopathy that can be triggered by infections such as pneumonia, sepsis and urinary tract infections or inadequate insulin therapy in a patient with underlying diabetes mellitus. Signs and symptoms of hyperglycemia include polydipsia, polyurea, nausea, vomiting, dehydration, lethargy and mental status changes. Typical laboratory findings include abnormalities in electrolytes, renal function, dehydration and compromised immune function [2, 3].

Diabetic ketoacidosis (DKA) is characterized by metabolic acidosis and high glucose levels typically above 800 mg/dL. DKA can be distinguished from hyperosmolar hyperglycemic states (HHS), another acute complication of diabetes in which patients can develop neurologic symptoms without ketoacidosis in the presence of high glucose levels that can exceed 1000 mg/dL [4]. Treatment protocols for both conditions focus on correcting fluid and electrolyte abnormalities with concomitant insulin administration for DKA. Isotonic saline infusion is used to expand intravascular volume, lower the plasma osmolality and reduce vasoconstriction, which is important for stabilizing cardiovascular perfusion. Most patients with DKA or HHS have a total body potassium deficit and replacement is initiated in patients with serum potassium below 5.3 mEq /L when there is adequate renal function and urinary output. Insulin therapy is another cornerstone of treatment that is critical for normalizing hyperglycemia but requires potassium monitoring so that patients do not develop hypokalemia and cardiac conduction abnormalities from intracellular potassium uptake [5]. Serial monitoring of glucose, basic chemistry profiles, pH levels and ketoacids is also important to ensure patients are improving with gradual correction of fluid and electrolyte abnormalities [4].

Adrenal Insufficiency and Excess

Adrenal hormones play a critical role in mobilizing a systemic response when patients have a life-threatening illness. Primary adrenal insufficiency occurs when cortisol biosynthesis in the adrenal glands is impacted by autoimmune disease, infectious processes, hemorrhage, metastatic disease or medications [5, 6]. Secondary adrenal insufficiency is due to deficient secretion of hormones in the anterior pituitary and tertiary disease is due to disruption of hormonal signaling at the hypothalamic level. Acute adrenal insufficiency can be life-threatening, and patients can present with fatigue, weight loss, decreased appetite, nausea, pain, delirium, confusion and coma [5, 7]. Clinical examination may reveal hypotension, fever and tachycardia [5].

While levels of cortisol, ACTH, aldosterone and renin levels as well as stimulation testing can be diagnostically useful for adrenal insufficiency, rapid treatment is of utmost importance when adrenal crisis is suspected. Immediate treatment strategies for ICU patients with probable adrenal insufficiency are administration of intravenous glucocorticoids, electrolyte repletion, vasopressors depending on hemodynamics and urine output, and supportive care [5].

Pheochromocytoma

Pheochromocytoma is a rare neuroendocrine tumor that can arise in the adrenal medulla, causing multiorgan failure due to excessive catecholamine release. Patients develop headaches or other signs of encephalopathy, sweating from hyperthermia and palpitations, or other manifestations of hemodynamic instability. Surgical resection is a first-line treatment but should be performed after stabilization of the patient's hemodynamics [5].

Thyroid Function

Regulation of the hypothalamic-pituitary-thyroid axis can be affected by infections, malignancy, surgery and medications as well as cardiac, renal and liver disease, and these factors complicate the evaluation of underlying thyroid disorders in critically ill patients [8, 9]. Although low serum thyroid hormones are often seen with elevated TSH in patients with primary hypothyroidism, severely ill patients with non-thyroidal illness syndrome (NTIS) can have low thyroid hormones with low or normal-range TSH. Peripheral tissues also exhibit a lack of responsiveness to thyroid hormone due to decreases in thyroid hormone-binding proteins, transporters, deiodinases and receptors [9]. While increasing thyroid hormone levels into the normal range is of benefit for patients with primary hypothyroidism, studies showing whether thyroid replacement improves outcomes in critically ill patients have yielded conflicting results, and replacement is not currently recommended for NTIS patients [2].

Myxedema coma is a rare, life-threatening form of severe hypothyroidism that can present with altered mental status, hypothermia, bradycardia, hypoventilation, edema, hyponatremia and low blood pressure in the setting of low or undetectable thyroid hormone levels [2, 5]. It is more common during the winter months in older patients with a past medical history of hypothyroidism and can be triggered by hypothermia, trauma, infections, stroke, surgery or medications. The condition is treated by supportive care and intravenous replacement of thyroid hormones along with intensive monitoring of blood glucose, hemodynamic and respiratory status and cardiac function in the ICU. Concurrent administration of corticosteroids may be of benefit in patients with adrenal insufficiency. [2]

Thyrotoxicosis or "thyroid storm" is a rare syndrome that can cause life-threatening multiorgan failure. Patients exhibit thermoregulatory dysfunction such as fever or heat intolerance, cardiovascular abnormalities, gastrointestinal symptoms and mental status changes in the context of acute systemic stress from infection, stroke, DKA, surgery, burns or thyroid dysfunction. Treatment varies depending on the patient's symptoms and the nature of the underlying precipitating factors. Cornerstones of patient management include hemodynamic monitoring in the ICU, supportive treatment with intravenous fluids, oxygen supplementation, management of hyperthermia with cooling blankets and acetaminophen, beta-blockers, or diltiazem to manage sympathetic response, propylthiouracil or methimazole and glucocorticoids to decrease synthesis of active thyroid hormone, and bile acid sequestrants such as cholestyramine to prevent enterohepatic recycling of thyroid hormones. After the patient's acute illness is resolved, longer-term treatment for hyperthyroidism can be pursued [5].

Pituitary Disorders

Pituitary apoplexy occurs when patients have hemorrhage or sudden infarction of the pituitary gland that can be caused by a previously undetected adenoma [2, 5]. Due to the vasculature of the anterior and posterior pituitary, this gland is more likely to bleed relative to other types of brain tumors, and patients with this condition experience a severe headache with sudden onset and visual changes due to the compression of the optic nerve. Patient management includes diagnostic imaging, pituitary hormone testing, visual field testing, monitoring of electrolyte levels, supportive management to stabilize hemodynamic and cardiopulmonary parameters, high-dose corticosteroids and neurosurgical consult for transsphenoidal surgery if indicated. Patients require long-term management after the acute illness is resolved.[5]

BASIC LABORATORY AND POINT-OF-CARE TESTS (WITH TIMELINE AND CLINICAL COURSE)

Blood Glucose Testing

The accurate and timely measurement of blood glucose is critical in the management of these patients. The three principal enzymatic reactions utilized by currently available glucometers include glucose oxidase, glucose dehydrogenase and hexokinase.

Several studies in critically ill patients have compared fingerstick glucose to glucose values on a chemistry lab analyzer as well as the blood gas analyzer, and results have been varied [10]. The blood gas/chemistry analysis represents the safer approach since hypoglycemia appears to be overestimated, while glucometer analysis of capillary or arterial blood underestimates hypoglycemia. It is recommended that values above or below the reportable range should be repeated in the central laboratory to ensure accuracy. The reliability of results depends on several factors, as listed in Table 19.1.

Endocrine Tests

Laboratory methods including immunoassay and mass spectrometry can also be used to assess endocrine abnormalities. These include thyroid function tests, adrenal hormones, catecholamines, metabolites and other hormones. Testing is usually done on blood, but in certain cases, urine and saliva are also used. Immunoassays are mostly used as they are available with minimal preparation on most chemistry analyzers with a fast turnaround time. However, immunoassays have limitations that can cause potential interferences in the assay. The result can be either a false elevation or a false lowering of results. Some of the interferences include the presence of heterophile antibodies, auto-antibodies and biotin when the assay is biotin-streptavidin-based. [11]

Due to the limitations of immunoassay platforms, mass spectrometry is gaining more popularity among laboratorians. However, the challenges in this case include complex and costly instrumentation that is out of reach for small- to medium-sized clinical laboratories, and turnaround time is an issue, as it often takes two to three days to obtain a result. Due to these methodological limitations, the reality is that in the ICU, prompt initiation of treatment usually takes precedence over diagnostic testing.

ADVANCED POINT-OF-CARE AND LABORATORY TESTS

Continuous Glucose Monitoring

In April 2020, during the COVID-19 pandemic, the Food and Drug Administration approved the use of continuous glucose monitoring (CGM) devices in the inpatient setting. Continuous glucose monitoring from the interstitial fluid can evaluate the pharmacology, nutritional therapy, physical activity, education and adhesion to therapy and thus improve glycemic control. There have been several studies on the benefits of continuous glucose monitoring in ICU patients [12]. The unique benefits include tracking real-time glucose levels to detect often unrecognized severe hypo- or hyperglycemic events while reducing the frequency of point-of-care testing during clinically tenuous states and continuous insulin infusion.

The real-time CGM system consists of a biosensor, transmitter and monitor. The biosensor is a tiny cannula that penetrates the skin and needs to be changed every 7–14 days, though some biosensors can be used for 90 days. The signal from the sensor is received by the monitor, which can display glucose levels and indicate if the interstitial fluid level is too high or too low.

Table 19.1 Pre-Analytical and Analytical Challenges in Point-of-Care Blood Glucose Testing

Condition of the Patient

Not recommended if patient is dehydrated, in shock, has anemia/decreased hematocrit, polycythemia/ increased hematocrit or hypertriglyceridemia.

Operational Issues

Test strip not completely inserted, patient sample site contaminated with sugar, squeezing fingertip too hard, not enough blood applied to the strip, other site sampled instead of finger, strip reused.

Drug Interference

Maltose, acetaminophen, ascorbate, mannitol, dopamine.

Reagent Storage

Storage of test strips/controls at extreme temperatures; vials cracked during shipping.

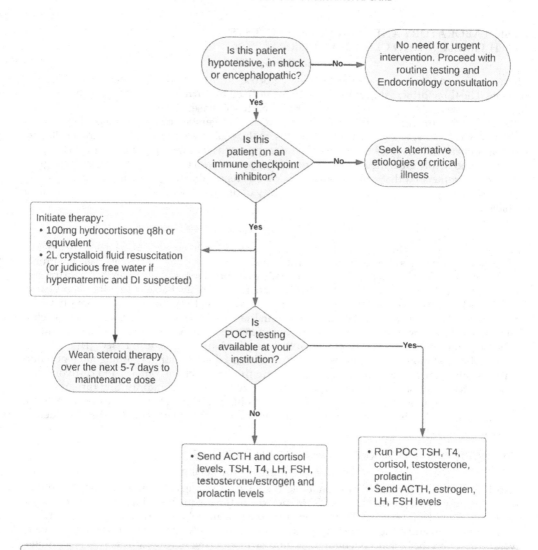

Figure 19.1 Diagnosis and initial management of a critically ill patient with endocrine toxicity immune checkpoint inhibitor toxicity (ICI). Adapted from "Acute management of the endocrine complications of checkpoint inhibitor therapy," by C. E. Higham et al, 2018 Endocrine Connections 7(7), G1–G7.

Some monitors can send the glucose readings directly to clinicians through a smartphone application which can streamline clinical intervention. Before implementing CGM in the ICU, it is advisable to have an interdisciplinary team of physicians, nurses, midlevel practitioners, pharmacists and laboratorians for a safe and effective rollout.

Innovative Technologies

Several new and promising technologies are entering the field of laboratory diagnostics. These include microfluids, magnetic sensors and point-of-care mass spectrometry. Advances in assay development, microfluidics and consumer electronics are enabling hormones and metabolites in endocrinology to be available on point-of-care platforms and even in the home setting. In the future, this will impact the management of patients in the ICU.

CLINICAL PEARLS

- Awareness of local abilities is vital. If POCT is not available at your institution or there may be a delay, initiating therapy in the appropriate clinical context prior to waiting for lab results is vital.

- A scenario where this approach is vital is suspected immunotherapy-related adverse effects (irAE). In these cases, deferring empiric treatment for test results can lead to increased morbidity or mortality and exposure to unnecessary medications.

- In patients with multiple comorbidities, the diagnosis of DKA may be confounded by other etiologies of ketosis such as starvation or alcoholic ketosis. As no definitive testing exists to discriminate between these entities and the consequences of untreated DKA can be catastrophic, it is prudent in these cases to proceed with DKA treatment.

- Similarly, treatment of DKA in a patient with underlying heart failure may be challenging. Though there is no optimal predefined volume management strategy, fluid resuscitation should not be omitted from the care plan. Consider incorporating point-of-care ultrasound to help guide resuscitation.

- Measurement of serum calcium is affected by serum albumin levels. Though a formula exists to correct for albumin, it is advisable to send an ionized calcium level (available on the blood gas analyzer) and use this to guide treatment.

FUTURE DIRECTIONS

Although, historically, endocrine crises in the ICU were often triggered by an infectious or other insult [7], the increasing use of immune checkpoint inhibitors (ICI) is changing this landscape. Among patients who are treated with ICIs, approximately 10–20% can be expected to develop an endocrine-related complication, most likely hypothyroidism [13]. There is some evidence to suggest that rates of endocrinopathies vary with the particular drug being used. Similarly, the prevalence of unusual endocrinopathies such as panhypopituitarism is much higher among patients being treated with ICIs than the general population. In fact, panhypopituitarism, with or without hypophysitis, is the second most common endocrinopathy associated with ICI treatment [13].

Because of the unusual way that irAE may present as a constellation of endocrinopathies, it is suggested that once this pathology is suspected in a critically ill patient, therapy for adrenal insufficiency should be initiated, and laboratory testing for primary adrenal insufficiency (serum cortisol and ACTH), hypophysitis (prolactin, testosterone/estradiol, LH, FSH) and thyroiditis (TSH, T4) all be done simultaneously. Additionally, as adrenal insufficiency may mask diabetes insipidus (DI), if a patient develops polyuria after initiation of steroid therapy, testing for DI should be performed with baseline serum and urine osmolarity, serum sodium and urine osmolality after administration of desmopressin. Unfortunately, acute illness may lead to hypothalamic suppression of the gonadotrophin or thyroid axis and may lead to difficulty with diagnosis (Figure 19.1) [14]. Follow-up with an endocrinologist would be beneficial in these complex cases.

Another more recent area of concern is metabolic manifestations of COVID-19 infection. Both in-vitro studies and examination of post-mortem tissue have identified infiltration of pancreatic tissue with immune cells as well as signs of necroptosis, leading to the suggestion that the SARS-CoV-2 virus may directly infect pancreatic cells [15]. This, in combination with the hyperinflammatory response, has led to a state of severe insulin resistance and higher rates of diabetic ketoacidosis and other metabolic complications of preexisting diabetes. In fact, it is suspected that COVID-19 itself may be a trigger for new-onset diabetes. [15] In light of this, ICU practitioners need to be aware of this extra-pulmonary aspect of providing complete care to patients with COVID-19 infection.

REFERENCES

1. Kerr DE, Wenham T, Newell-Price J. Endocrine problems in the critically ill 2: endocrine emergencies. *BJA Edu.* 2017;17:377–382.

2. Goldberg PA, Inzucchi SE. Critical issues in endocrinology. *Clin Chest Med.* 2003;24(4):583-+.

3. Bajwa SJ, Jindal R. Endocrine emergencies in critically ill patients: Challenges in diagnosis and management. *Ind J Endocrinol Metab.* 2012;16(5):722–727.

4. Hirsch IB, Emmett M. Diabetic ketoacidosis and hyperosmolar hyperglycemic state in adults: Treatment. 2022, 6/5/2023. Available from: https://www.uptodate.com/contents/diabetic-ketoacidosis-and-hyperosmolar-hyperglycemic-state-in-adults-treatment/.

5. Nasrullah A, *et al.* Endocrine emergencies in the medical intensive care unit. *Crit Care Nurs Q.* 2022;45(3):266–284.

6. Nieman KL. Causes of primary adrenal insufficiency (Addison's disease). 2023, 6/6/2023. Available from: https://www.uptodate.com/contents/causes-of-primary-adrenal-insufficiency-addisons-disease/https://www.uptodate.com/contents/causes-of-primary-adrenal-insufficiency-addisons-disease/.

7. Van den Berghe G. Adrenal function/dysfunction in critically ill patients: a concise narrative review of recent novel insights. *J Anesth.* 2021;35(6):903–910.

8. Economidou F, *et al.* Thyroid function during critical illness. *Hormones (Athens).* 2011;10(2):117–124.

9. Fliers E, *et al.* Thyroid function in critically ill patients. *Lancet Diabet Endocrinol.* 2015;3(10):816–825.

10. Deng T, *et al.* A comparison of arterial blood glucose and peripheral blood glucose levels in critically ill patients: measurements using the arterial blood gas analyzer and the rapid glucose meter. *Ann Palliat Med.* 2021;10(3):3179–3184.

11. Haddad RA, Giacherio D, Barkan AL. Interpretation of common endocrine laboratory tests: technical pitfalls, their mechanisms and practical considerations. *Clin Diabetes Endocrinol.* 2019;5:12.

12. Krinsley JS, *et al.* Continuous glucose monitoring in the ICU: clinical considerations and consensus. *Crit Care.* 2017;21(1):197.

13. Wright JJ, Powers AC, Johnson DB. Endocrine toxicities of immune checkpoint inhibitors. *Nat Rev Endocrinol.* 2021;17(7):389–399.

14. Higham CE, *et al.* Society for endocrinology endocrine emergency guidance: acute management of the endocrine complications of checkpoint inhibitor therapy. *Endocr Connect.* 2018;7(7):G1–G7.

15. Steenblock C, *et al.,* COVID-19 and metabolic disease: mechanisms and clinical management. *Lancet Diabetes Endocrinol.* 2021;9(11):786–798.

20 Pregnancy and Puerperium

Manju Mathew and Kannan Vaidyanathan

INTRODUCTION

Worldwide, major obstetric hemorrhage (MOH) remains the most common cause of maternal mortality, with a higher incidence in low- and lower-middle-income countries. In India, the leading causes of maternal death are obstetric hemorrhage (47%; higher in poorer states), pregnancy-related infection (12%), and hypertensive disorders of pregnancy (7%) [1]. Cardiovascular, neurological (epilepsy and stroke) and mental health causes, thromboembolism, and hypertensive disorders of pregnancy are the common causes of maternal death in the Western world [2].

PHYSIOLOGICAL VARIATIONS IN PREGNANCY

Biochemical Tests

Serum glutamic-oxaloacetic transaminase (SGOT) and serum glutamate pyruvate transaminase (SGPT) are markers of hepatocellular damage. Serum alkaline phosphatase (ALP) and γ-glutamyl transferase (GGT) are suggestive of cholestasis. However, an overlap between the two classes of LFTs is very common in many disease conditions [3]. During pregnancy, the concentrations of the transaminases, the bilirubin, the bile acids, and GGT remain in the normal range, as with non-pregnant women. Unlike this, ALP increases and may reach two times the normal adult upper reference value due to the production of the placental isoenzyme. Pregnant women with isolated raised alkaline phosphatase in this range do not need further investigation. After delivery, the ALP level falls, reaching non-pregnant values within 2 weeks. Serum albumin level falls by about 25% and is thought to be related to the increase in total plasma volume. Similarly, serum creatinine values also fall during pregnancy, and a value of 1mg/dl may suggest worsening renal function.

Hematological Tests

Hematological changes in pregnancy include physiological anemia, thrombocytopenia, and hypercoagulopathy. The definition of anemia in pregnancy is a hemoglobin (Hb) less than 11.0 g/dL in the first trimester or immediate postpartum period [4]. In the majority of cases, iron deficiency is the etiological factor. Pre-existing anemia is found to be a risk factor for transfusion requirement at the time of delivery and might possibly be a risk for PPH as well.

Levels of clotting factors increase and levels of natural anticoagulants decline in pregnancy, contributing to a relative hypercoagulable state and higher risk of thromboembolism. On the other hand, antepartum and postpartum bleeding is a major cause of maternal mortality. Fibrinogen levels increase from 2–5 g/L in the normal population to 3–6 g/L by the third trimester. Hence, in a bleeding obstetric patient, the aim should be to keep fibrinogen at > 2 g/L. Furthermore, platelet counts decline as pregnancy progresses. In pregnant women, 6% to 12% have platelet counts less than 150,000/cmm at term. As the blood volume is much higher, a blood loss of 1.5 L or more (at term) may occur before signs of hypovolemia develop, at which point there is an increased risk of death.

Both ESR and C-reactive protein are elevated in pregnancy. Procalcitonin increases at the end of the third trimester and the first few postpartum days. Hence, the utility of these tests for diagnosis becomes debatable.

Urinalysis

In the absence of any discernible organic causes, microscopic hematuria during pregnancy may be considered idiopathic. The physiological renal changes during pregnancy such as the rupture of small veins around the dilated renal pelvis may be the reason. The various anatomic and physiological genitourinary changes associated with pregnancy lead to a three- to four-times higher rate of progression of asymptomatic bacteriuria to symptomatic infection. Symptoms of frequency and urgency of urination are also common during pregnancy, which makes clinical signs and symptoms of urinary tract infections in pregnant patients less reliable.

Apart from the changes seen in the routine biochemical and hematological blood analysis, specific tests used in common practice for the diagnosis of disease conditions may become unreliable in pregnancy. The cut-off values of these tests in pregnancy are often different from non-pregnant values. The treating physician should be aware of these variations.

D-Dimer

The levels of D-dimer, a fibrin degradation product, rise steadily throughout pregnancy. Only a few may have a normal D-dimer value during the third trimester. Unlike non-pregnant patients, where negative D-dimer is used to rule out venous thromboembolism, it is not helpful during pregnancy.

Cardiac Enzymes

Creatinine kinase from the myocardium has been shown to be elevated with uterine contraction. Troponin levels tend to be unaffected by uterine contraction but may be elevated in cases of pre-eclampsia and gestational hypertension. While in non-pregnant women, **brain natriuretic peptide** (BNP) < 100 pg/ml has an excellent negative predictive value for heart failure, and > 500 has a good positive predictive value, in pregnancy 100–500 pg/ml levels are non-diagnostic. NT-proBNP is elevated in preeclampsia.

Thyroid Hormones

Thyroid-stimulating hormone (TSH) levels during pregnancy are lower in comparison to the non-pregnant state. With the increase in estrogen-stimulated thyroid binding globulin, total T4 (TT4) and total T3 (TT3) levels significantly increase in pregnancy. FreeT4 (FT4) and FreeT3 (FT3) only represent ~ 0.05% to 0.5% of sampled serum by the end of the first trimester and are preferred for diagnostic purposes (Table 20.1).

Thromboelastography

Point-of-care coagulation tests such as thromboelastography (TEG)
(Thrombelastograph Hemostasis Analyzer System, Haemonetics, Braintree, Massachusetts) and rotational thromboelastometry (ROTEM) can identify patients with decreased fibrinogen levels and increased fibrinolysis, enabling appropriate management with blood products in massive hemorrhage. It is worth noting that measures of clot firmness are higher and the time to clotting onset is shorter in laboring women than non-laboring women in TEG. Similarly, ROTEM reference ranges are also different [5].

LAB INVESTIGATIONS DURING PREGNANCY

Common laboratory investigations like complete blood count, basic biochemistry, and urine analysis are indicated in pregnant females. Additional tests are required in specific situations. The battery of investigations depends on the epidemiology and distribution of diseases as per the geographical region (Table 20.2).

Urinalysis
Blood Sugar

Perform a 2-hour 75 g oral glucose tolerance test in all pregnant patients at first antenatal contact (ANC). If negative, repeat at 24 to 28 weeks of gestation (Tables 20.3 and 20.4).

LABORATORY INVESTIGATIONS IN COMMON PATHOLOGICAL CONDITIONS IN PREGNANCY AND PUERPERIUM

Pregnant females often present with medical conditions such as bleeding, jaundice, pelvic and urogenital infections, and cardiac, neurologic, and endocrine complications. In these cases, tests specific to the diagnosis and follow-up of the suspected disease must be performed. Along with biochemical and microbiological tests, other investigations like ECG, imaging, etc. may be required. Discussion in this chapter is focused on lab parameters.

Table 20.1   Trimester-Specific Normal Range for TSH in Uncomplicated Pregnancy

Trimester-specific Normal Range for TSH in Uncomplicated Pregnancy	mIU/L
First trimester	0.1–2
Second trimester	0.2–3
Third trimester	0.3–3

Table 20.2   Basic Investigations During Pregnancy

Basic Investigations*

Hematology

Hb

Total WBC count

Platelet count

Peripheral smear: look for malaria or features
    of hemolysis

BT/CT

PT/APTT/INR

Blood group/Rh type

Biochemistry

Serum hCG

Oral glucose tolerance test

Blood urea   (Done in preeclampsia)

Serum creatinine

Serum uric acid   (in preeclampsia)

Serum sodium

Serum potassium

Serum calcium

Serum total protein/albumin

Serum bilirubin: total/indirect/direct

SGPT/SGOT

Alkaline phosphatase

Gamma GT

LDH

Serum fibrinogen

Urine analysis

Arterial blood gas, lactate

HIV/HBsAg

VDRL/RPR/POC test for syphilis   Done at first ANC visit.
                                                  Those with a high risk of syphilis or with a history of
                                                      adverse outcomes in previous pregnancies are to be
                                                      screened again in the third trimester. Spouse of syphilis-
                                                      positive woman should be tested.

Microbiology

Blood and urine culture
Wound/vaginal swab

Stool for ova/cyst

Serum hCG

   Additional Investigations**

Sickling index

TSH and FT4

S ammonia

Troponin

HbA1C

Antibody screen   (at 28 weeks if D(Rh)negative and unsensitized)

Pap smear

Rubella serology

Gonococcal screening

(Continued)

Table 20.2 (Continued)

Basic Investigations*

Chlamydial screening	
Group B streptococcus rectovaginal culture	35–37 weeks
Genetic tests	
Fetal aneuploidy screening	(10–14 weeks)
Neural tube defect screening maternal serum alfa-foetoprotein level. If increased, additional tests like amniocentesis	
Cystic fibrosis carrier screening	
Screening for spinal muscular atrophy	

*https://nhm.gov.in/images/pdf/programmes/maternal-health/guidelines/Operational_Guidelines_for_
Obstetric_ICUs_and_HDUs.pdf
**Adapted from Table 10-1. Williams Obstetrics. 26th ed.
**ACOG Publications: January 2020. Obstetrics & Gynecology 135(1): pp. 239–240, January 2020.

Table 20.3 Urinalysis in Pregnancy

Urinalysis	Normal range for first, second, and third trimester of uncomplicated pregnancy	
Protein in 24 h urine	< 150 mg/24 hr	≥ 300 mg/24 hr in Preeclampsia
Protein creatinine ratio		≥ 0.3 in preeclampsia
Glucose	None	
Blood (microscopic) red blood cells (RBC) per high power field	May be seen	Seen in acute cystitis, acute pyelonephritis
RBC casts	Absent	
Hemoglobin	Absent	Seen in HELLP, TTP

Bleeding in Pregnancy

MOH may be antepartum or postpartum. The etiology of MOH are pregnancy-related conditions, trauma, or bleeding disorders. Pregnancy-related conditions are:

- Ectopic pregnancy
- Abruptio placenta
- Placenta previa
- Abortion
- Postpartum hemorrhage (PPH)

Lab Tests In Bleeding
Serum hCG
Grouping and crossmatching
Hemoglobin,
Haptoglobin
Peripheral blood smear for schistocytes
LDH
LFT
RFT
ABG
Lactate
Coagulation parameters PT, APTT, INR, platelet count, fibrinogen/ FDP

During First Trimester

Bleeding may be because of ectopic pregnancy or abortion. Successful management of ectopic pregnancy relies on early diagnosis using quantitative serum human chorionic gonadotropin

Table 20.4 Blood Sugar Levels in Pregnancy

Fasting plasma glucose	92 to 125 mg/dL	Diagnostic of gestational diabetes
	126 mg/dL or higher	Diagnostic of overt diabetes
Random plasma glucose	200 mg/dL or higher	Diagnostic of overt diabetes
HbA1C test		Not recommended in gestational diabetes. Early pregnancy levels between 5.7% and 6.4% may predict subsequent development of gestational diabetes
	6.5% or higher	Diagnostic of overt diabetes
75-g oral glucose tolerance test (OGTT) (irrespective of fasting state)		
Two-hour postprandial glucose level	≥ 140 mg/dl	

https://pmsma.mohfw.gov.in/wp-content/uploads/2016/10/High-Risk-Conditions-in-preg-modified-Final .pdf

[hCG] assays and vaginal ultrasonography. Medical treatment for ectopic pregnancies with a serum hCG level less than 5000 IU/L, and surgical treatment for the rest may be provided.

During Second and Third Trimesters

Abnormal placental implantation may present with bleeding. Preeclampsia, HELLP syndrome (hemolysis, elevated liver enzymes, and low platelet count), intra-uterine death, and acute fatty liver of pregnancy (AFLP) may have coagulopathy before bleeding is observed. Coagulopathy associated with hemorrhage is caused by the consumption of clotting factors and hemodilution secondary to fluid administration. Disseminated intravascular coagulation (DIC), a stage of widespread thrombosis, consumption coagulopathy, and fibrinolysis can occur as a result of several obstetric complications. Diffuse bleeding from venepuncture sites and uterus associated with suggestive lab abnormalities confirm the diagnosis of DIC (Tables 20.5 and 20.6). Placental abruption during labor manifests as bleeding and DIC. Amniotic fluid embolism presents at the time of labor or cesarean section with sudden cardiovascular collapse, and pulmonary edema followed by DIC.

Hypothermia and acidosis impair coagulation. Therefore, hypoperfusion should be aggressively treated to avoid acidosis. Fibrinogen levels decrease early and rapidly during hemorrhage. A fibrinogen level < 2 g/L has been shown to have a 100% positive predictive value for severe PPH.

Postpartum hemorrhage: Blood loss of > 500 ml in 24 hrs is primary PPH. Bleeding after 24 hrs is secondary PPH and is usually caused by infection. Continued bleeding from various sites may be the initial manifestation of DIC.

Jaundice in Pregnancy

Abnormal liver tests occur in 3–5% of pregnancies. The first step is to differentiate between physiological changes and alterations related to the presence of liver disease. The physiological changes in LFT in pregnancy are commonly mild and transient. In contrast, severe liver dysfunction in pregnancy may be due to pregnancy-related liver diseases and represents a severe threat to fetal and maternal survival. The next step is to rapidly differentiate between liver diseases related or unrelated to pregnancy in these women (Figure 20.1).

Table 20.5 Lab Abnormalities Suggesting DIC in Pregnancy and Puerperium

PT, APTT, INR	Increase
Platelet count	Decrease
Fibrinogen	< 2 g/L
Fibrin degradation product	Increase
Microangiopathic hemolysis	Present

Table 20.6   Lab Abnormalities Suggesting Microangiopathic Hemolysis

Hemoglobin	Decrease
Haptoglobin (reduced)	< 2 g/L
Peripheral blood smear	Shows schistocytes, reticulocytes
LDH	Increase
Indirect bilirubin	Increase
Red cell distribution width	Increase

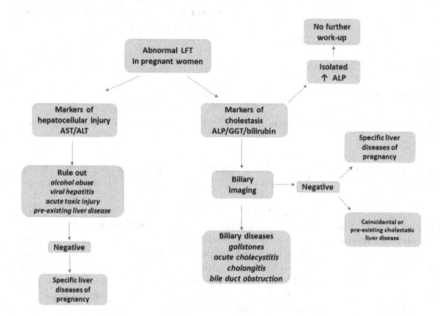

Figure 20.1   Workup of abnormal liver function test (LFT) in pregnant women. Guarino M, Cossiga V, Morisco F. The interpretation of liver function tests in pregnancy. Best Pract Res Clin Gastroenterol. 2020 Feb-Apr;44-45:101667.

Pregnancy-Related Liver Diseases

Intrahepatic cholestasis of pregnancy

Preeclampsia and eclampsia

Hemolysis elevated liver enzymes and low platelet syndrome (HELLP)

Acute fatty liver of pregnancy (AFLP)

Hyperemesis gravidarum

Pregnancy-Unrelated Liver Diseases

Viral hepatitis A, B, C, and E

Autoimmune hepatitis Wilson's disease

Cirrhosis and portal hypertension

Biliary disease

Budd Chiari syndrome

Drug-induced hepatotoxicity

Lab tests in pregnant with jaundice:

Table 20.7 Differential Diagnosis of Liver Diseases Unique to Pregnancy

Specific Liver Diseases of Pregnancy	Suggestive Features	ALT and AST	ALP	Bilirubin	Gestational Age
Hyperemesis gravidarum	Dehydration, ketosis	1–2x in most of the patients	Normal	Normal	First trimester
AFLP	Fulminant hepatic failure, ↓ platelets, ↑ INR, hypoglycemia. Liver biopsy: microvesicular steatosis, foamy hepatocytes, hepatic necrosis	1–10x	1–2x	increased	Third trimester
Eclampsia/ preeclampsia	Proteinuria, renal failure, pulmonary edema	1–100x	1–2x	normal	After 20 weeks or postpartum
HELLP syndrome	↓ platelets, hemolysis, ↑ LDH, proteinuria,↑ creatinine and uric acid, pulmonary edema ABG Abnormal coagulation parameters: DIC (with evidence of elevated fibrin degradation products and D-dimer, low fibrinogen, and a secondary rise in the prothrombin time)	1–100x	1–2x	normal	Third trimester or postpartum
ICP	↑bile acids	1–4x	1–2x	normal	Third trimester

Adapted from Table 1. Differential diagnosis of liver diseases unique to pregnancy. Guarino M, Cossiga V, Morisco F. The interpretation of liver function tests in pregnancy. Best Pract Res Clin Gastroenterol. 2020 Feb–Apr; 44–45:101667.

- CBC, LFT, RFT, urine analysis, blood sugar, ABG, lactate, serum uric acid, coagulation profile, fibrinogen, serum ammonia
- Serum magnesium at baseline before starting treatment with MgSO4 IV infusion, and subsequently, if serum creatinine is > 1 mg/dl, repeat magnesium levels. Maintain levels at 4–7 mEq/L to avoid magnesium toxicity (Table 20.7).

Preeclampsia

Preeclampsia is characterized by hypertension and proteinuria (≥ 300 mg per 24-hour collection) with or without edema after 20 weeks of gestation or postpartum [6].

Lab abnormalities suggestive of severe preeclampsia are:
Progressive renal insufficiency (serum creatinine concentration >1.1 mg/L or doubling of the serum creatinine concentration in the absence of other renal disease
Elevated liver enzymes to twice normal concentration
Platelet count <100,000/μL

HELLP Syndrome

In HELLP syndrome, 70% of cases occur between the 27th and 30th gestational weeks. It is seen in approximately 2% to 12% of women with preeclampsia and is considered a severe form of the latter. However, approximately 12% to 18% of women who develop HELLP syndrome do so without developing hypertension or proteinuria, suggesting that the entity may be at least partially distinct from preeclampsia.

Lab criteria for the diagnosis of HELLP syndrome published by Sibai and colleagues include evidence of hemolysis (see Table 20.6 on hemolysis), abnormal findings on peripheral blood smear, lactate dehydrogenase [LDH] level of > 600 U/L, bilirubin level of > 1.2 mg/dL, SGOT levels > 70 U/L, or platelet count of < 100,000/μL. Serious maternal morbidities include DIC (21%), abruptio placentae (16%), acute renal failure (8%), pulmonary edema (6%), subcapsular liver hematoma (1%), and maternal mortality of 1%.

Acute Fatty Liver of Pregnancy (AFLP)

The condition is rare, with an incidence of 1 in 20,000 pregnancies with a high mortality. Deranged liver and kidney function with low fibrinogen is characteristic. Morbidities include PPH, sepsis, stroke, seizures, and multisystem organ failure. AFLP has overlapping features with HELLP syndrome, but the presence of hyperbilirubinemia and abnormal coagulation test results are the distinguishing features.

The Swansea criteria for AFLP include lab parameters:
Elevated bilirubin > 0.8 mg/dl
Glucose < 72 mg/dl
Urea and creatinine increased
WBC > 11000/μL
Elevated transaminase levels
Ammonia > 47 μmmol/L
Prothrombin time > 14 sec
Microvesicular steatosis on liver biopsy specimens

In addition, raised lactate, RFT, and ABG suggestive of respiratory failure, acute pancreatitis, or DIC may be seen.

Intrahepatic Cholestasis of Pregnancy (ICP)

This is one of the most common liver diseases specific to pregnancy. The typical feature of ICP is elevated serum bile acid level. The cut-off values, used during pregnancy, range between 10 and 14 μmol/L. Higher bile acid levels (> 40 μmol/L) have been found to be associated with higher rates of fetal complications like spontaneous preterm delivery and asphyxia events, which were found in a large cohort of Swedish women with ICP. The liver transaminases are commonly elevated in ICP, and bilirubin levels can increase up to 10% of pregnancies.

ICP is a diagnosis of exclusion, and differential diagnoses include preeclampsia, HELLP, and AFLP. Rarely, women have persistent symptoms and develop a cholestatic disease after delivery. These cases may be related to MDR3 deficiency, and it should be suspected in young women with cholestasis of unknown origin who develop a severe ICP (Table 20.8).

DIFFERENTIATION BETWEEN SEVERE HELLP SYNDROME, AFLP, AND TTP

Urogenital Infections

The risk of developing **acute cystitis and acute pyelonephritis** during pregnancy is much higher and associated with complications. In order to prevent this, all pregnant women should be screened for bacteriuria and treated appropriately. Asymptomatic bacteriuria is defined as the presence of > 10^5 colony-forming units (CFU) of a single pathogen per milliliter of urine in a properly collected specimen without concomitant symptoms[1]. However, bacterial counts as low as 10^2 CFU should also be considered significant in pregnant women and treated accordingly. Urinary

Table 20.8   Differentiation between Severe HELLP Syndrome, AFLP and TTP

Lab Parameter	HELLP	AFLP	TTP
Proteinuria	++	–	+ and hematuria
↓ Hemoglobin	+	+	++
↑ LDH level	++	+/–	++(very high)
↓ Platelets	++	+	++
↑ SGPT/ SGOT	++	++	+/–
↑ Creatinine level	+/–	+/–	++
↑ Uric acid level	+	++	+
↑ Bilirubin level	+	+	–
↑ PT/PTT	–	++	–
↓ Glucose level	+/–	++	–

Pourrat O et al. Differentiation between severe HELLP syndrome and thrombotic microangiopathy, thrombotic thrombocytopenic purpura and other imitators. Eur J Obstet Gynecol Reprod Biol. (2015).

tract pathogens in pregnant women can be caused by *Escherichia coli* (most common), *Klebsiella*, and *Enterobacter*. Follow-up cultures should be done to ensure adequate treatment and to rule out recurrent or persistent infections.

Pelvic infections, chorioamnionitis, and endometritis require antibiotics after sending cultures to cover gram-positive cocci, GNB, and anaerobes. Enterobacteriaceae like *Escherichia coli* is the most common cause. Others include *aerobic and anaerobic streptococci, bacteroides,* and *clostridium* species. *Staphylococcus aureus* and *beta-hemolytic streptococci* can cause **toxic shock syndrome**.

Endocrine Abnormalities

Diabetic ketoacidosis may present as euglycemic ketoacidosis during pregnancy with blood sugars < 200 mg/dl. Investigations include blood sugar, ketones, sodium, potassium, magnesium, phosphorous, RFT, and lactate.

Hyperthyroidism may present in pregnancy. Subclinical hyperthyroidism should never be treated in pregnancy (because it has been shown that maternal-fetal outcomes are just as favorable with a suppressed TSH) [7]. In case of overt hyperthyroidism (elevated T4 and/or T3 for pregnancy), antithyroid drugs should be titrated to maintain T4 at the upper level of the normal pregnancy range to avoid fetal hypothyroidism. FT4 may be used for titration of antithyroid drugs because it is reasonably accurate and the normal range does not require adjustment for pregnancy.

In thyroid storm, severe thyrotoxicosis with a completely suppressed TSH and very elevated FT4 and FT3 is seen. Additional laboratory abnormalities that often coexist in thyroid storms include leucocytosis, hyperglycemia, hypercalcemia, elevated liver enzymes, and electrolyte disturbances. Graves antibodies cross the placenta and should be measured. Graves antibody levels, measured by either a thyroid-stimulating immunoglobulin or TRAb assay and found to be three times higher than the normal range, place the fetus at risk for developing fetal or newborn Graves' disease.

ADDITIONAL TESTS IN SPECIFIC MEDICAL CONDITIONS

There are a few medical conditions that present more frequently in pregnancy compared to the general population like thrombotic thrombocytopenic purpura (TTP), antiphospholipid antibody (APLA) syndrome, thromboembolism, etc., which need specific diagnostic tests. Advanced point-of-care tests such as thromboelastography, if available, are shown to guide the choice of specific blood products in case of major obstetric hemorrhage.

Thromboelastography

Major bleeding requires monitoring of Hb and coagulopathy repeatedly. Point-of-care monitors are quick and allow more timely estimation of transfusion requirements compared to laboratory testing when rapid bleeding is ongoing. Thromboelastography and thromboelastometry give results from whole blood within 30 min. These tests show a high degree of sensitivity and specificity and improve management of coagulopathy during obstetric haemorrhage [5].

Cardiopulmonary Emergencies

D-dimer test is not reliable in pregnant patients with suspected pulmonary embolism. Some society guidelines do not recommend the testing of D-dimer levels in pregnant patients to assess for VTE, while others believe that a negative D-dimer using standard thresholds is still reliably negative in pregnant patients with low pre-test probability, especially in the first trimester [8]. Lab evaluation for cardiac emergencies including acute coronary syndrome and postpartum cardiomyopathy includes troponin and BNP, which may also have abnormal thresholds in pregnancy.

Thrombotic Conditions

Thrombotic thrombocytopenic purpura (TTP) can be precipitated by pregnancy, albeit rarely. TTP presents with thrombocytopenia, microangiopathic hemolytic anemia, neurologic symptoms, and renal insufficiency. HELLP syndrome and AFLP may also be associated with similar manifestations, which make their distinction from TTP-HUS difficult. If a patient with this constellation of signs and symptoms does not improve after delivery, or deteriorates after delivery, TTP may be the diagnosis. **ADAMTS-13 activity** levels of less than 10% are diagnostic of congenital TTP. However, acquired TTP with antibodies is more common than this congenital type (Table 20.8).

Heparin-induced thrombocytopenia (HIT) may be diagnosed in a patient initiated on heparin if thrombocytopenia and/or thrombosis develops within a 5–10 daytime period. Platelets drop to >

50% and reach a nadir of 40000–80000/μL. **Platelet-activating HIT antibodies** should be checked for diagnosis. In both TTP and HIT, platelet transfusion is contraindicated.

For suspected antiphospholipid antibody syndrome, look for **lupus anticoagulants, anticardio-lipin IgG and IgM, antibeta2glycoprotein-1 IgG, and IgM antibodies.** If any of these is positive, then a confirmatory test should be performed 12 weeks later, and anticoagulation should be initiated.

SUMMARY

Pregnancy results in physiological changes in the body along with variations in the normal range of biochemical parameters. At the same time, pregnancy and puerperium predispose women to many pathological disease conditions that need to be attended to urgently. Interpretation of both clinical signs, as well as lab investigations, needs sound awareness of the diagnostic possibilities and risks associated with pregnancy. Undue delay in diagnosis and initiation of treatment should be avoided to prevent maternal and fetal compromise.

CLINICAL PEARLS

- It is important to consider that the fetus is vulnerable to hypoxia and reduced placental perfusion.

- Physiological changes in pregnancy lead to decreased cardiac output in the supine position, anemia, thrombocytopenia, and hypercoagulability.

- The normal ranges for biochemical tests in pregnant women differ from non-pregnant women.

- Pregnancy and puerperium predispose women to diseases like cerebral thromboembolism, pulmonary thromboembolism, peripartum cardiomyopathy, preeclampsia, liver diseases of pregnancy, and acute pyelonephritis.

- The physiological and biochemical variations result in diagnostic challenges to clinicians.

FREQUENTLY ASKED QUESTIONS

1. What is anemia during pregnancy? What is the reason for anemia in pregnancy?

Anemia in pregnancy is defined as hemoglobin levels < 11 gm/dl. It is the result of hemodilution. Plasma volume increases more than the RBC mass, leading to hemodilution.

2. Does pregnancy result in changes in the coagulation system?

Yes. Hypercoagulopathy is seen in pregnancy as a result of increased clotting factors and decreased natural anticoagulants. Deep vein thrombosis, pulmonary thromboembolism, stroke, and cerebral venous thrombosis are more common in pregnancy and puerperium. At the same time, a higher risk for severe bleeding is also seen in pregnant women.

3. How does pregnancy affect the management of infections?

Pregnancy results in increased vulnerability to infections. However, many of the markers are non-specifically elevated in pregnancy, resulting in diagnostic challenges. Blood, urine, and rectovaginal cultures may be helpful. Asymptomatic bacteriuria should be treated.

4. How should you interpret ABG in pregnancy?

Mild respiratory alkalosis is seen in pregnancy due to increased respiratory rate and minute ventilation. There is an associated mild compensatory metabolic acidosis. High normal PaCO2 is an indication of hypoventilation. Also, the lower bicarbonate values increase the risk of severe acidosis in disease states like DKA or renal failure.

5. How are LFT abnormalities interpreted in pregnancy and puerperium?

Serum alkaline phosphatase increases of up to two times need not be investigated in this group. However, SGOT, SGPT, and S bilirubin changes are always abnormal and should alert the clinician to look out for preeclampsia, HELLP, AFLP, or other liver diseases. These conditions can lead to fatal complications including DIC and warrant aggressive management.

REFERENCES

1. Meh C, Sharma A, Ram U, Fadel S, Correa N, Snelgrove J, *et al.* Trends in maternal mortality in India over two decades in nationally representative surveys [Internet]. *BJOG: Int J Obstet Gynaecol.* 2022 [cited 2023 May 14];129:550–561.

2. Gary Cunningham F. *Williams Obstetrics.* 26th ed. McGraw-Hill Education, 2022.

3. Guarino M, Cossiga V, Morisco F. The interpretation of liver function tests in pregnancy. *Best Pract Res Clin Gastroenterol.* 2020;44:101667.

4. High risk factors of pregnancy and their management at an ANC clinic [Internet]. [cited 2023 May 14]. Available from: https://pmsma.mohfw.gov.in/wp-content/uploads/2016/10/High -Risk-Conditions-in-preg-modified-Final.pdf.

5. Bolton S, Harkness M, Thompson S. ROTEM thromboelastometry identifies blood product requirements during major obstetric hemorrhage. *Int J Obstet Anesth* [Internet]. 2011 [cited 2023 May 14]:S22. Available from: http://researchrepository.napier.ac.uk/id/eprint/9270.

6. Gestational hypertension and preeclampsia: ACOG Practice Bulletin, Number 222. *Obstet Gynecol.* 2020;135:e237-60.

7. Hamidi OP, Barbour LA. Endocrine emergencies during pregnancy: diabetic ketoacidosis and thyroid storm. *Obstet Gynecol Clin N Am.* 2022;49:473–489.

8. Borhart J, Palmer J. Cardiovascular emergencies in pregnancy. *Emerg Med Clin North Am.* 2019;37:339–350.

21 Pediatric Diseases

R. Saxena and U.D. Bindal

> *"Without diagnostics, medicine is blind."*

> *– Garcia-Basteiro*

INTRODUCTION

In the pediatric intensive care unit (PICU), laboratory investigation provides valuable insights into diagnosis and severity assessment of illnesses, and aids in therapeutic interventions. The response to laboratory abnormalities is integral in achieving and maintaining stable physiologic status. Over the years, there has been an explosion of laboratory tests including biochemical, pathological, and genetic. In order to avoid prescription of unecessary or duplication of tests, it is important that the clinicians practice diagnostic stewardship and know the inherent fallacies, presumptions and interpretation of each test that they prescribe (e.g., specificity, sentivity, positive predictive value, etc.). Tests also should not become a replacement of clinical skill, and should only complement them [1, 2]. In this chapter, we shall explore a few common investigations that are commonly performed in a PICU.

A. Infections

Infections are one of the most common reasons, why clinicians need to perform multiple and serial diagnostic tests. This depends on the site of the suspected infection, and may include inflammatory markers, cultures among others. One of the most common infections, that an intensivist come across is a urinary tract infection. It is not just at presentation, but also as part of investigation of new onset fever in Picu, for excluding catheter associated urinary tract infection.

1. Urinary tract infections

Urinary tract infection (UTI) is a common bacterial infection in infants and children. The risk of having a UTI before the age of 14 years is approximately 1–3% in boys and 3–10% in girls [3, 4]. The diagnosis of UTI is often missed in infants and young children, as urinary symptoms are minimal and often non-specific. Rapid evaluation and treatment of UTI is important to prevent renal parenchymal damage and renal scarring that can cause hypertension and progressive renal damage [4].

Point-of-care testing (POCT) is ideally suited for PICU and pediatric emergency setups, as it decreases the turnaround time substantially (Table 21.1 and Figures 21.1 and 21.2).

2. Sepsis

In 2017, an estimated 48.9 millioexperienced sepsis worldwide, leading to more than 11 million deaths (19.7% of all cause mortality) [5]. Many pediatric survivors of sepsis have ongoing physical, cognitive, emotional, and psychological sequelae, which may have long-term effects on them and their families. Since the symptoms are multifaceted and overlap with other disease types, more clues are often needed to pinpoint the diagnosis. This is described in Table 21.2.

2. ROLE OF PROCALCITONIN

This has been further elaborated in Table 21.3.

B. Hematological tests

Other tests that are commonly done in PICU include hemoglobin and coagulation profiles, including PT/INR. This is a test that is often feared by residents since it requires a lot of blood samples, and pediatric samples are hard to extract, especially in sick children.

1. Approaches to Prothrombin Time/INR In PICU

Coagulation disorders are quite rampant in PICU, with the disturbance of pro- and anticoagulation cascades. It is important to identify where in the coagulation cascade the defect lies in order to diagnose and treat the same, with appropriate blood product if needed. In this section, we shall be discussing prothrombin time. Conditions like liver failure, disseminated intravascular coagulation, and the addition of warfarin in post-op cardiac patients are the various indications where patients require sampling during ICU stay and on out-patient follow-up. Table 21.4 describes how PT/INR is used in a PICU setup (Figure 21.3 and Table 21.4).

DOI: 10.1201/9781003449713-21

Table 21.1 Approach to UTI

Definitions[4]	Significant pyuria	>10 leukocytes per mm3 in a fresh uncentrifuged sample, or >5 leukocytes per high power field in a centrifuged sample.
	Significant bacteriuria	Colony count of >10⁵/mL of a single species in a midstream clean catch sample.
	Asymptomatic bacteriuria	Significant bacteriuria in the absence of symptoms of urinary tract infection (UTI).
	Simple UTI	UTI with low-grade fever, dysuria, frequency, and urgency, and absence of symptoms of complicated UTI.
	Complicated UTI	Presence of fever >39°C, systemic toxicity; persistent vomiting, dehydration, renal angle tenderness, and raised creatinine.

Role of POCT

Urine dipsticks are a quick, inexpensive bedside screening tool. The reagent strips change color in the presence of leucocyte esterase and nitrites which generally appear in the urine in response to UTI. Although most uropathogens convert dietary nitrates into urinary nitrites, some like Enterococcus and Klebsiella species do not do so. Dipsticks are also less reliable in young infants, where frequent voiding flushes substrates out of the bladder [6,7].

Neither leucocytes nor nitrites are fully sensitive or specific for UTI, but they are a useful screening test, particularly when used in combination. If UTI is unlikely, dipsticks have a good negative predictive value to exclude the diagnosis [8]. In the presence of suggestive symptoms and either leucocytes or nitrites, empirical antibiotics while awaiting culture are indicated (Figures 21.1 and 21.2).

Type of analysis	POC device used	Manufacturer
Albumin, bilirubin, creatinine, glucose, ketone, leukocytes, nitrite, pH, protein, specific gravity, and urobilinogen	Clinitek status+ analyzer	Siemens Healthcare
Leukocyte, nitrite, protein, blood, glucose, ketone, bilirubin, urobilinogen, pH, specific gravity, creatinine, and protein-to-creatinine ratio	Clinitek Advantus Urine Chemistry Analyzer	Siemens Healthcare
Urea nitrogen/urea, creatinine	i-STAT Handheld using CHEM8+ cartridge	Abbot India Limited

Role of microbiological test

Method of collection colony count (per mL) [4, 9]	
Suprapubic aspiration	Any number
Urethral catheterization	>10⁴
Midstream void	>10⁵

False +ve leucocyte detection

Leukocyturia might occur in conditions such as fever, glomerulonephritis, renal stones or presence of other foreign bodies in the urinary tract. The detection of leukocyturia in absence of significant bacteriuria is not sufficient to diagnose a UTI.

Diagnosis

- Diagnosis of UTI in young children is made in presence of symptoms such as fever, dysuria, urgency, frequency, abdominal/flank pain in older children and fever, vomiting, diarrhea, and poor weight gain in infants
  PLUS
- Positive dipstick for leukocyte esterase and nitrite (as a screening tool)
- Abnormal urinalysis with significant pyuria and bacteriuria
  AND
- Isolation of a single species of microorganism in significant numbers in a properly collected urine sample prior to starting antimicrobial therapy and tested for urine culture (gold standard)

Sample

Ideal sample of urine for urine culture for diagnosis of UTI in young children:
- Toilet-trained children: Midstream collected by clean catch method (most preferred, non-invasive practical method). Genital area should be cleaned properly with soap and water before collecting midstream urine sample.
- Non-toilet-trained children: Simple urethral catheterization OR suprapubic aspiration
- Note: Urine samples should never be collected from urobag or minicom in neonates, infants, and older children.
- Urine sample should be processed as soon as possible ideally within 30 minutes of collecting the sample to avoid contamination and incorrect result [4, 9].

Follow-up [4, 9]

Further follow-up and monitoring:
- Aim for symptomatic improvement, complete and sustained resolution of fever, and return to normal well-being
- Document normal urine analysis at the end of treatment of current UTI
- Do not repeat urine culture unless there is a new UTI/breakthrough UTI
- Periodic monitoring of growth
- Urine analysis during further febrile episodes in presence of a known risk factor for UTI
- Blood pressure evaluation once in 6–12 months
- Assess renal function once a year in a child who had severe complicated UTI or recurrent UTI
- Watch for proteinuria after successful treatment of UTI; it may be associated with pyelonephritic renal scarring and would need medical intervention

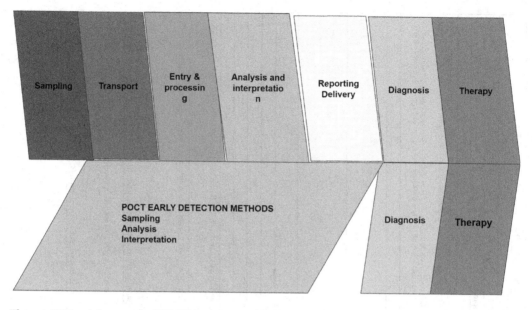

| Sampling | Transport | Entry & processing | Analysis and interpretation | Reporting Delivery | Diagnosis | Therapy |

POCT EARLY DETECTION METHODS
Sampling
Analysis
Interpretation

Diagnosis | Therapy

Figure 21.1   Advantage of POCT in cutting the turn around time.

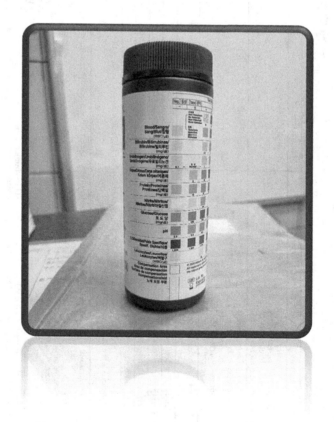

Figure 21.2   POCT: urine multistrips used in PICU and pediatric emergency.

Table 21.2   Approach to Pediatric Sepsis: Role of CRP

Diagnosis [10]	International Consensus Criteria for Pediatric Sepsis and Septic Shock, revised the criterion for pediatric sepsis and gave the new Phoenix Sepsis Score as a composite four-organ system model including criteria for cardiovascular, respiratory, neurological, and coagulation dysfunction. As per this score, any child who is unwell with suspected infection should be screened for sepsis, with institutionally available procedures. If screened positive, the child should be screened for organ dysfunction. If the child has a Phoenix sepsis score of ≥2, the child is deemed to meet the criterion for sepsis. If the child further meets Phoenix sepsis score cardiovascular criterion ≥1, the child is considered to meet the criterion for septic shock/sepsis with cardiovascular dysfunction. These criteria were not designed for screening pediatric sepsis or identification of children at risk for sepsis. There is a need for sepsis screening tools and early warning scores and systems. Various models have been proposed over the years, with various tests such as CRP and procalcitonin. They have been described below.
CRP	A CRP is an acute phase reactant and a sensitive marker when an individual has inflammation. When there is an acute infection or inflammation, the concentration of CRP in the blood can be measured, which can be elevated as early as two hours after the triggering event, reaching peak values in 48 hours [11]. Increased CRP concentration occurs much earlier than other acute phase reactants, In addition, CRP levels return to normal quickly at the end of an acute episode making CRP useful for both detection of acute episode as well as in monitoring treatment [12]. There are different CRP assays in internal medicine, including cardiology, gastroenterology, rheumatology, infectious diseases, and oncology.
Principles behind the test	• CRP is an acute-phase reactant protein that is primarily induced by the IL-6 action on the gene responsible for the transcription of CRP during the acute phase of an inflammatory/infectious process. • C-reactive protein is an acute-phase reactant produced by hepatocytes. The concentration of CRP increases 4 to 6 hours after acute tissue injury or inflammation and declines rapidly with resolution of the injurious process [13]. • CRP has both proinflammatory and anti-inflammatory properties. It plays a role in the recognition and clearance of foreign pathogens and damaged cells [14]
CRP POCT Vs lab tests	Studies have shown similar values, with lesser turnaround time for POCT as compared to lab tests [15].
Lab values [13, 14]	• Less than 0.3 mg/dL: Normal (level seen in most healthy adults). • 0.3 to 1.0 mg/dL: Normal or minor elevation (can be seen in obesity, pregnancy, depression, diabetes, common cold, gingivitis, periodontitis, sedentary lifestyle, cigarette smoking, and genetic polymorphisms). • 1.0 to 10.0 mg/dL: Moderate elevation (Systemic inflammation such as RA, SLE, or other autoimmune diseases, malignancies, myocardial infarction, pancreatitis, bronchitis). • More than 10.0 mg/dL: C-reactive protein levels. 10 mg/L is often associated with infection, some inflammatory diseases, or malignancy; some patients have levels in this range on a purely genetic basis [13]. Marked elevation (acute bacterial infections, viral infections, systemic vasculitis, major trauma). • More than 50.0 mg/dL: Severe elevation (acute bacterial infections).
False reactions [13, 14]	• Certain medications, such as non-steroidal anti-inflammatory drugs (NSAIDs), will falsely decrease CRP levels. • Statins are known to decrease hs-CRP levels in a manner largely unrelated to the reduction of low-density lipoprotein cholesterol (LDL-C). • Recent injury or illness can falsely elevate levels, particularly when using this test for cardiac risk stratification. Magnesium supplementation also can decrease CRP levels.
Interpretation [14, 16–18]	Very high levels of CRP, greater than 50 mg/dL, are associated with bacterial infections about 90% of the time. In multiple studies, CRP has been used as a prognostic factor in acute and chronic infections, including hepatitis C, dengue, and malaria.

2. Approaches to Hemoglobin in PICU

One of the most important and common tests done in PICU and the ward is hemoglobin, which is used for screening and diagnosis of the underlying etiology that has led to anemia, if RBC indices, peripheral smear, etc. are available alongside. This is further detailed in Table 21.5.

C. Dyselectrolytemia in PICU

Fluid and electrolyte balance is crucial in maintaining homeostasis within the body. Body fluids are composed of water and solutes. These solutes are electrically charged electrolytes (e.g., Na+, K+, and Cl-) and nonelectrolytes (e.g., glucose, urea). Fluid and electrolyte homeostasis occurs when fluid and electrolyte balance is maintained within narrow limits, despite a wide variation

Table 21.3   Approach to Pediatric Sepsis: Role of Procalcitonin

Procalcitonin

Principle	The synthesis of PCT can be increased up to 100 to 1000 fold due to circulating endotoxins or cytokines such as interleukin (IL)-6, tumor necrosis factor (TNF)-alpha, and IL-1b, which act on various tissues [19, 20]. The extra-thyroid synthesis of PCT occurs in the liver, pancreas, kidney, lung, intestine, and leukocytes; notably, the synthesis of PCT is suppressed within these tissues in the absence of bacterial infection [20, 21]. In contrast, cytokines released following viral infection, such as interferon (INF)-gamma, will lead to the down-regulation of PCT, thus highlighting another advantage of PCT assays [20, 22].
	Though the studies on the kinetics of PCT are limited, the biomarker has been shown to rise two to four hours after a bacterial stimulus, peak in 24–48 hours, and achieve a half-life of 2436 hours. Serial PCT measurements at 24-hour intervals for three to five days may be more beneficial than stand-alone PCT tests [20].
Procalcitonin Vs CRP	Few studies have done head ot head comparison of CRP and Pct. One such study, showed that the diagnostic accuracy of PCT with respect to CRP, was higher (75% Vs 72.6%) with greater specificity of Pct (72% Vs 33.3%), and negative predictive values (50 Vs 42.8). However, sensitivity of CRP was higher (76% Vs 85.5%). [23].
Current role in sepsis and infections	The United States Food and Drug Administration has approved using PCT assays for initiating or discontinuing antibiotics in lower respiratory tract infections (LRTIs) and for discontinuing antibiotics in patients with sepsis. The commonly used PCT cut points for withholding or stopping antibiotics in adults and children are 0.1 µg/L (very low risk of bacterial etiology) or 0.25 µg/L (low risk of bacterial etiology) [20, 24].
False reactions with PCT	• PCT assay may exhibit interference when a sample is collected from a person consuming a supplement with a high dose of biotin (also termed as vitamin B7 or B8, vitamin H, or coenzyme R) [24, 25]. • False decreased levels maybe observed in Mycoplasma pneumonia and localized infections (osteomyelitis, abscess, subacute endocarditis, empyema). Elevated levels may be observed in systemic vasculitis and acute graft vs host disease. • Treatment with agents that stimulate cytokines (OKT3, anti-lymphocyte globulins, alemtuzumab, IL-2, granulocyte transfusion), newborns <48–72 hours of age, end-stage renal disease, and paraneoplastic syndromes due to medullary thyroid and small cell lung cancer [20].

in dietary intake, metabolic rate, and kidney function. Water is one of the most significant components of the human body, and accounts for approximately 50% to 80% of total body weight. Total body water (TBW) varies from one individual to another. The percentage of TBW varies with age, gender, skeletal muscle mass, and fat content. In the average adult, water accounts for approximately 50% to 60% of total weight. The body weight of children who are less than 1 year of age has a significantly higher percentage of body water; premature infants and neonates have the highest percentages. At birth, TBW is 70% to 75% of body weight. This decreases dramatically in the first year of life. At puberty, more changes occur. Because of the lower water content of adipose tissue, TBW as a percentage of body weight is less in women than it is in men. TBW is distributed in two compartments: intracellular fluid (ICF) and extracellular fluid (ECF). In addition to the changes in the percentage of TBW as body weight, infants and young children have higher percentages of ECF as compared with adults. More than half of the newborn infant's body weight is ECF. This changes rapidly over the first 6 to 8 weeks of life. By 3 years of age, body fluid components more closely resemble those of the adult, with an ECF of approximately 20% to 23% and an ICF of 40% to 50% [45].

In this section, we shall look at some specific electrolytes and their lab testing and interpretation in PICU

1. Approaches to Potassium Testing and Management of Dyskalemia in PICU

Derangements in serum potassium levels can be life threatening .Flame Photometry and Ion Selective electrode method (ISC) are the two mainstays in potassium assays. These methods are simple, fast and reproducible. In estimation of potassium, it should be remembered that potassium gets redistributed in the body, intracellular potassium concentrations are nearly forty fold higher than extracellular concentration (K is predominantly intracellular), hence, any procedure that leads to releaseof intracellular contents as hemolysis can falsely elevate the potassium levels. This is particularly important is squeezed samples as those from NICU. This has been further elaborated in Table 21.6. Figure 21.4 shows the effect of hemolysis on potassium values.

Table 21.4 Approach to Prothrombin Time

Indications of doing INR [26, 27]	• Bleeding diathesis in patients with coagulation factors deficiency (fibrinogen and factors II, V, VII, or X, or a combined deficiency) in the extrinsic pathway. • Disseminated intravascular coagulation (DIC). • Baseline sample collection before starting anticoagulation. • Monitoring the efficacy and safety while the patients are on warfarin due to clinical conditions with an increased risk of thrombosis such as mechanical heart valves, persistent atrial fibrillation, venous thromboembolism, stroke, and peripheral arterial disease. • Test for liver synthetic function and to calculate the model for end-stage liver diseases (MELD) score in end-stage liver disease.
Principle	Prothrombin time is used to evaluate the extrinsic and common pathways of coagulation, which helps detect deficiencies of factors II, V, VII, and X and low fibrinogen concentrations [28–30]. Prothrombin time measures the time, in seconds, for plasma to clot after adding thromboplastin (a mixture of tissue factor, calcium, and phospholipid) to a patient's plasma sample [28, 30]. The principle of the test is as follows: The venous blood samples are collected in plastic tubes with a light blue top that contains 3.2% sodium citrate [31]. Sodium citrate chelates the calcium in the blood sample and prevents the activation of the coagulation cascade [32]. This chelation keeps the blood sample in stasis until it is ready to be tested. Tube filling must be within 90% of the full collection volume with a blood-to-sodium citrate ratio of 9 to 1 [30, 33]. The tube is then gently inverted a few times to mix the sodium citrate solution with the blood. The tube should not be shaken to avoid hemolysis, which would lead to inaccurate results. Once the blood sample is ready to be tested, calcium chloride is added to restore the calcium required for coagulation activation [32]. Clot formation can be detected mechanically or optically, depending on the instrumentation used [30, 34]. The time required for the formation of a stable clot is recorded in seconds and represents the actual PT result. INR is calculated from the PT and allows for worldwide standardization of results [35].
Values [26]	For normal patients who are not on anticoagulation, the INR is usually 1.0 regardless of the ISI or the particular performing laboratory [8]. For patients who are on anticoagulant therapy, the therapeutic INR ranges between 2.0 to 3.0. INR levels above 4.9 are considered critical values and increase the risk of bleeding
Interpretation	Different preparations of thromboplastin reagents are available but can give different prothrombin time results even when using the same plasma. Due to this variability, the World Health Organization (WHO) introduced the international normalized ratio (INR), the standard reporting format for prothrombin time results [30, 36, 37]. The INR represents the ratio of the patient's prothrombin time divided by a control prothrombin time value obtained using an international reference thromboplastin reagent developed by the WHO, it was initially developed by Kirkwood in 1983 [27, 28, 30, 37]. The reference values for INR consider, in PT measurement, device-related variations, type of reagents used, and sensitivity differences in the TF activator. INR value is dimensionless and ranges from a score of 2.0 to 3.0 [27].
POCT INR [37]	Capillary whole blood can be obtained from POC-PT systems by a fingerstick which is then applied to a test strip or cartridge. The INR value from POCT is considered acceptable if it does not exceed plus or minus 0.5 INR units by the reference laboratory INR value [27]. TTR has been employed to verify the quality of the oral anticoagulation in the control groups, i.e., that of patients treated with warfarin. One meta-analysis [31] shows an increase in the TTR of 8% in patients who carry out self-monitoring or self-management of therapy [37, 39]. The meta-analysis showed that POCD INR testing reduced the risk of major thromboembolic events (odds ratio [OR] = 0.51; 95% confidence interval [CI] 0.35–0.74), was associated with fewer deaths (OR = 0.58; 95% CI = 0.38–0.89), and resulted in better INR control compared with laboratory INR testing [39]. The various POCTs available are as follows

Type of analysis	POC device used	Manufacturer
Prothrombin time/international normalized ratio (PT/INR)	Xprecia stride coagulation analyzer	Siemens Healthcare
PT/INR, activated clotting time (ACT) kaolin, ACT celite	i-STAT Handheld using CG8+ cartridge	Abbot India Limited
PT and activated partial prothrombin time (aPTT)	CoaguCheck Pro II	Roche Diagnostics India Pvt. Ltd.
PT/INR	CoaguCheck XS system	Roche Diagnostics India Pvt. Ltd.

(Continued)

Table 21.4 (Continued)

Interactions	The following are the drugs that cause prolongation of INR: Antibiotics, especially cotrimoxazole, macrolides, metronidazole, and fluoroquinolones; Antifungals: azoles (fluconazole); Chemotherapeutics: imatinib, Fluorouracil (5-FU); Amiodarone; Allopurinol; Serotonin reuptake inhibitors (fluoxetine, sertraline)
	Several medications may decrease INR value, for example: Antibiotics: Dicloxacillin, nafcillin; Azathioprine; Antiepileptics (Carbamazepine, phenobarbital, phenytoin); Saint John's Wort and Vitamin K [27].

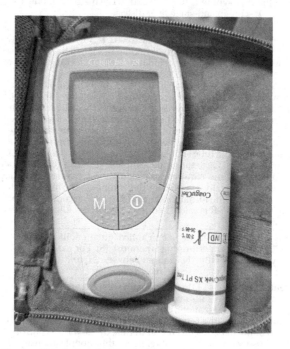

Figure 21.3 POCT CoagucCheck for checking INR with minimal blood sample requirement with lower turnaround time.

2. **Approach to Sodium Testing and Dysnatremia in PICU**

- Sodium absorption occurs almost quantitatively in the distal small bowel and the colon.

- Kidneys: Sodium filtered by the glomeruli is reabsorbed in a proportion ranging from 0.5% to 10% according to the needs at the tubular level. Na 2/3rd absorbed in PCT. 20% in ascending limbs secondary to Cl (active transport). 7% in DCT and 5% in CD – aldosterone dependent exchange for K or H.

- Angiotensin II, norepinephrine, aldosterone, and insulin stimulate reabsorption, whereas dopamine, cAMP, the cardiac natriuretic peptides, and prostaglandins exert a natriuretic effect.

- Small losses of sodium occur through feces and sweat; these losses increase with increasing sodium intake, although part of them are obligatory [53]. Approach to dysnatremia in PICU has been further elucidated in Table 21.7.

3. **Approach to Calcium in PICU**: Calcium is the most abundant mineral in the body. It plays an important role in bone metabolism and maintaining body homeostasis. Calcium homeostasis is maintained in our bodies by vitamin D levels, parathyroid harmone, phosphate, and magnesium. It is predominantly measured by automated colorimetric method, but in some resource limited settings manual methods are still being used. The clinicians must be aware whether the lab has reported ionized (the term ionized calcium is used for free ionic calcium fraction that is physiologically active in our blood) or total calcium, and interpret accordingly. Total calcium

Table 21.5   Approach to Hemoglobin in PICU

Ground picture and prevalence of anemia in India	The highest spike in anemia was reported among children (659 months) with a rise to 67.1% (NFHS-5) from 58.6% (NFHS-4, 2015–16) followed by girls aged 15–19 years [40, 41]. The Comprehensive National Nutrition Survey (CNNS) conducted in 2016–2018, revealed that 41% of preschoolers (1–4 years), 24% of school-age children (5–9 years), and 28% of adolescents (10–19 years) in India have anemia [40, 41].			
Definition of anemia	Anemia is defined as a hemoglobin concentration below a specified cut-off point; that cut-off point depends on the age, gender, physiological status, smoking habits, and altitude at which the population being assessed lives. WHO defines anemia in children aged under 5 years and pregnant women as a hemoglobin concentration <110 g/L at sea level, and anemia in non-pregnant women as a hemoglobin concentration <120 g/L [42]. However, a recent study based on CNNS Data showed that anemia cutoffs in children and adolescents from African and Asian regions were substantially lower (1–2 g/dL) in several datasets compared with WHO-recommended cutoffs [43].			
Blood test [43]	Capillary fingerpick blood usually produces higher Hb concentrations compared with venous blood			
Blood test principles [44]	**Method**	**Laboratory**	**Blood volume (mcgL)**	**Time required for test (in sec)**
	Copper sulphate technique	Clinical laboratory	10	20
	Cyanmethemoglobin method	Clinical laboratory	10	5–10 min prep time and 60 s for the test, with Drabkin's reagent as control
	Automated hematology analyzers (AHA)	Clinical laboratory	200	30 sec
	Invasive photometric point-of-care analyzers (e.g., HemoCue, Hemo-Control, Hb-Quick, DiaSpect, URIT, and TrueHb)	Clinical laboratory and field settings	10	20 sec
	Paper- or color-based analytical devices (e.g., μPADs and color-based filter test)	Clinical laboratory	20	45–60 min
	Available POCTs include the following			
	Test type	**Product**	**Company**	
	Hemoglobin and whole blood CBS	HemoCue Hb 201+ system	HemoCue India	
	Low levels of hemoglobin	HemoCue Plasma/Low Hb system	HemoCue India	
	Low levels of hemoglobin	HemoCue Plasma/Low Hb system	HemoCue India	
Treatment [45]	• Depending upon the clinical condition and degree of anemia, the treatment can vary from the requirement of transfusion to conservative nutritional rehabilitation and finding the inherent cause of anemia.			

(Continued)

Table 21.5 (Continued)

	• In the recently published TAXI guidelines, the authors recommend prior to transfusion, the clinicians consider not only the Hb concentration, but also the overall clinical context (e.g., symptoms, signs, physiological markers, laboratory results) and the risks, benefits, and alternatives to transfusion. • In critically ill children with respiratory failure who do not have severe acute hypoxemia, a chronic cyanotic condition or hemolytic anemia, and whose hemodynamic status is stable, the Pediatric Critical Care Transfusion and Anaemia Expertise Initiative (TAXI) consensus recommendations do not recommend administering an RBC transfusion if the Hb concentration is ≥7 g/dL. They recommend RBC transfusion for critically ill children with respiratory failure who have an Hb concentration <5g/dL. • In critically ill children with acute brain injury (e.g., trauma, stroke), the TAXI authors recommend that an RBC transfusion be considered if the Hb concentration falls between 7 and 10 g/dL. • In hematological diseases, as children with sickle cell disease who are critically ill or those at risk of critical illness, TAXI authors recommend RBC transfusion to achieve a target Hb concentration of 10 g/dL.

Table 21.6 Approach to Potassium Values in PICU

Underlying physiology	The vast majority of potassium is in the intracellular compartment with a small amount in the extracellular space. Normal serum potassium is 3.5 to 5.5 mEq/L; however, plasma potassium is 0.5 mEq/L lower.
Principle [47, 48]	Serum potassium is measured by the use of a flame photometer or ion-selective electrode. The procedure is rapid, simple, and reproducible. It is usually measured using an Ion-selective electrode (ISE), which converts the activity (or effective concentration) of the ion dissolved in solution into an electric potential measured by a voltmeter. Both plasma and serum can be used to measure potassium. Samples can be collected in plain silicone-coated glass/plastic tubes, gel separator tubes with or without clot activator for serum estimations (with thrombin-based clot activator for stat estimations), or in tubes containing lithium/sodium/ammonium heparin as an anticoagulant for plasma estimations with or without gel separator.
Approach to Hyperkalemia	
Effect of hemolysis	Hemolysis is known to have a significant impact on values of potassium. HI≥136.97 is known to have a significant impact [49] (Figure 21.4). In addition, hemolysis is of concern in neonatal samples, as neonatal sampling is difficult, and squeezing increases the possibility of hemolysis.
False high values	• Tight tourniquet; (2) vigorous exercise of the extremity during blood drawing; (3) hemolysis due to vigorous shaking of the test tube; (4) thrombocytosis (platelet count greater than 600,000); and (5) leucocytosis (WBC greater than 200,000) • The problem of hemolysis due to squeezing out a sample is particularly pronounced in pediatrics, especially in small children where taking out a sample is very difficult. • If ethanol-containing antiseptics are not allowed to dry completely before venipuncture, the solution can enter the blood stream and disrupt cell membranes. • Delayed processing results in exhaustion of available glucose to generate ATP. Since ATP fuels the sodium-potassium pump and maintains the gradient across the cell membrane, failure of the pump results in leakage of potassium out of the cell, resulting in pseudohyperkalemia. • Fear of imminent venipuncture or crying associated with hyperventilation (even for 3–6 min) is associated with acute respiratory alkalosis, which results in a significant hyperkalemic response mediated by enhanced alpha-adrenergic activity. • Carryover and backflow of potassium salts of tube additives such as ethylenediamine tetra-acetic acid (EDTA) or oxalate can elevate measured potassium.
Values	The normal range for serum potassium is narrow (3.5 to 5.5 mEq/L),
ECG changes	• Elevated potassium causes ECG changes in a dose-dependent manner: • K = 5.5 to 6.5 mEq/L ECG will show tall, peaked t-waves • K = 6.5 to 7.5 mEq/L ECG will show loss of p-waves • K = 7 to 8 ECG mEq/L will show widening of the QRS complex • K = 8 to 10 mEq/L will produce cardiac arrhythmias, sine wave pattern, and asystole It should be noted that the rate of rise in serum potassium is a greater factor than the level. Patients with chronic hyperkalemia may have relatively normal EGCs even at high levels, and significant ECG changes may be present at much lower levels in patients with sudden spikes in serum potassium. ECG features of hyperkalemia include small or absent P wave; prolonged PR interval; augmented R wave; wide QRS and peaked T waves.

(Continued)

Table 21.6 (Continued)

Additional testing	Additional laboratory testing should include serum blood urea nitrogen and creatinine to assess renal function, and urinalysis to screen for renal disease. Urine potassium, sodium, and osmolality may also be helpful in evaluating the cause. In patients with renal disease, the serum calcium level should also be checked because hypocalcemia may exacerbate the cardiac effects of hyperkalemia. Complete blood count to screen for leucocytosis or thrombocytosis may also be helpful. Serum glucose and blood gas analysis should be ordered in diabetics and patients with suspected acidosis. Lactate dehydrogenase should be ordered in patients with suspected hemolysis. Creatinine phosphokinases and urine myoglobin should be ordered in patients with suspected rhabdomyolysis. Uric acid and phosphorus should be ordered in patients with suspected tumor lysis syndrome. Digoxin toxicity may cause hyperkalemia so serum levels should be checked in patients on digoxin. If no other cause is found, consider cortisol and aldosterone levels to assess for mineralocorticoid deficiency [50].
Pathophysiology	• Pseudohyperkalemia signifies an in vitro phenomenon (i.e., the in vivo serum potassium is normal). This is caused by the release of potassium from cellular components of blood during the process of clotting and, less commonly, by the release of potassium from ischemic muscle cells due to tight tourniquet or hand/arm exercise during the blood-drawing process. If the latter is suspected, blood should be drawn in a proper manner again and serum potassium repeated. • Hyperkalemia with normal total body potassium is caused by the shift of potassium out of the cell and is commonly seen in acidemia, a sudden increase in plasma osmolality. In patients with relatively normal GFR, hyperkalemia is usually due to a defect in the renin-angiotensin-aldosterone axis or to a defect in the renal tubular responsiveness to aldosterone [47]. • On the other hand, hypokalemia with normal total body potassium, by definition, is due to a shift of potassium into the cell. This shift could occur in alkalemia, states of high endogenous or exogenous insulin or catecholamines, and, in very rare situations, for unknown reasons (hypokalemia periodic paralysis).
Treatment of hyperkalemia	• Step 1: Evaluate patient for potential toxicities and initiate ECG monitoring. If patient has severe hyperkalemia or shows ECG changes, transfer to intensive care unit (ICU) immediately. Ca-Gluconate 10% can be used in patients with cardiac symptoms to stabilize membrane potential and positively influence bradycardia and ECG changes. Contraindications: digoxin-intoxication, hypercalcemic states. • Step 2: Identify and immediately eliminate sources of potassium intake. Review prescriptions and stop oral or parenteral potassium supplements. Stop all drugs that might cause or aggravate hyperkalemia. Input from dieticians might be needed to identify potassium-rich foods (check for "special diets"), especially in patients with chronic renal failure. • Step 3: Increase potassium shift from extra- to intracellular space. Dextrose and/or insulin infusion. An effect can often be seen immediately but response remains unpredictable. Close electrolyte and blood glucose monitoring is needed, hypoglycemia being the main side-effect. Aim to maintain blood glucose 10–15 mmol/l. Beta-adrenergic agonists (salbutamol, reproterol) stimulate potassium to shift from extra to intracellular space via Na^+/K^+-ATPase as described above. Salbutamol can be applied via a nebulizer or given intravenously. If given IV, the lowering effect of salbutamol is quite predictable with a mean decrease of 1.6–1.7 mmol/l after 2 h. It can cause tachycardia. Salbutamol has been shown to be safe and even superior to rectal cation-exchange resin in nonoliguric preterm with hyperkalemia. Sodium bicarbonate is preferably given to patients who are acidotic. In hemodialysis patients with hyperkalemia, it has only a moderate effect if given as prolonged infusion. • Step 4: Increase potassium excretion. Loop diuretics (furosemide) inhibit the inward transport of potassium via NKCC2 channel in the TAL. Even in chronic hemodialysis patients, treatment with loop diuretics may be of value if the patient has some residual renal function. Ion-exchange resins (containing calcium or sodium) aim to keep enteral potassium from being resorbed. More effective if given orally. Enemas should be retained for at least 30–60 min. Onset within 1–2 h, lasting 4–6 h. Renal replacement therapy (RRT) is the ultimate measure of severe hyperkalemia. Hemodialysis (HD) provides a substantially higher potassium clearance (removal of 50–80 mmol of K^+ in a 4 h session) than continuous forms of RRT. Continuous veno-venous hemofiltration (CVVH) can more satisfactorily provide long-term control of potassium. Choice of method depends on local circumstances and hemodynamics of the patients, as critical ill patients will rarely tolerate HD sessions [51]

(Continued)

185

Table 21.6 (Continued)

Treatment of hypokalemia [52]	Clinical manifestations do not occur with mild to moderate hypokalemia; thus, repletion is not urgent. Mild to moderate hypokalemia is typically treated with oral potassium supplements. Replacement therapy must be given more rapidly with severe hypokalemia or when clinical symptoms are present. Rapid correction can be provided via oral and/or IV formulation. IV administration is preferred in the setting of cardiac dysrhythmias, digitalis toxicity and recent or ongoing cardiac ischemia. The goal of potassium replacement in the context of renal or GI losses is to immediately raise serum potassium concentration to a safe level and then replace the remaining deficit over days to weeks [52].

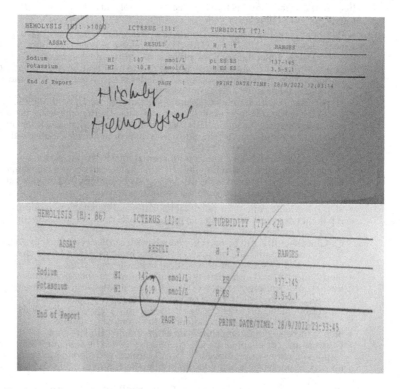

Figure 21.4 Sample reports illustrating the effect of hemolysis (as demonstrated by hemolytic index) on potassium values (the machine used is Vitros 5600).

should be interpreted with reference to albumin values, as most of the calcium is protein bound (predominantly albumin bound) in blood. This has been further elaborated in Table 21.8.

D. Acute liver failure

Acute hepatitis is an inflammatory disease of the liver, grossly subdivided into infectious and non-infectious. The condition can be self-limiting or can progress to fibrosis (scarring), cirrhosis, or liver cancer. This has been further elucidated in Table 21.9.

Some Clinical Pearls

1. Diagnostic stewardship is important in PICU as pediatric samples are precious.

2. The time lag between sampling, processing, transport from the sampling site to the lab, and lab diagnosis needs to be as quick as possible.

Table 21.7 Approach to Sodium Values in PICU

Sodium is an essential nutrient involved in the maintenance of normal cellular homeostasis and in the regulation of fluid and electrolyte balance and blood pressure (BP). Its role is crucial for maintaining ECF volume because of its important osmotic action and is equally important for the excitability of muscle and nerve cells and for the transport of nutrients and substrates through plasma membranes. Sodium absorption occurs almost quantitatively in the distal small bowel and the colon. Sodium balance in the body is closely linked to that of water and is finely maintained by the kidneys. Here, the sodium filtered by the glomeruli is reabsorbed in a proportion ranging from 0.5% to 10% according to the needs at the tubular level, in which angiotensin II, norepinephrine, aldosterone, and insulin stimulate reabsorption whereas dopamine, cAMP, the cardiac natriuretic peptides, and prostaglandins exert a natriuretic effect. Generally, small losses of sodium occur through feces and sweat; these losses increase with increasing sodium intake, although part of them are obligatory [53].

Hypernatremia	
What it is	• Defined as s. sodium >145meq/l. • Acute hypernatremia: hypernatremia of <48 hrs duration • Chronic hypernatremia >48 hrs. duration • Symptoms of hypernatremia appear in most children at s. sodium >158 meq/l • Life-threatening hypernatremia commonly due to salt poisoning, at s. sodium >180 meq/l • However, a crucial factor in determining the occurrence of cerebral lesions is hyperosmolality rather than actual s. sodium.
Severity of clinical manifestations	

Osmolarity (mOsm/kg)	Manifestations
350–375	Restlessness/irritability
375–400	Tremulousness/ataxia
400–430	Hyperreflexia/twitching/spasticity
>430	Death

• Severe symptoms are usually evident only with acute and large increases in plasma sodium concentrations above 158–160 mmol/l.
• If s. osmolality >350 mOsm/kg, mortality rate is >50%

Etiology	Classified into four categories. The first is pseudohyponatremia, in which the sodium level is low due to hyperproteinemia, hyperlipidemia, or hyperglycemia. The other three categories are based on overall patient fluid status and include hypovolemic (commonly due to fluid loss), hypervolemic (most often because of the syndrome of inappropriate secretion of antidiuretic hormone). Hypovolemic hyponatremia is managed by rehydration with isotonic saline. Hypervolemic hyponatremia is managed by addressing the underlying cause. Euvolemic hyponatremia is managed by restricting free water intake, addressing the underlying cause, and occasionally with drugs (e.g., vasopressin receptor antagonists). Patients with severe or acutely symptomatic hyponatremia (e.g., altered mental status, seizures), including those with acute symptomatic exercise-induced hyponatremia, require urgent treatment. This should consist of hypertonic saline administration along with monitoring of sodium levels to avoid overly rapid correction. Hypernatremia most often occurs because of water loss or inadequate water intake. Depending on severity, management involves oral or intravenous hypotonic fluids and addressing the underlying cause [54].

(Continued)

Table 21.7 (Continued)

Treatment

The primary goal in the treatment of patients with hypernatremia is the restoration of serum tonicity. In patients with hypernatremia that has developed over a period of hours, rapid correction of plasma sodium (falling by 1 mmol/L per hour) improves the prognosis without the risk of convulsions and cerebral edema). Management of a shocked patient needs specialist input and close monitoring, preferably in a high-dependency unit. Intravenous normal saline should be used to correct the extracellular fluid depletion, with calculation of the free water deficit to determine how much 5% dextrose to give. In patients with hypernatremia of longer or unknown duration, reducing the sodium concentration more slowly; with desmopressin, either as intranasal spray or tablets, with careful monitoring to avoid the complications of water intoxication (delaying one dose each week to allow polyuria and thirst to "breakthrough" in patients susceptible to hyponatremia with desmopressin may be prudent). Treatment of nephrogenic diabetes insipidus includes removal of precipitating drugs (if possible) and sometimes initiation of thiazide diuretics, non-steroidal anti-inflammatory drugs, or both. The following discussion primarily applies to the majority of patients in whom hypernatremia is induced by water loss [53, 55].

Method of fluid replacement: For stable/asymptomatic patients oral/NG, but, for persistent vomiting/high purge rate/altered sensorium is indication for IV correction.

Water deficit can be calculated from various equations.

Rate of correction: There are no definitive clinical trials, but data in children suggest that the maximum safe rate at which the plasma sodium concentration should be lowered is by 0.5 mEq/L per hour and no more than 12 mEq/L per day. Overly rapid correction is potentially dangerous in hypernatremia (as it is in hyponatremia). Hypernatremia initially causes fluid movement out of the brain and cerebral contraction that is primarily responsible for the associated symptoms. Within one to three days, however, brain volume is largely restored due to water movement from the cerebrospinal fluid into the brain and to the uptake of solutes by the cells). Rapidly lowering the plasma sodium concentration once this adaptation has occurred causes osmotic water movement into the brain, increasing brain size above normal. This cerebral edema can then lead to seizures, permanent neurologic damage, or death [55].

Hyponatremia

Pathophysiology

Acute hyponatremia is characterized by onset of symptoms <48h. Patients with acute hyponatremia develop neurologic symptoms resulting from cerebral edema induced by water movement into the brain. These may include seizures, impaired mental status, or coma and death.

Chronic hyponatremia: Hyponatremia developing over >48 h should be considered "chronic." Most patients have chronic hyponatremia. The serum sodium concentration is usually above 120meq/L. Brain adapts itself to hyponatremia by generation of idiogenic osmoles. This is a protective mechanism that reduces the degree of cerebral edema; it begins on the first day and is complete within several days. Hence, chronic hyponatremia patients may appear asymptomatic. Mild hyponatremia is characterized by gastrointestinal tract symptoms of nausea, vomiting, and loss of appetite. Sometimes, subtle neurologic abnormalities may be present when the serum sodium is between 120 and 130 meq/L [56]

Classification of hyponatremia by plasma tonicity

Classification	Serum sodium concentration (mmol/L)	Plasma osmolarity (mOsm/kg water)	Typical causes
Hypotonic	<135	Low <280	SIADH, heart failure, cirrhosis
Isotonic	<135	Normal (285–295)	Hyperglycemia, pseudohyponatremia (hyperlipidemia, hyperproteinemia)
Hypertonic	<135	High (>295)	Severe hyperglycemia with dehydration, mannitol

188

Investigations

1. Step 1: Measurement of serum sodium Ideally by ion-specific electrode (ISE) using direct potentiometry (IB)
2. Step 2: Serum osmolality: It differentiates true, pseudo, or translocational hyponatremia
3. Step 3: Urine osmolality: Urine osmolality can be used to distinguish between impaired water excretion and hyponatremia with normal water excretion
4. Step 4: Urine sodium: Determination of source of sodium loss-renal or non-renal is the next step. This is done by measuring the urinary sodium losses. In patients with hyperosmolar hyponatremia and inappropriate urine concentration, the urine sodium and urine chloride concentrations can be used to distinguish between hypovolemic and euvolemic hyponatremia
5. Step 5: Urine to serum electrolyte ratio
   It is the sum of the urine sodium plus potassium concentrations divided by the serum sodium concentration.
   Ratio <0.5 (high urine electrolyte-free water): fluid restriction is adequate.
   Ratio >1 (urine is hypertonic compared to the serum. Water restriction is not sufficient and other therapeutic measures are necessary to correct the hyponatremia.
6. Step 6: Fractional excretion of sodium: Fractional excretion of sodium (FENa) provides an accurate assessment of volume status than the urine sodium alone because it corrects for the effect of variations in urine volume on the urine sodium.
7. Step 7: In patients with normal renal function and hyponatremia cut off for FENa is <0.1%.
   <0.1%: hypovolemic hyponatremia
   >0.1%: hypervolemic and normovolemic hyponatremia.
8. Step 8: Serum uric acid and urea concentrations: Low serum uric acid and urea in SIADH, hypopituitarism, hypervolemia (V1a receptor stimulation), and thiazide diuretic-induced hyponatremia
9. Step 9: Acid-base and potassium balance: Evaluation of acid-base and potassium balance may be helpful in some patients
   Metabolic alkalosis and hypokalemia – diuretic use or vomitingMetabolic acidosis and hypokalemia – diarrhea or laxative abuseMetabolic acidosis and hyperkalemia primary adrenal insufficiency in patients without renal failureNormal acid-base and potassium – in the SIADHMild metabolic alkalosis and normal K – seen in hypopituitarism because of higher plasma aldosterone levels.

Treatment

1. Euvolemic hyponatremia [56]
General treatment Acute hyponatremia is generally symptomatic. The risk of brain herniation is high and rapid correction is needed.
   Acute hyponatremia is common in marathon runners, patients with primary polydipsia, and users of ecstasy. These patients have not had time for the brain adaptations to occur.Chronic hyponatremia: It is generally asymptomatic or has mild symptoms. However; it may present with seizures if hyponatremia is very severe. In chronic hyponatremia the brain undergoes adaptation and hence the risk of cerebral herniation is very low, unlike the risk in acute hyponatremia. Instead, very rapid correction can lead to osmotic demyelination syndrome (ODS).Equation to estimate efficacy of initial therapy: The degree to which one liter of a given solution initially raises the serum sodium concentration (SNa) in a hyponatremic patient, without any water or sodium losses in the urine, is estimated from the Adrogué-Madias formula.   2.   Hypervolemic hyponatremia [56]
Hypervolemic hyponatremia is seen in CHF and cirrhosis.Salt administration or 3% NaCl is generally contraindicated for chronic therapy in edematous patients, however may be needed in case of acute symptomatic hyponatremia and can be given as per management of acute symptomatic hyponatremia discussed above.Water restriction is the mainstay of therapy. Cirrhotics may need severe water restriction (<750 ml/day) which is difficult.Loop diuretics are the cornerstones of therapy in hypervolemic hyponatremia.In CHF. other therapies used include neurohormonal blockade, angiotensin-converting enzyme inhibitors, and β-adrenergic antagonists. 3.   Hypovolemic hyponatremia
Presentation may be acute or chronic. Mostly it is chronic.Sodium chloride, usually as 0.9% NaCl (11 provides 154 meq of Na+). Patients need administration of sodium chloride to correct the volume deficit. 3%/normal saline is not indicated. K may be added if required. 0.9% NaCl corrects the hyponatremia by two mechanisms: It slowly raises the serum sodium by approximately 1 meq/L for every liter of fluid infused since 0.9% NaCl has a higher sodium concentration (154 meq/L) than the hyponatremic plasma and by correcting the hypovolemia, it removes the stimulus to ADH release.Gastrointestinal losses: may be acute or chronic. Urine Cl is a better marker for volume status in patients with vomiting instead of Urine Na. Both K and bicarbonate deficits should be corrected along with volume correction [56].

Table 21.8   Approach to Calcium Values in PICU

Calcium homeostasis	Calcium homeostasis is largely regulated through an integrated hormonal system that controls calcium transport in the gut, kidney, and bone. It involves two major calcium-regulating hormones and their receptors – PTH and the PTH receptor (PTHR) [19] – and 1, 25(OH)$_2$D and the vitamin D receptor (VDR) [20] as well as serum ionized calcium and the calcium-sensing receptor (CaR). Serum calcium homeostasis has evolved to simultaneously maintain extracellular ionized calcium levels in the physiologic range while allowing the flow of calcium to and from essential stores. A decrease in serum calcium inactivates the CaR in the parathyroid glands to increase PTH secretion, which acts on the PTHR in the kidney to increase tubular calcium reabsorption, and in bone to increase net bone resorption. The increased PTH also stimulates the kidney to increase secretion of 1,25(OH)$_2$D, which activates the VDR in the gut to increase calcium absorption, in the parathyroid glands to decrease PTH secretion, and in bone to increase resorption. The decrease in serum calcium probably also inactivates the CaR in the kidney to increase calcium reabsorption and potentiate the effect of PTH. This integrated hormonal response restores serum calcium and closes the negative feedback loop. With a rise in serum calcium, these actions are reversed, and the integrated hormonal response reduces serum calcium. Together, these negative feedback mechanisms help to maintain total serum calcium levels in healthy individuals within a relatively narrow physiologic range of ~10% [57]. Approximately 50% of the calcium is free, 40–45% is protein bound mainly associated with albumin, and between 5–10% is complexed. Calcemia measures total calcium but only free calcium is biologically active [58].
Hypercalcemia	
Clinical manifestations	Severe hypercalcemia inhibits neuromuscular and myocardial depolarization leading to muscle weakness and arrhythmias. Cardiovascular effects include prolonged PR interval, short QT interval, widened QRS complex, and bradycardia. Increased thirst with polydipsia and polyuria is seen initially, progressing to nephrolithiasis and nephrocalcinosis in chronic cases. Neurologic features include impaired concentration and altered mental status ranging from confusion to irritability. Levels of more than 14 mg/dL can cause encephalopathy, and levels above 15 mg/dL are a medical emergency. Severe acute abdominal pain should be a clue to evaluate for pancreatitis. Osseous changes can lead to bone pain, gait abnormalities, and fractures and are seen radiologically as subperiosteal and endosteal bone resorption. In infants and young children, hypercalcemia can cause poor weight gain and failure to thrive [59]. Glucocorticoids are effective in hypercalcemia due to lymphoma or granulomatous diseases. Dialysis is generally reserved for those with severe hypercalcemia complicated with kidney failure [60].
Lab investigations	Hypercalcemia can be classified into 1. Mild hypercalcemia: 10.5 to 11.9 mg/dL 2. Moderate hypercalcemia: 12.0 to 13.9 mg/dL 3. Hypercalcemic crisis: 14.0 to 16.0 mg/Dl
Treatment	Treatment for hypercalcemia is required if the patient is symptomatic or if the calcium level is more than 15 mg/dL, even in asymptomatic patients. The goals of treating hypercalcemia include increased elimination from the extracellular fluid, reduced gastrointestinal (GI) absorption, and decreased bone resorption. Immediate therapy is directed at restoring intravascular volume and promoting calcium excretion in the urine with an infusion of 0.9% saline at twice the maintenance rate until any fluid deficit is replaced and diuresis occurs. Calcitonin can be administered subcutaneously but in most cases, the effects are mild and limited to a few days. Patients with hyperparathyroidism require surgical exploration and removal of the source of increased PTH secretion. Postoperatively, patients need to be monitored closely for the development of hypocalcemia and tetany. Bisphosphonates such as etidronate, pamidronate, and alendronate are the drugs of choice for hypercalcemia of malignancy as they inhibit osteoclastic activity [59].

(Continued)

Table 21.8 (Continued)

Hypocalcemia	
Manifestations	The history and physical exam of patients with suspected hypocalcemia should be conducted with two underlying principles in mind. First, the potential manifestations of hypocalcemia must be uncovered. • Seizures: Can be the sole manifestation or a part of the whole myriad of clinical presentation. • Tetany: Generally induced by a rapid decline in serum ionized calcium. Tetany is usually the most dangerous and most commonly seen in the presence of respiratory alkalosis causing hypocalcemia. • Paresthesia: Can be perioral or otherwise. • Psychiatric manifestations: Can be associated with anxiety/depression/emotional lability. • Carpopedal spasm: Also referred to as Trousseau's sign. It represents increased neuromuscular excitability which may be related to the gating function of calcium ion for ion channels at a cellular level (particularly in neurons). This manifests as a spasm of hand upon routine BP check. • Chvostek's sign: Another manifestation of heightened neuromuscular excitability. It is the spasm of facial muscles in response to tapping the facial nerve near the angle of the jaw. • QTc prolongation: Can lead to Torsade's de pointes although extremely rare, it can be fatal. • The second part of history and physical should focus on determining the cause of hypocalcemia such as recent head and neck surgery, family history of similar problems, history of kidney disease, alcohol abuse (hypomagnesemia), psychiatric history, etc.
Workup	Work up of hypocalcemia is discussed as follows: Confirming hypocalcemia: The first part of the evaluation should focus on confirming the hypocalcemia and requires checking a serum albumin level to correct the total calcium, or measuring directly the ionized calcium level (where available). An EKG should also be obtained for all suspected cases of hypocalcemia to look for QTc prolongation which if present is a risk factor for Torsade's de pointes. Etiology of hypocalcemia: This part can be driven by the clinical picture obtained during previous steps. Usually entails checking electrolytes such as serum magnesium and phosphorus levels and at least a serum PTH level. If suspicion for vitamin D deficiency is high based on history then Vitamin D2 level should be measured as vitamin D3 can be affected by PTH levels. Other biomarkers may be obtained as indicated by history and physical, e.g., serum lipase in suspected pancreatitis [61].
Management	Management of hypocalcemia can be divided into two broad categories: Symptomatic hypocalcemia: intravenous calcium is recommended for rapid repletion if there is any evidence of neuromuscular excitability. If the symptoms are mild such as paresthesia or psychiatric oral calcium can be attempted. Calcium gluconate is the preferred solution and can be given over 10–30 minutes depending on the severity of symptoms. Calcium chloride can be used if central venous access is available. Alkaline solutions like bicarbonate and phosphorus-containing solutions need to be avoided through the same IV to avoid the precipitation of calcium salts. Asymptomatic hypocalcemia: if corrected total serum calcium is below 7.5mg/dL, IV calcium should still be the preferred method. However, if corrected serum calcium is >7.5 mg/dL and the patient is asymptomatic, oral calcium can be used. Vitamin D supplementation is often recommended with calcium to promote absorption because vitamin D deficiency is commonly encountered in most clinical scenarios leading to hypocalcemia. It is also important to address disease-specific problems and correct co-exiting electrolyte disturbances, e.g., hypomagnesemia [61].

Table 21.9 Approach to Various Lab Tests in the Context of Acute Liver Failure

Definition	PALFSG definition of ALF in children [62, 63] (1) No known evidence of chronic liver disease (2) Biochemical evidence of acute liver injury, (3) Hepatic-based coagulopathy defined as a prothrombin time (PT) ≥ 15 seconds or INR ≥ 1.5 not corrected by Vitamin K in the presence of clinical hepatic encephalopathy (HE) or a PT ≥20 seconds or INR ≥2.0 regardless of the presence or absence of clinical hepatic encephalopathy (HE).

(Continued)

Table 21.9 (Continued)

Other definitions	O'Grady *et al.* [64, 65]. (King's College Hospital data, 1972–1985)	Sub-classification: interval between jaundice and HE [64, 65] • Hyper-acute liver failure: 0 to 7 days • Acute liver failure: 8 to 28 days (high incidence of cerebral edema) • Subacute liver failure 5 to 12 weeks of the onset of jaundice (low incidence of cerebral edema but a poor prognosis) • Late-onset acute liver failure: 56 to 182 days
	Bernuau *et al.* (Paris, 1986) [66] FHF defined by temporal relationship between jaundice and encephalopathy	1. ALF: Rapidly developing impairment of hepatocyte function 2. Severe ALF: a. Without hepatic encephalopathy b. ≥ 50% decrease in hepatic coagulation factors Particularly prothrombin and factor V (proaccelerin). 3. FHF: a. ALF complicated by hepatic encephalopathy b. <2 weeks after the onset of jaundice 4. Sub-fulminant liver failure: a. ALF complicated by encephalopathy b. 2 weeks to 3 months after the onset of jaundice
	Acute liver failure [67] (AASLD position paper) (2005)	1. Evidence of coagulation abnormality (INR ≥1.5) 2. Any degree of mental alteration (encephalopathy) 3. Patient without pre-existing cirrhosis 4. An illness of <26 weeks duration
General tests	(a) General laboratory/organ-specific investigations, followed by serial hepatic re-assessments. (b) Etiological investigations: Should be prioritized according to age and history. (c) Liver Tests: Ammonia should preferably be an arterial sample. (d) Radiological: Ultrasound abdomen is essential to look at liver parenchyma (nodularity, texture, etc.), varices, splenomegaly, and portal hypertension. Doppler helps assess patency of hepatic veins, portal veins, and hepatic artery.	
Liver function tests	1. Tests Reflecting Hepatocellular Necrosis: LFT: Serum NH3, AST (aspartate aminotransferase (AST) and ALT (serum alanine aminotransferase (ALT). Serum ALT values are higher than serum AST values unless cirrhosis already is present. AST and ALT can be derived from muscle, the clinician should verify that serum creatine kinase values are within the normal range 2. Tests reflecting cholestasis: Total bilirubin, direct bilirubin, S.GGT(gamma-glutamyl transferase) (GGT is found in hepatocytes and biliary epithelial cells), S.ALP (serum alkaline phosphatase) 3. Tests reflecting liver failure: PT (prothrombin time), albumin, A:G ratio. Always do PT for all patients who come with hepatitis; it helps identify the severity of liver cell dysfunction. 4. Other organ systems: KFT/SE, urea, blood, and urine culture. 5. Blood group/cross matching: Arrange blood (for possibility of bleeding) 6. Radiological: Ultrasound abdomen is essential to look at liver parenchyma (nodularity, texture, etc.), varices, splenomegaly, and portal hypertension. Doppler helps assess patency of hepatic veins, portal veins, and hepatic artery. Ultrasound abdomen: not routinely indicated, important, if persistence of fever with tender hepatomegaly and other atypical features as referred pain or firm hepatomegaly, among others, to rule out conditions such as liver abscess. It can also help identify liver echotexture, and intrahepatic biliary radicle dilation to rule out features of obstruction.	

(Continued)

Table 21.9   (Continued)

Specific lab investigations for workup [65, 67–69]	Hematological and coagulation	Complete blood cell count with platelets PT-INR, aPTT, fibrinogen, D-dimer, blood group, cross-match
	Biochemistry	Serum sodium, potassium, chloride, bicarbonate, calcium, magnesium, phosphate, glucose, AST, ALT, alkaline phosphatase, GGT, total bilirubin, albumin, creatinine, blood urea nitrogen, serum osmolarity. Blood gas with pH
	Liver synthetic function	Ammonia, PT, aPTT, lactate, LFT
	Sepsis screening	Procalcitonin, urinalysis and microscopic analysis, blood cultures, urine cultures, tracheal cultures (if intubated)
	Radiological	USG abdomen (focusing on liver)/Doppler of hepatic vasculature/chest radiograph, electrocardiogram
	Additional monitoring	EEG, BIS, ICP monitor as indicated
	Etiological Workup	
	INFECTIVE (Paediatric Acute Liver Failure study group incidence: 8%) [70]	
	Viral hepatitis; A, B, C, E	Hepatitis A infection Anti-HAV antibody (IgM) Hepatitis B infection HbsAg, anti-core antibody (HbcAb IgM) Hepatitis D infection Anti-hepatitis D virus antibody (IgM) Hepatitis C infection Anti-hepatitis C virus antibody (IgM)
	EBV, Adenovirus, Parvovirus, HSV, CMV	Viral serology
	Other infection	Malaria; dengue; leptospirosis
	Autoimmune hepatitis Paediatric Acute Liver Failure study group incidence 9% [70]	
	Autoantibodies ANA, ASMA, anti-LKM1, immunoglobulins IgG	
	Hematological: includes familial lymphohistiocytosis, macrophage activation syndrome, leukemia	
	Hemophagocytic Lymphohistiocytosis	Bone marrow aspiration (typical cells), raised ferritin, raised triglycerides, low/absent NK cell activity
	Leukemia/lymphoma	Blood film, bone marrow
	Toxicology screen and drug panel	
	Acetaminophen, opiates, barbiturates, cocaine, alcohol, sodium valproate, sulfasalazine, halothane, amanita phalloides, chemotherapy	
	Metabolic	
	Galactosemia	Urine positive for non-glucose reducing substances while on lactose feeds; confirmation by blood Galactose-1 phosphatase uridyl transferase enzyme assay
	Neonatal hemochromatosis/ Congenital alloimmune hepatitis	Buccal mucosal biopsy, raised ferritin, high transferrin saturation
	Urea cycle disorders	Plasma aminoacidogram. Orotic acid estimation in urine to diagnose supplementation OTC deficiency, blood gas, lactate/pyruvate ratio, urine organic acids, ammonia
	Tyrosinemia	Tyrosinemia urinary succinylacetone, tandem mass spectroscopy
	Hereditary Fructose Intolerance	History, enzyme analysis
	Neonatal hemochromatosis	*Transferrin saturation, iron, *ferritin, *lip biopsy
	Niemann Pick Type C	Bone marrow

(Continued)

Table 21.9 (Continued)

Wilson's Disease [68]	Serum ceruloplasmin, 24-hour urinary copper estimation, KF ring. Clue to etiology: alkaline phosphatase/bilirubin ratio <4.0, AST/ALT ratio >2.2 ± evidence of Coombs negative hemolysis/24-hour urine penicillamine challenge; mutational analysis
Mitochondrial cytopathies	Muscle biopsy, skin biopsy for fibroblasts, acylcarnitines, MRI head/plasma lactate >2.5 mmol/L, molar ratio of plasma lactate/pyruvate >20:1, paradoxical increase in plasma ketone bodies or lactate after meals Urinary analysis by mass spectroscopy; Genetic mutational analysis for respiratory chain disorders and tandem mass spectrometry for fatty acid oxidation defects.
Reye syndrome and fatty acid oxidation disorders	Urinary and blood organic acid chromatography, carnitine and fatty-acid level Carnitine – acylcarnitine profile
Vascular/Ischemic	
Budd Chiari Syndrome	Doppler US/CT/MRI
Acute circulatory failure	History/ischemic
Cardiomyopathy	History/ECG/ECHO
Sepsis	Blood/urine cultures/D-dimers
Impaired Adrenal Function	Cortisol, short synacthen test
Miscellaneous	Pancreatitis (amylase), myositis (CK)

The components of the management strategy are:
Etiological determination
Severity assessment and prognostication
Prevention or treatment of complications and monitoring for further organ deterioration
Liver transplantation when spontaneous survival is considered unlikely
Possible use of liver support devices and ammonia salvage

Summary of management strategies [71]

Ensuring airway: to monitor the GCS of the child and secure airway if clinically indicated (GCS<8 or rapidly falling).

It is important to ensure oxygenation and carbon dioxide elimination, in keeping with neuroprotective strategies.

Continuous monitoring including: vital signs, heart rate, respiratory rate, blood pressure, continuous oxygen saturation, and ETCO2 monitoring are recommended. Frequent neurological observations/coma grading and keeping an eye on clinical features of increased intracranial pressure are imperative.

Regular electrolytes, arterial blood gases, blood sugar (more frequently in an unstable child), ammonia and prothrombin time should also be monitored. It is also helpful to monitor the liver function tests and kidney function tests periodically [72, 73].

Securing IV access: If vasopressor support and high glucose infusion rates are required central venous access may be required [74].

Coagulopathy: Vitamin K may be given. Blood products may be required in discussion with specialist center, if the child is actively bleeding, if he requires invasive procedures, or has severe coagulopathy [74, 75].

Regular monitoring of blood glucose is recommended.

Prophylactic administration of proton pump inhibitors/H2 blockers is recommended in acute liver failure (ALF) [74, 76, 77].

IV fluids: Intravenous fluids should be adjusted as per patient's clinical condition, electrolyte, glucose, and renal parameters of the patient [74]. Restriction of fluids to 2/3rd maintenance is generally advisable [78]. 0.9% NaCl +10% Dextrose, with added potassium as per lab potassium values, is a good alternative for maintenance.

N-Acetylcysteine: This may be further discussed with specialist center and instituted as required [74, 79].

Antibiotics.

(Continued)

Table 21.9 (Continued)

Etiology specific management	Cause	Target-specific therapy of underlying ALF
	Acetaminophen poisoning [65, 67]	1. NAC may be given orally (140 mg/kg by mouth or nasogastric tube diluted to 5% solution, followed by 70 mg//kg by mouth q4hrly X 17 doses). Side effects include nausea, vomiting, urticaria, or bronchospasm. 2. In patients when oral administration is difficult as GI bleeding Intravenously (loading dose is 150 mg/kg in 5% dextrose over 15 minutes; maintenance dose is 50 mg/kg given over 4 hours followed by 100 mg/kg administered over 16 hours). Watch for allergic reactions.
	HSV	Acyclovir 10 mg/kg 8 hourly or 150 mg/m²/day IV
	Neonatal hemochromatosis(NH)	1. Certain centers recommend one dose of IVIG while NH is being considered. 2. If NH is proven, and the infant has not improved, an exchange transfusion should be performed followed by administration of a second dose of IVIG [80] 3. "Cocktail" composed of vitamin E (25 IU/kg/day, orally), N-acetylcysteine (100 mg/kg/day, intravenously), prostaglandin-E1 (0.4 µg/kg/h, intravenously, for a maximum of two weeks), selenium (3 micrograms/kg/day, intravenously), and desferrioxamine (30 mg/kg/day, intravenously until the ferritin level falls to 500 ng/mL) [81].
	Mushroom poisoning(usually Amanita phalloides) [67]	1. Gastric lavage and activated charcoal via nasogastric tube. 2. Fluid resuscitation 3. Penicillin G 300,000–1 million units/kg/day IV 4. Silymarin (silibinin or milk thistle) 30–40 mg/kg/day IV or orally 5. N-acetylcysteine
	Autoimmune hepatitis [65]	1. Methyl prednisolone 1–2 mg/kg IV (max 60mg) 2. Azathioprine may be added to steroids
	Metabolic disorders	
	Tyrosinemia type 1 (HT1, fumarylacetoacetase deficiency)	1. Nitisinone (NTBC, Orfadin®,): Dose of 1 mg/kg/d once a day as the half-life is 54 hrs. A dose of 2 mg/kg/d should be given for 48 hours for those in acute severe liver failure [82, 83]. 2. A diet low in phenylalanine and tyrosine.

3. Interpret samples in the context of the possibility of hemolysis, turbidity, and lipemia. Look out for hemolytic indices in the report, when feasible.

4. Ensure appropriate diagnostic algorithm is followed in the context of disease diagnosis.

5. Understand that tests are only there to supplement clinical history and examination, and are not a replacement of the same.

6. Ensure that due precautions are undertaken when sampling is done to avoid needle pricks.

REFERENCES

1. Fatemi Y, Bergl PA. Diagnostic stewardship: appropriate testing and judicious treatments. *Crit Care Clin.* 2022;38(1):69–87.

2. Sick-Samuels AC, Woods-Hill C. Diagnostic stewardship in the pediatric intensive care unit. *Infect Dis Clin North Am.* 2022;36(1):203–218.

3. Chon CH, Lai FC, Shortliffe LM. Pediatric urinary tract infections. *Pediatr Clin North Am.* 2001;48(6):1441–1459.

4. Indian Society of Pediatric Nephrology, Vijayakumar M, Kanitkar M, Nammalwar BR, Bagga A. Revised statement on management of urinary tract infections. *Indian Pediatr.* 2011;48(9):709–717.

5. Rudd, Kristina E *et al*. Global, regional, and national sepsis incidence and mortality, 1990–2017: analysis for the Global Burden of Disease Study. *Lancet*.2020;395(10219):200–211.

6. Kaufman J, Temple-Smith M, Sanci L. Urinary tract infections in children: an overview of diagnosis and management. *BMJ Paediatrics Open*. 2019;3(1):e000487.

7. Cyriac J, Holden K, Tullus K. How to use… urine dipsticks. *Arch Disease Childhood Edu Pract*. 2017;102(3):148–154.

8. Fritzenwanker M, Imirzalioglu C, Chakraborty T, Wagenlehner FM. Modern diagnostic methods: for urinary tract infections. *Exp Rev Anti-Infective Therapy*. 2016;14(11):1047–1063.

9. Ekambaram S, Jahan A, Sathe KP. Urinary tract infection in children. In: *Standard Treatment Guidelines* 2022 [Internet]. IAP Action Plan 2022, IAP Standard Treatment Guidelines Committee, Indian Academy of Pediatrics (IAP); Available from: https://iapindia.org/pdf/STG-06-Urinary-Tract-Infection-in-Children.pdf.

10. Schlapbach LJ, Watson RS, Sorce LR, Argent AC, Menon K, Hall MW, *et al*. International consensus criteria for pediatric sepsis and septic shock. *JAMA*. 2024 [cited 2024 Feb 6]. Available from https://doi.org/10.1001/jama.2024.0179.

11. Anush MM, Ashok VK, Sarma RI, Pillai SK. Role of C-reactive protein as an indicator for determining the outcome of sepsis. *Indian J Crit Care Med*. 2019;23(1):11–14.

12. Hansson LO, Lindquist L. C-reactive protein: its role in the diagnosis and follow upof infectious diseases. *Curr Opin Infect Dis*. 1997;10:196–201.

13. Windgassen EB, Funtowicz L, Lunsford TN, Harris LA, Mulvagh SL. C-reactive protein and high-sensitivity C-reactive protein: an update for clinicians. *Postgrad Med*. 2011;123(1):114–119.

14. Nehring SM, Goyal A, Patel BC. C Reactive protein. In: *StatPearls*. Treasure Island (FL): StatPearls Publishing; 2024 [cited 2024 Feb 8]. Available from http://www.ncbi.nlm.nih.gov/books/NBK441843/.

15. Prince K, Omar F, Joolay Y. A comparison of point of care C-reactive protein test to standard C-reactive protein laboratory measurement in a neonatal intensive care unit setting. *J Trop Pediatr*. 2019;65(5):498–504.

16. Bhardwaj N, Ahmed MZ, Sharma S, Nayak A, Anvikar AR, Pande V. C-reactive protein as a prognostic marker of Plasmodiumfalciparum malaria severity. *J Vector Borne Dis*. 2019;56(2):122–126.

17. Vuong NL, Le Duyen HT, Lam PK, Tam DTH, Vinh Chau NV, Van Kinh N, *et al*. C-reactive protein as a potential biomarker for disease progression in dengue: a multi-country observational study. *BMC Med*. 2020;18(1):35.

18. de Souza Pires-Neto O, da Silva Graça Amoras E, Queiroz MAF, Demachki S, da Silva Conde SR, Ishak R, *et al*. Hepatic TLR4, MBL and CRP gene expression levels are associated with chronic hepatitis C. *Infect Genet Evol*. 2020;80:104200.

19. Lippi G, Sanchis-Gomar F. Procalcitonin in inflammatory bowel disease: drawbacks and opportunities. *World J Gastroenterol*. 2017;23(47):8283–8290.

20. Katz SE, Sartori LF, Williams DJ. Clinical progress note: procalcitonin in the management of pediatric lower respiratory tract infection. *J Hosp Med*. 2019;14(11):688–690.

21. Schuetz P, Albrich W, Mueller B. Procalcitonin for diagnosis of infection and guide to antibiotic decisions: past, present and future. *BMC Med*. 2011;9:107.

22. Christ-Crain M, Müller B. Biomarkers in respiratory tract infections: diagnostic guides to antibiotic prescription, prognostic markers and mediators. *Eur Respir J.* 2007;30(3):556–573.

23. Nargis W, Ibrahim M, Ahamed BU. Procalcitonin versus C-reactive protein: Usefulness as biomarker of sepsis in ICU patient. *Int J Crit Illn Inj Sci.* 2014;4(3):195–199.

24. Cleland DA, Eranki AP. Procalcitonin. In: *StatPearls*. Treasure Island (FL): StatPearls Publishing, 2024 [cited 2024 Feb 8]. Available from http://www.ncbi.nlm.nih.gov/books/NBK539794/.

25. Rodrigo J, Bullock H, Mumma BE, Kasapic D, Tran N. The prevalence of elevated biotin in patient cohorts presenting for routine endocrinology, sepsis, and infectious disease testing. *Clin Biochem.* 2022;99:118–121.

26. Lange N, Méan M, Stalder O, Limacher A, Tritschler T, Rodondi N, *et al.* Anticoagulation quality and clinical outcomes in multimorbid elderly patients with acute venous thromboembolism. *Thromb Res.* 2019;177:10–16.

27. Shikdar S, Vashisht R, Bhattacharya PT. International normalized ratio (INR). In: *StatPearls*. Treasure Island (FL): StatPearls Publishing, 2024 [cited 2024 Feb 8]. Available from http://www.ncbi.nlm.nih.gov/books/NBK507707/.

28. Levy JH, Szlam F, Wolberg AS, Winkler A. Clinical use of the activated partial thromboplastin time and prothrombin time for screening: a review of the literature and current guidelines for testing. *Clin Lab Med.* 2014;34(3):453–477.

29. Triplett DA. Coagulation and bleeding disorders: review and update. *Clin Chem.* 2000;46(8 Pt 2):1260–1269.

30. Yang R, Moosavi L. Prothrombin time. In: *StatPearls*. Treasure Island (FL): StatPearls Publishing, 2024 [cited 2024 Feb 8]. Available from http://www.ncbi.nlm.nih.gov/books/NBK544269/.

31. Kamal AH, Tefferi A, Pruthi RK. How to interpret and pursue an abnormal prothrombin time, activated partial thromboplastin time, and bleeding time in adults. *Mayo Clin Proc.* 2007;82(7):864–873.

32. Winter WE, Flax SD, Harris NS. Coagulation testing in the core laboratory. *Lab Med.* 2017;48(4):295–313.

33. Bolliger D, Tanaka KA. Point-of-care coagulation testing in cardiac surgery. *Semin Thromb Hemost.* 2017;43(4):386–396.

34. Lippi G, Plebani M, Favaloro EJ. Interference in coagulation testing: focus on spurious hemolysis, icterus, and lipemia. *Semin Thromb Hemost.* 2013;39(3):258–266.

35. Ignjatovic V. Prothrombin time/international normalized ratio. *Methods Mol Biol.* 2013;992:121–129.

36. van den Besselaar AMHP, Chantarangkul V, Tripodi A. Thromboplastin standards. *Biologicals.* 2010;38(4):430–436.

37. Barcellona D, Fenu L, Marongiu F. Point-of-care testing INR: an overview. *Clin Chem Lab Med.* 2017;55(6):800–805.

38. Luppa PB, Müller C, Schlichtiger A, Schlebusch H. Point-of-care testing (POCT): current techniques and future perspectives. *TrAC Trends Anal Chem.* 2011;30(6):887–898.

39. Wells PS, Brown A, Jaffey J, McGahan L, Poon MC, Cimon K. Safety and effectiveness of point-of-care monitoring devices in patients on oral anticoagulant therapy: a meta-analysis. *Open Med.* 2007;1(3):e131–e146.

40. National Family Health Survey (NFHS-5) INDIA Report | International Institute for Population Sciences (IIPS). [cited 2024 Feb 8]. Available from https://www.iipsindia.ac.in/content/national-family-health-survey-nfhs-5-india-report.

41. Comprehensive National Nutrition Survey (2016–18) reports: National Health Mission. [cited 2024 Feb 8]. Available from https://nhm.gov.in/index1.php?lang=1&level=2&sublinkid=1332&lid=713.

42. World Health Organisation. Anaemia: Nutrition Landscape Information System (NLiS). Nutrition and nutrition-related health and development data. [cited 2024 Feb 8]. Available from https://www.who.int/data/nutrition/nlis/info/anaemia.

43. Sachdev HS, Porwal A, Acharya R, Ashraf S, Ramesh S, Khan N, *et al.* Haemoglobin thresholds to define anaemia in a national sample of healthy children and adolescents aged 1–19 years in India: a population-based study. *Lancet Global Health.* 2021;9(6):e822–e831.

44. Whitehead RD, Mei Z, Mapango C, Jefferds MED. Methods and analyzers for hemoglobin measurement in clinical laboratories and field settings. *Ann NY Acad Sci.* 2019;1450(1):147–171.

45. Valentine SL, Bembea MM, Muszynski JA, Cholette JM, Doctor A, Spinella PC, *et al.* Consensus recommendations for red blood cell transfusion practice in critically Ill children from the pediatric critical care transfusion and anemia expertise initiative. *Pediatr Crit Care Med.* 2018;19(9):884–898.

46. Roberts KE. Pediatric fluid and electrolyte balance: critical care case studies. *Crit Care Nurs Clin North Am.* 2005;17(4):361–373, x.

47. Rastegar A. Serum potassium. In: Walker HK, Hall WD, Hurst JW, editors. *Clinical Methods: The History, Physical, and Laboratory Examinations.* 3rd ed. Boston (MA): Butterworths; 1990 [cited 2024 Feb 8]. Available from http://www.ncbi.nlm.nih.gov/books/NBK307/.

48. Asirvatham JR, Moses V, Bjornson L. Errors in potassium measurement: a laboratory perspective for the clinician. *N Am J Med Sci.* 2013;5(4):255–259.

49. Liu S, Li J, Ning L, Wu D, Wei D. Assessing the influence of true hemolysis occurring in patient samples on emergency clinical biochemistry tests results using the VITROS® 5600 Integrated system. *Biomed Rep.* 2021;15(5):1–7.

50. Simon LV, Hashmi MF, Farrell MW. Hyperkalemia. In: *StatPearls.* Treasure Island (FL): StatPearls Publishing, 2020 [cited 2020 Feb 6]. Available from http://www.ncbi.nlm.nih.gov/books/NBK470284/.

51. Lehnhardt A, Kemper MJ. Pathogenesis, diagnosis and management of hyperkalemia. *Pediatr Nephrol.* 2011;26(3):377–384.

52. Castro D, Sharma S. Hypokalemia. In: *StatPearls.* Treasure Island (FL): StatPearls Publishing, 2020 [cited 2020 Feb 6]. Available from http://www.ncbi.nlm.nih.gov/books/NBK482465/.

53. Strazzullo P, Leclercq C. Sodium1. *Adv Nutr.* 2014;5(2):188–190.

54. Braun MM, Mahowald M. Electrolytes: sodium disorders. *FP Essent.* 2017;459:11–20.

55. Kim SW. Hypernatemia: successful treatment. *Electrolyte Blood Press.* 2006;4(2):66–71.

56. Sahay M, Sahay R. Hyponatremia: a practical approach. *Indian J Endocrinol Metab.* 2014;18(6):760–771.

57. Peacock M. Calcium metabolism in health and disease. *CJASN.* 2010;5(Supplement 1):S23–S30.

58. Wu AHB. *Tietz Clinical Guide to Laboratory Tests.* 4th ed. Edited by Alan H.B. Wu. St Louis (MO): Saunders/Elsevier, 2006, li, 1798.

59. Sadiq NM, Naganathan S, Badireddy M. Hypercalcemia. In: *StatPearls.* Treasure Island (FL): StatPearls Publishing, 2020 [cited 2020 Feb 6]. Available from http://www.ncbi.nlm.nih.gov/books/NBK430714/.

60. Assadi F. Hypercalcemia: an evidence-based approach to clinical cases. *Iran J Kidney Dis.* 2009;3(2):71–79.

61. Goyal A, Singh S. Hypocalcemia. In: *StatPearls.* Treasure Island (FL): StatPearls Publishing, 2020 [cited 2020 Feb 6]. Available from http://www.ncbi.nlm.nih.gov/books/NBK430912/.

62. Squires RH, Shneider BL, Bucuvalas J, Alonso E, Sokol RJ, Narkewicz MR, *et al.* Acute liver failure in children: the first 348 patients in the pediatric acute liver failure study group. *J Pediatr.* 2006;148(5):652–658.

63. Lutfi R, Abulebda K, Nitu ME, Molleston JP, Bozic MA, Subbarao G. intensive care management of pediatric acute liver failure. *J Pediatr Gastroenterol Nutr.* 2017;64(5):660.

64. O'Grady JG, Schalm SW, Williams R. Acute liver failure: redefining the syndromes. *Lancet.* 1993;342(8866):273–275.

65. Dhaliwal M, Raghunathan V, mohan N, Deep A. Acute liver failure in children – a constant challenge for the treating intensivist. *J Pediatr Criti Care.* 2016;3(4):37.

66. Bernuau J, Rueff B, Benhamou JP. Fulminant and subfulminant liver failure: definitions and causes. *Semin Liver Dis.* 1986;6(2):97–106.

67. Polson J, Lee WM. AASLD position paper: the management of acute liver failure. *Hepatology.* 2005;41(5):1179–1197.

68. Bhatia V, Yachha SK, Bavdekar A. Management of acute liver failure in infants and children: consensus statement of the pediatric gastroenterology chapter, *Indian Acad Pediatr. Indian Pediatr.* 2013;50:477–482.

69. Devictor D, Tissieres P, Durand P, Chevret L, Debray D. Acute liver failure in neonates, infants and children. *Expert Rev Gastroenterol Hepatol.* 2011;5(6):717–729.

70. Ng VL, Li R, Loomes KM, Leonis MA, Rudnick DA, Belle SH, *et al.* Outcomes of children with and without hepatic encephalopathy from the pediatric acute liver failure (PALF) study group. *J Pediatr Gastroenterol Nutr.* 2016;63(3):357–364.

71. Saxena R, Dhaliwal M, Ramnarayan P, Deep A. Transport Of Critically Sick Children To Transplant Centres. *J Pediatr Criti Care.* 2018;5(3):81–90.

72. Deep A, Saxena R, Jose B. Acute kidney injury in children with chronic liver disease. *Pediatr Nephrol.* 2019;34(1):45–59.

73. Saxena R, Deep. Abstract PCCLB-19: acute kidney injury in pediatric liver F. *Pediatr Crit Care Med.* 2018;19(6S):249.

74. Bhatia V, Bavdekar A, Yachha SK. for the Pediatric Gastroenterology Chapter of Indian Academy of Pediatrics. Management of acute liver failure in infants and children: consensus statement of the pediatric gastroenterology chapter. Indian Pediatr. 2013;50(5):477–482.

75. Martí-Carvajal AJ, Solà I. Vitamin K for upper gastrointestinal bleeding in people with acute or chronic liver diseases. *Cochrane Database Syst Rev.* 2015;(6):CD004792.

76. Yang J, Guo Z, Wu Z, Wang Y. Antacids for preventing oesophagogastric variceal bleeding and rebleeding in cirrhotic patients. *Cochrane Database Syst Rev.* 2008;(2):CD005443.

77. Macdougall BR, Bailey RJ, Williams R. H2-receptor antagonists and antacids in the prevention of acute gastrointestinal haemorrhage in fulminant hepatic failure. Two controlled trials. *Lancet.* 1977;1(8012):617–619.

78. Dhaliwal M, Raghunathan V, Mohan N, Deep A. Acute Liver Failure in Children - A constant challenge for the treating intensivist. *J Pediatr Criti Care.* 2016;3(4):37.

79. Scott TR, Kronsten VT, Hughes RD, Shawcross DL. Pathophysiology of cerebral oedema in acute liver failure. *World J Gastroenterol.* 2013;19(48):9240–9255.

80. Feldman AG, Whitington PF. Neonatal hemochromatosis. *J Clin Exp Hepatol.* 2013;3(4):313–320.

81. Rodrigues F, Kallas M, Nash R, Cheeseman P, D'Antiga L, Rela M, *et al.* Neonatal hemochromatosis — medical treatment vs. transplantation: the king's experience. *Liver Transplant.* 2005;11(11):1417–1424.

82. de Laet C, Dionisi-Vici C, Leonard JV, McKiernan P, Mitchell G, Monti L, *et al.* Recommendations for the management of tyrosinaemia type 1. *Orphanet J Rare Dis.* 2013;8:8.

83. Hall MG, Wilks MF, Provan WM, Eksborg S, Lumholtz B. Pharmacokinetics and pharmacodynamics of NTBC (2-(2-nitro-4-fluoromethylbenzoyl)-1,3-cyclohexanedione) and mesotrione, inhibitors of 4-hydroxyphenyl pyruvate dioxygenase (HPPD) following a single dose to healthy male volunteers. *Br J Clin Pharmacol.* 2001;52(2):169–177.

22 Miscellaneous Diseases

Rahul Kumar Anand and Magesh Parthiban

WILSON'S DISEASE

Introduction

Wilson's disease (WD) is a rare autosomal recessive disorder (deficit or reduced function of the ATP7B protein) caused by abnormal copper accumulation in the body. It primarily affects the brain, liver, and cornea. Hepatocellular excretion of copper into bile decreases, resulting in copper buildup in the liver. Excess copper levels in the body lead to the formation of toxic hydroxyl groups, causing oxidative stress and cell damage. Copper is eventually released into the bloodstream and deposited in other organs, including the brain, kidney, and cornea. This damage manifests clinically as liver failure, behavioral problems, movement disorders, and the characteristic Kayser-Fleischer rings in the cornea. The onset of liver dysfunction typically occurs between the ages of 6 and 20 but can also manifest later in life. The severity of liver disease varies from mild biochemical abnormalities to fulminant hepatic failure.

Clinical Profile

Physical examination of individuals with Wilson's disease may reveal hepatosplenomegaly, isolated splenomegaly, and stigmata of chronic liver disease in advanced cases. Eye examinations often show icterus, and the presence of Kayser-Fleischer rings on the cornea. Skeletal involvement may resemble premature osteoarthritis, primarily affecting the axial skeleton and spine. The Leipzig criteria were developed to standardize the diagnosis and management of WD [1].

In **basic laboratory testing**, impaired liver function, Coombs-negative hemolytic anemia, and normal alkaline phosphatase levels in young patients should raise suspicion of Wilson's disease. Blood liver tests often reveal hepatocellular injury, indicated by elevated levels of alanine transaminase (ALT) and aspartate transaminase (AST), as well as increased bilirubin levels. Low values of serum alkaline phosphatase and an increased AST:ALT ratio are associated with fulminant WD. Combining an alkaline phosphatase (ALP) to total bilirubin (TB) ratio below 4 with an AST to ALT ratio above 2.2 offers high diagnostic sensitivity [2].

Advanced laboratory testing includes assessing serum ceruloplasmin levels, 24-hour urinary copper excretion, total serum copper, and liver biopsy. A low level of ceruloplasmin in the blood, usually below 0.2 g/L (normal range: 0.2–0.5 g/L) or below 50% of the lower limit of the normal range, may be indicative of WD. A 24-hour urinary copper excretion exceeding 100 μg/24h in adults and 40 μg/24h in children confirms the diagnosis. Total serum copper (TSC) measurement has limited diagnostic value, as it does not reflect tissue concentrations accurately. Free copper levels and the toxic fraction bound to non-ceruloplasmin proteins are more suitable markers for WD diagnosis. The liver histology findings are known as specific and depend on the presentation and stage of the disease.

In summary, Wilson's disease is a rare genetic disorder characterized by abnormal copper accumulation in the body, primarily affecting the brain, liver, and cornea. Recognizing clinical manifestations, conducting basic and advanced laboratory tests, and evaluating brain imaging findings contribute to the diagnosis and management of this condition.

HEREDITARY HEMOCHROMATOSIS

INTRODUCTION

Hemochromatosis is a disorder characterized by excess iron deposition and multiple organ dysfunction. Organs affected include the liver, pancreas, heart, thyroid, joints, skin, gonads, and pituitary. Hereditary hemochromatosis occurs in individuals with a mutation in the hemochromatosis gene (HFE), which causes increased iron absorption despite normal dietary intake. The most common mutations are C282Y and H63D. Hereditary hemochromatosis is the most common autosomal recessive disorder in whites, with a prevalence of 1 in 300 to 500 individuals. Types 2, 3, and 4 are seen worldwide, while type 1 is predominantly observed in people of northern European descent. Men are affected two to three times more frequently than women, with symptoms typically appearing later in women's lives due to iron loss during menstruation. Symptoms usually manifest in men during the fifth decade and in women during the sixth decade. Juvenile hemochromatosis can affect individuals aged 10–30 years.

DOI: 10.1201/9781003449713-22

Presentation

Hemochromatosis pathology affects the liver, pancreas, heart, thyroid, joints, skin, gonads, and pituitary. Alcohol intake and viral hepatitis can accelerate liver and pancreatic damage. Cirrhosis is present in 70% of patients, significantly increasing the risk of hepatocellular carcinoma. Pancreatic iron deposition primarily leads to diabetes, with a 50% incidence in symptomatic patients. Arthropathy presents as joint pain without joint destruction, often with calcium pyrophosphate crystals in synovial fluid. Cardiac symptoms result from iron accumulation in cardiac cells, causing abnormal electrocardiographic findings, congestive heart failure, and arrhythmias. Iron-induced hypothalamic or pituitary failure leads to hypogonadism and impotence. Skin hyperpigmentation occurs with iron stores exceeding five times normal levels.

Basic laboratory testing includes liver enzyme evaluation, with consistent elevations in aminotransferases. Fasting blood glucose levels should be checked for diabetes, but glycosylated hemoglobin may be unreliable in patients with high red cell turnover. Additional tests include echocardiography, hormone level assessment, and bone densitometry.

Advanced laboratory testing involves measuring serum transferrin saturation or ferritin concentration. Transferrin saturation testing may be less effective in erythropoietic hemochromatosis, and ferritin levels can be influenced by inflammation. Elevated ferritin (>200 mcg/L in women, >300 mcg/L in men) or transferrin saturation (>40% in women, >50% in men) warrants further testing. In regions with prevalent HFE mutations, genetic testing for C282Y and H63D confirms the diagnosis in over 90% of cases. Liver biopsy remains the most sensitive and specific test, revealing iron deposits primarily in hepatocytes and biliary epithelial cells. It is indicated in cases of elevated liver enzymes in diagnosed patients or when serum ferritin levels exceed 1000 mcg/L.

Radiography, such as echocardiography and chest radiographs, aids in diagnosing organ involvement, while MRI measures liver iron content non-invasively.

MULTIPLE MYELOMA

Introduction

Multiple myeloma (MM) is a clonal plasma cell proliferative disorder characterized by the abnormal increase of monoclonal immunoglobulins. Unchecked, the excess production of these plasma cells can ultimately lead to specific end-organ damage. Most commonly, this is seen when at least one of the following clinical manifestations is present: hypercalcemia, renal dysfunction, anemia, or bone pain accompanied by lytic lesions. The exact etiology of multiple myeloma is unknown. However, frequent alterations and translocations in the promoter genes, especially chromosome 14, are commonly found in multiple myeloma and likely play a role in disease development. Multiple myeloma occurs predominantly in the geriatric population with a median age at diagnosis of about 70 years and is slightly more commonly seen in males than females (1.4:1).

Clinical Profile

MM is essentially a stage in the spectrum of monoclonal gammopathy. It is thought to arise from a pre-malignant, asymptomatic phase of clonal plasma cell growth called monoclonal gammopathy of undetermined significance (MGUS). MGUS is defined as detecting monoclonal immunoglobulins in the blood or urine without evidence of end-organ damage. This is quite common and is known to be detectable in over 3% of persons above age 50. It appears that the cell of origin is a post-germinal center plasma cell. his is typically a benign condition, although as noted above, it has a risk of progression to MM of about 1% per year.

Multiple myeloma is simply a part of the spectrum of plasma cell proliferative disorders. This concept is restated on the National Comprehensive Cancer Network (NCCN) guidelines, where the disease is divided into MGUS, smoldering myeloma (asymptomatic), or multiple myeloma (symptomatic), as well as reiterated elsewhere [14]. As treatment and management of each category are vastly different, correct identification and diagnosis of MM are paramount.

Diagnosis: The revised International Myeloma Working Group (IMWG) criteria for the diagnosis of multiple myeloma and related disorders are shown in Table 22.1.

Table 22.1   Revised IMWG Criteria for the Diagnosis of Multiple Myeloma and Related Disorders

Multiple myeloma

Both criteria must be met:
- Clonal bone marrow plasma cells ≥10% or biopsy-proven bony or extramedullary plasmacytoma
- Any one or more of the following myeloma-defining events:

Evidence of end-organ damage that can be attributed to the underlying plasma cell proliferative disorder, specifically:
- Hypercalcemia: serum calcium >0.25 mmol/L (>1 mg/dL) higher than the upper limit of normal or >2.75 mmol/L (>11 mg/dL)
- Renal insufficiency: creatinine clearance <40 mL per minute or serum creatinine >177 μmol/L (>2 mg/dL)
- Anemia: hemoglobin value of >2 g/dL below the lower limit of normal, or a hemoglobin value <10 g/dL
- Bone lesions: one or more osteolytic lesions on skeletal radiography, computed tomography (CT), or positron emission tomography-CT (PET-CT)

Clonal bone marrow plasma cell percentage ≥60%
Involved: uninvolved serum free light chain (FLC) ratio ≥100 (involved free light chain level must be ≥100 mg/L)
>1 focal lesions on magnetic resonance imaging (MRI) studies (at least 5 mm in size)

TUMOR LYSIS SYNDROME

Introduction

Tumor lysis syndrome (TLS) is a metabolic and oncologic emergency that can occur spontaneously or after the initiation of chemotherapy. It is characterized by metabolic disorders such as hyperkalemia, hyperphosphatemia, hypocalcemia, and hyperuricemia, which can lead to end-organ damage. TLS is most commonly seen in patients with solid tumors and poses a significant risk to both adult and pediatric oncology patients undergoing chemotherapy. The release of intracellular chemical substances due to tumor cell destruction can adversely affect the functions of target organs, resulting in acute kidney injury, fatal arrhythmias, and even death.

Pathology

The exact incidence of tumor lysis syndrome is not known, but there are certain risk factors that can increase its occurrence. These factors include tumor burden, tumors with a high rate of proliferation, tumors sensitive to chemotherapy, and preexisting renal disease or impairment. The predisposition to tumor lysis syndrome is not related to race or sex. Non-Hodgkin lymphoma, solid tumors, acute myeloid leukemia, and acute lymphocytic leukemia are among the most common malignancies associated with tumor lysis syndrome.

The incidence of tumor lysis syndrome varies based on the specific malignancy and its risk stratification. For high-risk tumors such as acute lymphocytic leukemia, acute myeloid leukemia with a high white blood cell count, B-cell acute lymphoblastic leukemia, and Burkitt lymphoma, the reported incidences range from 5.2% to 26.4%. Intermediate-risk tumors, such as diffuse large B-cell lymphoma and acute myeloid leukemia with moderate white blood cell counts, have an incidence of around 6%. Low-risk tumors, including chronic lymphocytic leukemia, chronic myelogenous leukemia, and certain solid tumors, have a lower incidence of tumor lysis syndrome, ranging from 0.33% to 6%.

Basic Laboratory Investigations

The diagnosis of tumor lysis syndrome is based on criteria established by Cairo and Bishop. These criteria require the presence of two or more specific laboratory parameters within the same 24-hour period, occurring between 3 days before and 7 days after chemotherapy initiation. The criteria include:

- Uric acid increase of 25% from baseline or a level greater than or equal to 8.0 mg/dL

- Potassium increase of 25% from baseline or a level greater than or equal to 6.0 mEq/L

- Phosphorus increase of 25% from baseline or a level greater than or equal to 4.5 mg/dL (greater than or equal to 6.5 mg/dL in children)

- Calcium decrease of 25% from baseline or a level less than or equal to 7.0 mg/dL

Other Investigations

In addition to basic laboratory investigations, several other tests are necessary for the evaluation of tumor lysis syndrome. These include:

- Imaging: X-ray and CT scan of the chest can identify the presence of a mediastinal mass and pleural effusion. CT scan and ultrasound of the abdomen and retroperitoneal structures are required when the mass lesion is located in these areas.

- Electrocardiography (ECG): ECG is performed to evaluate findings associated with hyperkalemia and hypocalcemia, which can lead to fatal arrhythmias in tumor lysis syndrome.

- Complete blood count.

MYASTHENIA GRAVIS

Introduction

Myasthenia gravis (MG) is a prevalent disorder affecting the neuromuscular junction (NMJ) of skeletal muscles, characterized by fluctuating weakness, often more pronounced in the afternoon. This condition arises from the production of autoantibodies targeting specific postsynaptic membrane proteins, leading to impaired transmission of electrical impulses across the NMJ and subsequent muscle weakness. Various factors, including infections, immunizations, surgeries, and certain medications, can trigger the onset of MG.

Clinical Profile

The hallmark of MG is the formation of autoantibodies against postsynaptic membrane proteins, disrupting neuromuscular transmission. Extraocular muscle weakness is a common initial manifestation, presenting as diplopia and ptosis in around 85% of patients. Bulbar muscle involvement, seen in 15% of cases, leads to difficulties with chewing, dysphagia, hoarseness, and dysarthria. Limb weakness, primarily affecting proximal muscles more than distal muscles, typically manifests more prominently in the upper limbs. Myasthenic crisis, a severe complication, occurs due to the involvement of intercostal muscles and the diaphragm, posing a medical emergency.

Serologic Testing

Serologic tests serve as valuable tools in diagnosing MG. The anti-AChR antibody test, highly specific for MG, confirms the diagnosis in the majority of cases with classical clinical presentations. However, its sensitivity is lower in patients with pure ocular MG. Approximately 5–10% of patients exhibit anti-MuSK antibodies, and a small percentage are positive for both anti-AChR and anti-MuSK antibodies. For patients negative for these antibodies, about 3–50% will demonstrate anti-LRP4 antibodies. Additionally, anti-striated muscle antibodies are present in 30% of MG patients, particularly those with thymoma.

Electrophysiologic tests, including repetitive nerve stimulation (RNS) and single-fiber electromyography (SFEMG), are crucial for diagnosing MG, especially in seronegative cases. RNS testing involves stimulating nerves at 2–3 Hz to deplete acetylcholine (ACh) at the NMJ, with a 10% or greater decrease in excitatory postsynaptic potential (EPSP) between the first and fifth stimuli indicative of MG. SFEMG records action potentials from individual muscle fibers, revealing increased "jitter" due to reduced NMJ transmission in MG. The edrophonium (Tensilon) test, a short-acting acetylcholinesterase inhibitor, temporarily increases ACh availability, aiding in diagnosis, particularly for ocular MG. The ice-pack test, an alternative to edrophonium, involves placing an ice-pack over the eye for improvement assessment in ptosis, albeit limited to extraocular muscles.

AMYLOIDOSIS

Introduction

Amyloidosis encompasses a spectrum of disorders characterized by the deposition of insoluble beta-sheet fibrillar protein aggregates in various tissues. These deposits can lead to localized or systemic manifestations, affecting organs such as the liver, spleen, kidneys, heart, nerves, and blood vessels. Amyloidosis may arise through acquired or hereditary mechanisms, presenting a diverse array of clinical features.

Classification

Amyloidosis can be classified according to systemic, hereditary, central nervous system, ocular, and localized etiology. However, the most common types are AL, AA, ATTR (amyloid transport protein transthyretin), and dialysis-related amyloidosis (beta2M type). In AL amyloidosis, "A" represents amyloid followed by the associated fibrillar protein, and "L" means light chain fragment or immunoglobulin light chain. In AA amyloidosis, the second A stands for the serum amyloid A protein. The most common causes of amyloidosis are immunoglobulin-light-chain-related amyloidosis (AL), ATTR amyloidosis, and reactive amyloidosis (AA) due to chronic inflammatory diseases like chronic infections and rheumatoid arthritis. AL amyloidosis is acquired and is caused by a small plasma cell clone that produces misfolded amyloidogenic light chains that deposit in different organs and tissues.

Clinical Presentation

The clinical features of amyloidosis vary depending on which type of amyloid fibrils are responsible. Systemic amyloidosis can lead to heart failure with left ventricular hypertrophy on echocardiogram with standard or low voltage electrocardiogram. Hepatomegaly, nephrotic syndrome, macroglossia, orthostatic hypotension, ecchymosis, and autonomic and peripheral neuropathy can be present. Carpal tunnel syndrome, jaw claudication, and articular deposits of amyloid can also be a manifestations of systemic amyloidosis. In secondary amyloidosis, hepatosplenomegaly, proteinuria, renal failure, and orthostasis can be seen. ATTR amyloidosis onset is during midlife and presents with peripheral and autonomic neuropathy, cardiomyopathy, and vitreous opacities. Amyloid beta-amyloidosis is localized to the central nervous system and presents as sporadic Alzheimer's disease and aging.

Other physical exam findings that can lead to suspicion of amyloidosis are hypertrophied shoulder pads from amyloid deposition, amyloid purpura, and raccoon eyes secondary to factor-X deficiency in the case of AL amyloidosis and prolonged PT, PTT, that correct with mixing studies, pointing toward the involvement of factor deficiencies in the common pathway of coagulation.

Basic laboratory testing: Advanced laboratory investigations are essential for further evaluating organ involvement and disease staging. Cardiac evaluation includes echocardiography, NT-proBNP, troponins, ECG, Holter ECG, and cardiac MRI. Renal function is assessed with 24-hour urinary protein and eGFR, while liver function tests and imaging (ultrasound, MRI, or CT) aid in hepatic assessment.

Advanced and Specific Testing

The diagnosis of amyloidosis begins with clinical suspicion and is confirmed through tissue biopsy. Subcutaneous abdominal fat aspirate staining positive for Congo red with apple-green birefringence is sensitive for AL amyloidosis. When fat aspirates are negative, a biopsy of minor salivary glands aids in diagnosing systemic amyloidosis. However, liver biopsy should be performed cautiously due to bleeding risks. Assessment for plasma cell dyscrasia involves serum and urine electrophoresis, immunofixation, and free light chain assays. Tissue typing is accomplished through immunohistochemical staining and mass spectrometry. Transthyretin detection and gene sequencing are necessary for hereditary forms. Differentiating between AL and ATTR amyloidosis may involve cardiac biopsy or cardiac scintigraphy with bone tracers.

RARE AND BIOTERRORISM INFECTIONS

Anthrax

Introduction

The bacteria *Bacillus anthracis* causes anthrax. The bacteria is a small aerobic or facultatively-anaerobic, gram-positive or gram-variable, encapsulated, spore-forming rod. The organism produces toxins that are important for clinical virulence. It grows well on blood agar resulting in large, irregular-shaped colonies. The origin of the name comes from the Greek word "anthrakis," meaning black, in reference to the necrotic lesion seen in cutaneous anthrax.

Clinical Presentation

Inhalational anthrax presents following an incubation period of approximately 1 to 6 days post-exposure, with a non-specific prodromal phase including fever, sweats, nausea, vomiting, malaise, chest pain, and nonproductive cough. The second stage of illness occurs as bacterial replication in mediastinal lymph nodes results in hemorrhagic lymphadenitis and mediastinitis, and progression to bacteremia. Fever, dyspnea, and stridor from increasing lymphadenopathy impact the airways, and ultimately respiratory failure and hemodynamic collapse occur. Meningitis also occurs in up to 50% of inhalational cases, with a headache, confusion, and progression to coma. Chest x-rays classically demonstrate a widened mediastinum (the result of significant lymphade-nopathy) without pulmonary infiltrates, though pleural effusions and/or pulmonary infiltrates both of which may be hemorrhagic can also be seen. The time from onset of symptoms to death ranges from 1 to 10 days.

GI anthrax results from ingestion of contaminated, undercooked meat or ingestion of spores inhaled into the nasopharynx and can include oropharyngeal and/or intestinal symptoms. Patient with oropharyngeal anthrax develops ulcers of the posterior oropharynx and associated dyspha-gia, cervical swelling, and regional lymphadenopathy. Patients with intestinal anthrax develop fever, nausea, vomiting, and diarrhea. They can progress to an acute abdomen-like presentation with bloody diarrhea, hematemesis, and massive ascites. Intestinal involvement more frequently involves the terminal ileum and cecum. Untreated patients will progress to septicemia. Mortality ranges from 25% to 60%.

Cutaneous anthrax presents 1 to 10 days post-inoculation with a pruritic papular lesion that progresses over several days into a painless ulcer. The lesion may have associated satellite vesicles and will progress into a necrotic and blackened center with surrounding non-pitting edema. The painlessness of the lesion is characteristic of cutaneous anthrax and a distinguishing feature from other diagnoses. As the lesion heals, the eschar will dry and slough off after 1 to 2 weeks. Without appropriate treatment, the mortality rate can approach 20%.

Injection drug anthrax presents as a grouping of small vesicles or papules at the injection site, with progression to painless ulcerative lesions similar to cutaneous anthrax. Injection anthrax may make it more difficult to recognize and may progress more rapidly to systemic illness than cutane-ous anthrax

The procedures for the diagnosis of anthrax should be as follows: patient's history, clinical examination for signs and symptoms, routine laboratory examination, radiological examinations, and microbiological testing. A history of travel, residence in an endemic region, a job that involves working with animals, exposure to sick or dead animals; and the handling of contaminated ani-mal materials could indicate anthrax.

Basic Laboratory Testing

When biochemical and blood parameters are evaluated, the leukocyte count is usually less than 10×10.3 cells/μL in mild cutaneous cases. In complicated cutaneous infections, toxemic shock, systemic anthrax, leukocytosis with neutrophilia, hypoalbuminemia, hyponatremia, and rising aspartate aminotransferase (AST) and alanine aminotransferase (ALT) levels may be detected. If severe sepsis develops, leukopenia, thrombocytopenia, and disseminated intravascular coagula-tion (DIC) may occur.

Advanced and Specific Testing

The identification of the pathogen is based on a combination of microscopy and culture. The vegetative form of the bacteria appears as a gram-positive rod-shaped organism. Confirmation of the presence of a capsule that surrounds virulent forms of the bacterium can be confirmed using polychrome methylene blue or Indian ink. BACTEC™ FX40 device, an automated blood culture apparatus, is widely used in microbiology laboratories to recover pathogens from clinical samples. For specimens in which the bacteria are likely to present in the company of other microorganisms, a selective agar is recommended such as Polymyxin-Lysozyme-EDTA-Thallous acetate (PLET). It is based on heart infusion agar supplemented with polymyxin B, lysozyme, ethylenediaminetet-raacetic acid (EDTA), and thallus acetate. The use of DNA amplification-based PCR (polymerase chain reaction) and real-time PCR tests can be used for the definitive and rapid diagnosis of *B. anthracis* in clinical and environmental specimens.

REFERENCES

1. Ferenci P. Diagnosis of Wilson disease. *Handb Clin Neurol.* 2017;142:171–180.

2. Korman JD, Volenberg I, Balko J, Webster J, Schiodt FV, Squires RH Jr, Fontana RJ, Lee WM, Schilsky ML; Pediatric and Adult Acute Liver Failure Study Groups. Screening for Wilson disease in acute liver failure: a comparison of currently available diagnostic tests. *Hepatology.* 2008;48(4):1167–1174.

Index

A

ABG, *see* Arterial blood gas
ACR, *see* Acute cellular rejection
ACS, *see* Acute coronary syndrome
Activated partial thromboplastin time (aPTT), 32, 44, 109, 124, 152, 157
Acute cellular rejection (ACR), 74
Acute coronary syndrome (ACS), 95, 96, 173
Acute Fatty Liver of Pregnancy (AFLP), 111, 169, 172
Acute heart failure (AHF), 93, 95
Acute kidney disorders (AKD), 130, 131
Acute kidney injury (AKI), 124
    AACC (ADLM) guidance document, KDIGO 2012, 139–141
    alerts, 138
    basic laboratory investigations, 132
    biochemical investigations, 132
    biomarkers, 134
    causes, 133
    challenges in diagnosis, 131
    clinical use, 135
    definition, 130, 138
    diagnosis, 130
    electronic alerts, 140
    evaluation, 134, 136–137
    forms, 133
    limitations, 134
    point-of-care testing (POCT) assays
        biomarkers, 134–135
        combination of biomarkers, 135
        cystatin C, 131–132
        serum creatinine assay, 130–132
    staging criteria, 138–139
Acute liver failure (ALF), 111, 191
Acute myocardial infarction (AMI), 24, 93
Acute pancreatitis, 110–111, 116
Acute Physiology and Chronic Health Evaluation (APACHE), 93
Acute poisoning and toxicity
    advanced drug testing, 45–46
    analgesics-antipyretic drugs, 40–41
    antidepressants, 41–42
    antidotes, 40
    antipsychotics, 41–42
    basic laboratory and point-of-care tests, 44–45
    cardiac drugs, 42
    classification, 40
    drugs of abuse
        alcohols, 43
        hallucinogens, 42
        immunoassays, 45
        inhalants, 43
        NPS, 43
        opioids, 42
        sedative-hypnotics, 42
        stimulant drugs, 42
    drug tests, 39
    management of the poisoned patient, 43–45
    medical assessment, 39
Adenosine deaminase (ADA), 89
Advanced life support (ALS), 49
AF, *see* Atrial fibrillation
AFLP, *see* Acute Fatty Liver of Pregnancy
AHF, *see* Acute heart failure
AKI, *see* Acute kidney injury
Alanine aminotransferase (ALT), 111, 206
Albumin, 28, 78, 186
Alcohols, 39, 43
ALF, *see* Acute liver failure
Alkaline phosphatase (ALP), 111, 165, 174, 201
ALS, *see* Advanced life support
AMI, *see* Acute myocardial infarction
AMR, *see* Antibody-mediated rejection
Amyloidosis, 204–205
Analgesics-antipyretic drugs, 40–41
Anaphylactic shock, 2
ANAs, *see* Antinuclear antibodies
ANCA, *see* Anti-neutrophil cytoplasmic antibodies
Anemia, 2, 65, 78, 125, 165, 174, 183, 203
Anthrax, 205–206
Antibody-mediated rejection (AMR), 74
Antidepressants/antipsychotics, 41–42
Anti-neutrophil cytoplasmic antibodies (ANCA), 110
Antinuclear antibodies (ANAs), 118
Antiphospholipid syndrome (APS), 124, 157
Anti-Saccharomyces cerevisiae antibodies (ASCA), 110
APACHE, *see* Acute Physiology and Chronic Health Evaluation
APS, *see* Antiphospholipid syndrome
APTT, *see* Activated partial thromboplastin time
Arterial blood gas (ABG), 32, 48–49, 93, 111
ASCA, *see* Anti-Saccharomyces cerevisiae antibodies
Aspartate aminotransferase (AST), 111, 206
Atrial fibrillation (AF), 93
Automated notification systems, 84

B

Bacillus anthracis, 205
Benzodiazepines, 36, 42, 44
(1→3)-β-D-Glucan (BDG), 88
Bilirubin, 111, 165, 201
Bioterrorism infections, 205–206
Bleeding assessment tool (BAT), 4
Bleeding time (BT), 4, 152
Blood urea nitrogen (BUN), 52–53
BNP, *see* Brain natriuretic peptide
Bone and joint diseases
    anti-rheumatic drug therapy, 121
    connective tissue disorders, 119
    EULAR/ACR criteria, 120
    immune-mediated inflammatory myopathies, 122
    laboratory tests
        blood tests, 118

Printed in the United States
by Baker & Taylor Publisher Services